James F. Reinhardt

1961

CLINICAL USE *of* RADIOISOTOPES

A Manual of Technique

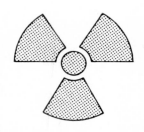

CLINICAL USE

of

RADIOISOTOPES

A Manual of Technique

Edited by

THEODORE FIELDS, M.S., F.A.C.R. (Assoc.)

Chief, Physics Section, Radioisotope Service, Veterans Administration Hospital, Hines, Illinois; Instructor in Radiology, Northwestern University Medical School; Attending Physicist, Cook County Hospital, Chicago, Illinois; Certified Medical Nuclear Physicist, American Board of Radiology

and

LINDON SEED, M.D.

Clinical Associate Professor of Surgery, University of Illinois College of Medicine; Director of Isotope Laboratories, Augustana Hospital, Chicago, Illinois, and Oak Park Hospital, Oak Park, Illinois; Consultant in Radioisotopes, Veterans Administration Hospital, Hines, Illinois

SECOND EDITION

THE YEAR BOOK PUBLISHERS · INC.

CHICAGO

© COPYRIGHT 1957 and 1961 by
THE YEAR BOOK PUBLISHERS, INC.

Second edition, 1961

Library of Congress Catalog Card Number: 60-8498

PRINTED IN U.S.A.

Contributors

SHELDON BERGER, M.D.

Assistant Director, Department of Metabolic and Endocrine Research, Medical Research Institute, Michael Reese Hospital, Chicago, Illinois; Physician-in-Charge, Radioisotope Laboratory, Michael Reese Hospital, Chicago, Illinois

WILLIAM R. BEST, M.D.

Assistant Professor of Medicine, University of Illinois College of Medicine; Attending Physician in Internal Medicine and Hematology, Research and Educational Hospitals, University of Illinois College of Medicine, Veterans Administration Hospital, Hines, Illinois, and Grant Hospital, Chicago, Illinois

JOHN A. D. COOPER, M.D., Ph.D.

Professor of Biochemistry, Northwestern University Medical School; Director, Radioisotope Service, Veterans Administration Research Hospital, Chicago, Illinois

THEODORE FIELDS, M.S., F.A.C.R. (ASSOC.)

Chief, Physics Section, Radioisotope Service, Veterans Administration Hospital, Hines, Illinois; Instructor in Radiology, Northwestern University Medical School; Attending Physicist, Cook County Hospital, Chicago, Illinois; Certified Medical Nuclear Physicist, American Board of Radiology

PATRICK J. FITZGERALD, M.D.

Professor and Chairman, Department of Pathology, State University of New York, College of Medicine at New York City, Brooklyn, New York

I. F. HUMMON, M.D., F.A.C.R.

Director, Department of Radiology, Cook County Hospital, Chicago, Illinois; Professor of Radiology, Cook County Graduate School of Medicine, Chicago, Illinois

JOHN J. IMARISIO, M.D.

Assistant Chief, Radioisotope Service, Veterans Administration Hospital, Hines, Illinois

ERVIN KAPLAN, M.D.

> Chief, Radioisotope Service, Veterans Administration Hospital, Hines, Illinois; Clinical Assistant Professor of Medicine, University of Illinois College of Medicine

JACK S. KROHMER, M.A., F.A.C.R. (ASSOC.)

> Assistant Professor of Radiology (Radiation Physics), University of Texas, Southwestern Medical School; Physicist, Parkland Memorial Hospital, Dallas, Texas, and The Radiation Center, Fort Worth, Texas; Consulting Physicist, Veterans Administration Hospital, Dallas, Texas, U. S. Naval Hospital, Portsmouth, Va., Brooke Army Medical Center, Fort Sam Houston, Texas

ROBERT S. LANDAUER, Ph.D., F.A.C.R. (ASSOC.)

> Assistant Professor in Radiology, Northwestern University Medical School; Physicist, Cook County Hospital, Chicago, Illinois; Attending Physicist, Veterans Research Hospital, Chicago, Illinois; Civilian Consulting Physicist, United States Naval Hospital, Great Lakes, Illinois

LOUIS R. LIMARZI, M.D., F.A.C.P.

> Associate Professor of Medicine and Hematologist, Research and Educational Hospitals, University of Illinois College of Medicine; Attending Physician and Hematologist, Augustana Hospital and West Side Veterans Administration Hospital, Chicago, Illinois

EUGENE F. LUTTERBECK, M.D., F.A.C.R.

> Professor of Radiology, Cook County Graduate School of Medicine, Chicago, Illinois; Associate in Radiology, Northwestern University Medical School

WILLIAM J. MACINTYRE, Ph.D.

> Associate Professor of Biophysics, Department of Medicine and Division of Psychiatry, Western Reserve University; Physicist, Highland View Hospital, Cleveland, Ohio

JAMES MAXFIELD, M.D.

> Director, Maxfield X-ray and Radium Clinic, Dallas, Texas; Radiologist, Texas Radiation and Tumor Institute; Regional Advisory Council of Nuclear Energy, Southern Governors' Conference; Area Consultant in Radiology, Veterans Administration

VINCENT J. O'CONOR, M.D.

> Professor and Head of the Department of Urology, Northwestern University Medical School; Chief of Urological Service, Chicago Wesley Memorial Hospital, Chicago, Illinois; Consultant Chief of Urology, Veterans Administration Research Hospital, Chicago, Illinois

NORMAN S. RADIN, Ph.D.

Research Biochemist, Mental Health Research Institute, University of Michigan

LINDON SEED, M.D.

Clinical Associate Professor of Surgery, University of Illinois College of Medicine; Director of Isotope Laboratories, Augustana Hospital, Chicago, Illinois, and Oak Park Hospital, Oak Park, Illinois; Consultant in Radioisotopes, Veterans Administration Hospital, Hines, Illinois

DONALEE L. TABERN, Ph.D.

Director of Radioisotope Education, Picker X-ray Corporation, White Plains, New York

Preface to the Second Edition

SINCE PUBLICATION OF THE FIRST EDITION in 1957, the specialty of Nuclear Medicine has advanced on many fronts. More reliable and new types of electronic devices have enabled more and better types of diagnostic procedures. The radioisotope pharmaceutical laboratories are now providing more convenient and more accurate packaging of radiopharmaceuticals. Indeed, during the intervening years since the first edition, the medical users of radioisotopes were being very materially assisted in their practice by the technical advances in their equipment and materials.

Problems of health, safety and physics consultations were reduced to a minimum with these advances. Even the regulations and controls of the Atomic Energy Commission were somewhat simplified.

Accordingly, we have added, subtracted and modified earlier sections to conform with modern nuclear medical practice. Sections on thyroid scanning, liver, and gastrointestinal function tests have been added.

Sections on ascetic fluid volume and AEC regulations have been eliminated. The balance of the chapters have received major alterations in line with accepted practice.

The editors wish to express their gratitude to their co-workers over many years who have contributed many suggestions, ideas and time to make such a text possible. In particular, they wish to emphasize that much of the techniques described have originated in laboratories under the jurisdiction of the Chief of the Radioisotope Division of the United States Veterans Administration, Division of Medicine and Surgery. This agency of the

Federal Government continues to be in the forefront in the development and application of atomic energy for the diagnosis, treatment and study of the diseases of man.

THEODORE FIELDS
LINDON SEED

Preface to the First Edition

THE SPECIALTY OF NUCLEAR MEDICINE is firmly established and warrants a manual describing currently accepted clinical procedures. The large number of published five-year reviews in this field justifies an attempt at presentation of preferred techniques by experienced users. In addition, the medical rationale, health physics precautions and government regulations which have been formalized and accepted require inclusion in a technical manual. It would not be practicable to report the multitudinous variations by which a single basic procedure can be performed. The editors have purposely selected those procedures which they consider to be most representative of the techniques giving the most accurate results in their experience. Comprehensive bibliographies (at the ends of chapters) supply sources of other descriptions of the same tests; for, it is emphasized, this is a manual for practical application, not a textbook of detailed compilation of all known techniques and their variations.

The chapters were assembled and edited for consistency of purpose and form. Any overlaps have been retained at a level believed necessary for better understanding of the material.

It is hoped that the appendixes—glossary, statistical data and examples of record and report sheets—will supply sufficient background information to enable the clinical scientist to accomplish recommended techniques without the prerequisite training of a nuclear physicist.

In order to pursue a program embodying the clinical use of radioisotopes, problems concerning acceptance by the Atomic Energy Commission, facilities, personnel, equipment and health physics must be considered along with their inevitable complications of procurement, standards, properties and finances. Recommendations and instructions have therefore been provided by scientists experienced in these areas.

The editors wish to acknowledge the assistance given them by Miss Ethel Davis in editorial review of the manuscript. We also are grateful to Dr. Arthur Jaffey for technical criticisms, to Dr. Leo Oliner for permission to reproduce his laboratory record forms, and to our wives for their endless patience.

Table of Contents

PART II. ROUTINE CLINICAL THERAPY TECHNIQUE

PART III. PLANNING AND OPERATING THE RADIOISOTOPE LABORATORY

PART IV. RADIATION SAFETY

APPENDIXES

(Appendixes A–D reprinted, with minor changes, by permission from *Radiological Health*, 1954, courtesy of the Robert A. Taft Sanitary Engineering Center of the U.S. Public Health Center, Department of Health, Education and Welfare, Cincinnati, Ohio; Radiological Health Training Section, Dr. Simon Kinsman, Chief. Appendix E, courtesy of Michael Reese Hospital, Radioisotope Unit, Chicago.)

PART I

ROUTINE CLINICAL
DIAGNOSTIC TESTS

CHAPTER 1

Thyroid Evaluation

IN TESTS OF THYROID FUNCTION utilizing radioiodine, various portions of the metabolic circuit of iodine are measured. In a normal person, thyroid accumulation (1)* of ingested iodine begins promptly; it is about 75 per cent complete within 12 hours and is almost 100 per cent complete at the end of 24 hours. The normal thyroid gland picks up approximately 30 per cent of a tracer dose, 60 per cent is excreted in the urine, and 10 per cent is distributed throughout the body. In hyperthyroidism due to toxic diffuse goiter or exophthalmic goiter, the thyroid gland clears iodine from the blood stream at an accelerated rate, accumulation is more rapid, is completed more quickly and is increased from a normal of 30 per cent to an average level of 70 per cent. The urinary excretion conversely diminishes from a normal of 60 per cent of the administered dose to as low as 10 per cent. On the other hand, in hypothyroidism the thyroid gland picks up less than a normal percentage of an administered dose at a slower rate, and the peak uptake may not be reached until after 24 hours. Most of the remainder is excreted in the urine within the first 24 hours, but excretion continues in smaller amounts for another day or two.

After the uptake of a tracer dose the thyroid gland immediately manufactures and releases a small quantity of radioactive hormone, which can be isolated as protein-bound iodine (PBI^{131}). The amount released varies according to the physiologic activity

---

* References in parentheses refer to bibliographical citations at end of chapter.

of the thyroid gland. If the gland is overactive, the PBI[131] in the plasma is increased in quantity and forms a greater percentage of the total plasma I[131]. During the process of iodine metabolism, an appreciable quantity is selectively secreted by the salivary glands, the concentration of which generally varies inversely with the thyroid activity.

The measurement of many aspects of this metabolic circuit can be used to evaluate thyroid function. It is not possible to describe here in detail all the methods which have been proposed and which have been found to be of clinical value; only a listing and brief description of the more important aspects are feasible. But a detailed description is presented of the recommended procedure for performing the three most important tests: the 24-hour thyroid uptake, the urinary excretion, and the determination of PBI[131]. There are many variations of these three tests, and the outline of a single technique for conducting each test can be varied to suit individual requirements.

A. TYPES OF TESTS

1. THYROID UPTAKE

The most useful single measurement, and the one most commonly used, is the 24-hour thyroid uptake of an ingested tracer dose. The method of determination is simple; it can be performed cheaply in both hospital and outpatient clinics and gives the approximate maximum thyroid uptake essential in calculating therapeutic doses. The 24-hour period, however, can be shortened without loss of accuracy in diagnosis. Crispell and his colleagues (2) have reported a 1-hour uptake with a dividing level between euthyroidism and hyperthyroidism at approximately 20 per cent. Similar results were obtained on oral and intravenous administration by Morton, Ottoman and Peterson (3) and by Kriss (4). Barrett and his co-workers (5) demonstrated a 6-hour thyroid uptake which has a normal spread of 7–23 per cent, as compared to a 24-hour uptake with a normal spread of 12–35 per cent. They used both a 6- and a 24-hour uptake. The 6-hour determination measured the rate of I[131] accumulation by the thyroid gland, and the 24-hour determination measured approximate maximum concentration. Greer (6) found that the 24-hour uptake in the euthyroid subject could be transformed into the 6- or 8-hour uptake by dividing by 1.67 or 1.43, respectively.

The 24-hour uptake is not necessarily the peak or maximum uptake, but it does approximate this value. In hyperthyroidism due to toxic diffuse goiter, the peak uptake is reached in 10–20 hours (7) and thereafter has a tendency to drop. In euthyroidism, uptake approaches the peak at 24 hours but does not finally reach this level until 48 hours or more (8). Using these differences as a basis, Lowry (7) devised an index by dividing the peak uptake by the time taken to reach the peak. Using the same physiologic principle, Adams and Purves (8) recommend making two uptake measurements—one at 8 hours and one at 48 hours—and also correlating these with the 48-hour urinary excretion. Meschan and his associates (9) believe that taking the percentage uptake at 1 and/or 2 hours is accurate enough for clinical application, but this method has a disadvantage in that the 1-hour test requires intravenous injection of the test dose. Friis and Christensen (10) think that the 4-hour measurement of the uptake combined with the PBI[131] serum level is superior to all other parameters. From a diagnostic point of view, Schultz and Zieve (11) found the uptake at 3 hours to be the best uptake measurement after an oral dose and also found it to be as effective as the more complicated measures.

The rate of uptake over short periods of time has diagnostic value. Larrson and Jonsson (12) and Taplits, Fine and Rosenberg (13) demonstrated that measurements over the neck made only 5–10 minutes after an intravenous injection of I[131] gave reliable information about the iodine-concentrating function of the gland provided that registration of the counting rates from the time of the injection was continuous. Astwood and Stanley (14) plotted 2-, 4- and 6-hour uptakes against the square root of time. This plotting results in a straight-line slope which they called the *accumulation gradient*. They found the method to have fair diagnostic reliability. Greer (6) found that a dose correlation of the accumulation gradient and the 6- and 8-hour uptake with the 24-hour uptake of radioactive iodine existed in euthyroid subjects, but he suggested that far less correlation might be found in thyrotoxic subjects.

2. RATES OF CLEARANCE AND EXCRETION

The physiologic basis of the determination of clearance rates has been succinctly set forth by Werner (15) as follows:

After intravenous administration, or ingestion and absorption, of stable iodine the material is distributed to all tissues by immediate diffusion. Complete equilibrium is achieved in 10–15 minutes after intravenous injection or at about 2 hours orally in the fasting state. During this time, uptake by the thyroid and excretion by the kidney have begun. After iodine has attained equilibrium with the tissues, the rates of uptake by the thyroid and excretion by the kidney become measurable and are proportional to the plasma concentration. Iodide returns gradually from the tissues to the blood as removal from plasma progresses; and by 24 hours the tissues, except for about 10–15 per cent, are freed of the isotope. The normal thyroid at this time has reached a plateau of accumulation and little is being excreted in the urine. The iodide in the gland becomes rapidly utilized and converted to organic form. Synthesized hormone is then stored as thyroglobulin or released into the blood stream as smaller fragments of thyroglobulin, to circulate in combination with the crude albumin fraction. Significant radioactivity does not appear in the organic fraction of the blood before 72 hours in euthyroidism, but considerable amounts may be detected in hyperthyroidism as early as 24 hours after administration of the tracer dose.

Thyroid clearance is defined as the volume of plasma cleared of I^{131} per minute by the thyroid gland. Myant, Pochin and Goldie (16) showed a normal range of 8–38 ml. of plasma cleared per minute, with a mean value of 16 ml./min.; and in thyrotoxic patients, a range of 198–1,300 ml./min. with a mean of 486 ml./min. Berson and his associates (17) showed a normal range of from 3.7 to 41 ml./min. with a mean of 17.7, compared to a hyperthyroid range of from 74.5 to 512 ml./min. with a mean of 210.5 ml./min.

A half hour is the minimum period of observation. A longer period is often used, and repeated tests may be made, for which Schultz and Zieve (11) give the following formula:

$$TC = \frac{U_2 - U_1}{(P_1 + P_2)/2} \times \frac{1}{t_2 - t_1}$$

where U_1 and U_2 are the percentage thyroid uptake at times t_1 and t_2, $(P_1 + P_2)/2$ is the average plasma I^{131} concentration in percentage of the dose per milliliter during the time interval $t_2 - t_1$, and TC is the milliliters of plasma cleared of I^{131} per minute.

There are many methods for simultaneously correlating the status of the I^{131} in the thyroid gland, in the blood and in the urine. Keating and his associates (18) computed the disappearance rate, renal excretion rate and collection rate on the basis of collections of urine every 6 hours for the first 24 hours and then 24-hour samples for two additional days. Berson and his colleagues (17) gave an intravenous injection of radioiodine and from a single 35-minute sitting were able to calculate a clearance rate from the assay of the neck and a single urine specimen. The method is based on an observed consistent relationship between the body weight and the space of I^{131} dilution during the first half hour following intravenous administration of the isotope. Nitowsky and Puck (19) checked each urine sample for 12 hours and calculated a specific rate constant for I^{131} uptake by the thyroid.

McAdams and Salter (20) developed an index called the "thyroid secretory rate," calculated from the maximal uptake within 8 hours, the rate of uptake in the first 21 hours and the final uptake at 24 hours. Foote and MacLagan (21) took a neck count every 10 minutes at a distance of 11 cm., immediately followed by a thigh count, and calculated a thigh-neck clearance rate after 1¼ hours. Ingbar (22) administered a 50 $\mu c.$ dose intravenously and made several measurements over the neck and thigh and several determinations of PBI^{131}. Pochin (23) devised a simple 2-hour neck/thigh ratio which has been found useful by others. In thyrotoxicosis the thyroid rapidly takes up radioiodine from the circulating plasma, so that the early neck counts become higher than normal and the early thigh counts become lower than normal, with a resulting great increase in the neck/thigh ratio.

3. URINARY EXCRETION

When renal function is normal, the 24-hour quantitative estimation of urinary excretion of I^{131} gives results of diagnostic value comparable to that derived from measurement of the 24-

hour thyroid uptake. The collection period can be extended to 48 hours with some diagnostic advantage. In the euthyroid subject, excretion of that portion of the dose not accumulated by the thyroid gland is virtually completed in 24 hours; in the hyperthyroid patient, it is accomplished in much less time; and in hypothyroidism there is some continued excretion for more than 24 hours.

Fraser (24) makes use of the changing rate of excretion with a diagnostic index T based on the 0–8-hour urinary output, the 8–24-hour output and the 0–48-hour output:

$$T = \frac{0\text{–}8 \text{ hr. activity}}{(8\text{–}24 \text{ hr. activity}) \times (0\text{–}48 \text{ hr. activity})}$$

The normal values are 2.8–13.

Mason and Oliver (25) measured the radioactivity of specimens passed between 0 and 6 hours, 6 and 24 hours and 24 and 48 hours. The amount of I^{131} excreted in the 0–6-hour sample was found to be nearly the same for normal and toxic patients. In the 6–24-hour sample, patients with hyperthyroidism excrete under 4 per cent of the dose; euthyroid subjects, 10–25 per cent; and hypothyroid patients, over 25 per cent. The Larrson (26) quotient is just as accurate an index and is by far the simplest way of using urinary excretion in diagnosis. With this index, the rate of excretion (T/U) is obtained by dividing the 24-hour thyroid uptake by the 24-hour urine output (T_{24}/U_{24}). The normal values are 0.4–1.6.

From a technical point of view, the quantitative estimation of urinary I^{131} is more accurate than a quantitative estimation of thyroidal I^{131}; but because of errors arising in the collection of urine and because of the inconvenience of collection, the estimation of urinary secretion is a less practical method than a neck survey. Thyroid-uptake and urinary-excretion tests performed simultaneously serve to check each other and diminish the possibility of error in measurement. If circumstances permit, this is the preferred routine for thyroid assay, especially in those cases involving a question of possible hypothyroidism.

4. PLASMA IODINE-131 AND PROTEIN-BOUND IODINE-131

With the introduction of the well-type scintillation counter,* the estimation of minute quantities of radioactivity in liquid solution or suspension has become relatively simple. This, in turn, has reduced the labor in measuring the amount of I^{131} in the blood stream.

New methods of determining the protein-bound fraction involving the use of an ion exchange column have further simplified the technique. The plasma is passed through a column which adsorbs the inorganic iodine, and the protein-bound fraction is contained in the filtrate. The quantitative variations in PBI^{131} are sufficient to be of diagnostic value.

Morton (27) separated out the thyroxin fraction of I^{131}, rather than just the protein-bound portion. The thyroxin fraction normally forms from 2 to 10 per cent of the total plasma I^{131}; from 50 to 70 per cent in hyperthyroidism, and 1 per cent or less in hypothyroidism. Silver and his associates (28) found that the PBI^{131} begins to rise at the eighth hour and continues to rise in hyperthyroid patients; whereas in euthyroid patients, it does not. At 72–96 hours the disparity between the two types is at its greatest.

Clark, Trippel and Sheline (29) have placed more emphasis on the 24-hour *conversion ratio* of PBI^{131} per total plasma I^{131}. They have found it to be more accurate diagnostically than the quantitative estimation of PBI^{131}. The ratio, as a rule, is above 0.30 in hyperthyroidism. Any figure below that is considered to be in the euthyroid or hypothyroid range. Barry and Pugh (30) obtained radioiodine concentrations 1 and 4 days after oral administration of 50 μc. tracer doses, and they described a statistical diagnostic index of the serum radioiodine level.

The PBI^{131} and the conversion ratio tests have definite diagnostic value and have continued to be used. The one serious objection to the routine use of these tests is the requirement of a tracer dose of 50 μc. Since it is desirable to reduce tracer doses to a minimum, blood determinations have either been abandoned

---

* See Chapter 16.

or been carried on only with the use of the most sensitive scintillation counters.

5. MISCELLANEOUS TESTS

Iodine-132, an isotope with a half-life of 2.3 hours, has been applied to tracer techniques by Hanbury and his co-workers (31), Goolden and Mallard (32) and Halnan and Pochin (33). Iodine-132 gives a lower total body dosage and about 1/30 the dosage to the thyroid gland as compared with I^{131}. With I^{132} one can do repeated tests at short intervals on either patients or volunteer subjects. Its short half-life makes it impractical to rely on obtaining I^{132} itself; but tellurium-132 (Te^{132}) (a fission product of uranium-235), with a half-life of 2.3 days, may be used as a source of I^{132}. The technical difficulties and expense of extracting the I^{132} from Te^{132}, either by distillation or by absorption on an alumina column, probably eliminate I^{132} from general usage. Berman, Becker and Benua (34) have used I^{133} with a half-life of 21 hours, average gamma energy of 0.581 Mev and average beta energy of 0.484 Mev. Iodine-133 has a usable half-life and might be a useful isotope, but it is not obtainable in the pure state. Eleven hours after radioiodine is removed from the atomic pile, it contains about 39 per cent I^{135} (6.7 hr. half-life), about 57 per cent I^{133} and about 4 per cent I^{131}. When the radioiodine is used 1–2 days later, the I^{135} content has become negligible, but the mixture contains an I^{131} content of 10–25 per cent.

Greer and Smith (35) have differentiated between thyrotoxic and euthyroid patients by the use of the suppressive effect of exogenous thyroid hormone on thyroidal radioiodine metabolism. After an uptake study the patients were given 180 mg. or more of USP desiccated thyroid, which they took daily for from 1 to 2 weeks, following which a second test was made. Almost without exception, the euthyroid patients showed a suppression of thyroidal uptake below 20 per cent following the administration of 540 mg. of desiccated thyroid daily for 1 or 2 weeks. In none of the thyrotoxic patients was suppression below 20 per cent.

Werner and Spooner (36) applied the same physiologic principle but used l-tri-iodothyronine (liothyronine) instead of desiccated thyroid. They found that 75 μg. administered daily by mouth for 8 days caused a sharp decrease in the 24-hour I^{131}

uptake in 48 euthyroid patients without thyroid disease and that no value exceeded 20 per cent. In contrast, no value under 35 per cent was obtained in patients with toxic goiter following tri-iodothyronine administration.

From a practical point of view, liothyronine is a better suppressive agent than desiccated thyroid, in that the result can be obtained in less time and the effect of the agent is dissipated much faster. Smollar (37) applied the test in 61 patients with excellent diagnostic differentiation.

Thode and his co-workers (38) studied the salivary excretion with I^{131}. The radioiodine level of the saliva was seen to rise steeply for all patients, reaching a maximum in about 4 hours. At that time there is a marked difference in values between hyperthyroid and hypothyroid patients, but a better result is obtained by correlating salivary concentration to PBI^{131}. This ratio gives an index of the state of thyroid function, being small in hyperthyroidism and high in hypothyroidism; but because of its variability and because of the practical difficulties in collecting sputum, it has not been accepted as a routine diagnostic test.

The iodide repletion test has been described by Burrell and Fraser (39). The patients, after an uptake study, were given 10 mg. of potassium iodide daily for 2 weeks and a second tracer study was performed. The test gave the following results: (1) persistently avid uptake in 24 out of 25 patients with mild thyrotoxicosis, (2) normal uptake in 29 out of 30 patients with anxiety states in whom thyroid uptake was initially high and (3) normal or low uptake in all 11 patients with nontoxic goiter who showed an initially high thyroid uptake and also in the other euthyroid patients tested. These investigators recommend the test where there is a high thyroid uptake of dubious clinical significance, and also for testing patients who have been receiving antithyroid drugs.

The in vitro red blood cell uptake of I^{131} l-tri-iodothyronine described by Hamolsky, Golodetz and Freedberg (40) presents a new approach to radioiodine diagnosis. (Because of as yet unknown variations in protein binding of the thyroid hormone, the red blood cells of a hyperthyroid patient will pick up more I^{131} than will the cells from a euthyroid person.) The method avoids the administration of radioactivity to the patient; and blood can be drawn at any time, stored for a week or more and shipped to distant points. The results are not greatly altered by the ingestion of iodine. The reliability of this method has been verified recently by Beary and Weiss.*

6. Conference on Standardization of Iodine-131 Thyroid Uptake

(Medical Division of Oak Ridge Institute of Nuclear Studies, September 24–29, 1956)

Dr. Marshall Brucer, Director of the Medical Division of the Oak Ridge Institute of Nuclear Studies, has made an exhaustive study of the factors influencing the accuracy of the thyroid-uptake test. As a part of this investigation, he sent representatives to approximately two hundred laboratories in the United States, Canada and England with a kit consisting of a standard dose of mock iodine and a dummy which contained a quantity of mock radioiodine in the region of the thyroid gland plus a suitable distribution of mock I^{131} in the other parts of the dummy. He found that the percentage uptake determined by the various laboratories varied considerably from the true amount and, furthermore, that the inaccuracies were as frequently encountered in well-supervised laboratories as in those less well supervised.

Dr. Brucer and his colleagues carried out an exhaustive study of the physiologic and physical aspects of thyroid uptake and, in order to discuss and present this material, held a week-long conference of fourteen pairs of workers in the field, each pair consisting of one clinician and one physicist. The following is a brief résumé of the material presented by him, and in a large part verified experimentally by the members of the conference.

a) MOCK IODINE.—A long life source with a spectrum approximately that of I^{131} can be simulated by about a 13.1:1 mixture of radiobarium (Ba^{133}) and radiocesium (Cs^{137}) surrounded by a babbitt metal shield 0.82 mm. thick. The Ba^{133} (9.5 yr. half-life) has a peak energy approximating the principal 360 Kev energy

---

* Beary, F. A., and Weiss, H. A.: "Comparison of Various Techniques Used to Determine Thyroid Iodine Uptake," speech given at the Annual Meeting of the Society of Nuclear Medicine, Chicago, 1959.

of I^{131}, and Cs^{137} (33 yr. half-life) has a single gamma peak almost identical to the 640 Kev of I^{131}. The useful life of the mixture is 10 years. Such a standard would be of inestimable value in a laboratory using I^{131}. On the other hand, calibration of the counters and scalers can also be accomplished by using the U. S. Bureau of Standards source, which is issued twice yearly, or by using the estimates on microcurie contents of the capsules issued by a secondary distributor. The latter are usually quite reliable.

b) DETECTOR AND COUNTING MECHANISM.—These mechanisms cannot be standardized. The inconvenience and expense of making necessary alterations would prevent changes in established laboratories. In new installations the choice of detector will be determined by four factors: (1) sensitivity, (2) flexibility, (3) maintenance and (4) reliability. A large (1½ in. O.D. by 1 in. thick) sodium iodide (Tl [thallium activated]) crystal gives a high degree of sensitivity and allows the use of the small doses required by present practices. Although a crystal of 1 in. diameter is sensitive enough to permit a 10 μc. tracer dose at a counting distance of 25 cm., an increase of crystal size to 1½ in. diameter allows the dose to be reduced by one half or the distance increased by 10 cm. Such crystal scintillation counters are, on the whole, reliable and easy to maintain. Although both binary and decade scalers are used, the latter offers considerable convenience in data calculation and has become reliable enough to offer no important problems. The medical spectrometer with a pulse-height analyzer is perhaps the ideal mechanism, in that it can be set to measure only the principal 360 Kev I^{131} peak. However, it is, at present, expensive, difficult to use and particularly difficult to maintain.

c) COLLIMATION.—Collimation should be standardized, but this is also impractical. Collimation reduces both room background and body scatter. A long collimator, 1 in. thick with sufficient flare to give an isoresponse field 10 cm. wide at 25 cm., is Brucer's preference. The members of the conference agreed to these principles but did not agree on the actual size of the collimator to be recommended.

d) DISTANCE.—The distance employed from the patient to the detector is critical. A short distance may give a large error, due to positioning, according to the inverse square law. A long distance (over 60 cm.) gives a large decrease in sensitivity. Dr. Brucer prefers 10 in. or 25.4 cm., measured from the neck to the front surface of the crystal. This is a reasonable distance, but the points of measurement do not allow accurate standardization or calculation. A measurement taken from the center of sensitivity of the crystal to the estimated center of the thyroid (2–3 cm. from front of neck) offers a more uniform and scientific approach. As Brucer emphasizes, however, the accurate measurement of the distance of the detector to the patient and of the detector to the standard is very important.

e) TRACER DOSE.—As a result of rules permitting the unrestrained use of quantities below 10 μc., the tracer dose for the thyroid uptake will ultimately reach a level of 10μc. But for the fact that from 25 to 50 μc. is necessary for the determination of the PBI[131], the 50 μc. dose would be outmoded. The capsule dose is more useful, being assayed more accurately than most laboratories can assay the dose. A group of capsules are very nearly alike, and it is quite simple to establish a reference standard. The kind of standard is of importance and may alter the results to an important degree. As indicated elsewhere, an I[131] capsule or testtube source placed 2 cm. within a 12.5 cm. O.D. lucite cylinder is a good standard source in a good phantom.

f) THE "A" FILTER.—Dr. Brucer recommends two filters: an "A" filter, consisting of a sheet of lead 1/16 in. thick, placed in front of the detector to reduce scatter; and a "B" filter, consisting of a 4 × 4 in. sheet of lead ½ in thick, placed in front of the neck to calculate soft-tissue radiation. The "A" filter acts as a low-energy cutoff and decreases the amount of scattered radiation that is measured. It makes the spectra of a point source and of the thyroid source of I[131] much more alike. Since it distorts the spectrum, it should be standardized. A sheet of lead 1/32 in. thick may be adequate, but 1/16 in. is a good compromise. The thickness of the "A" filter has been determined by counting a source in air and a source in a beaker of water, then placing increasingly thick filters in front of the counter until the counting rate in the air is the same as in the water. All counting mechanisms may be standardized empirically to these conditions. A capsule in air and in a phantom would also suffice. The "A" filter is a necessity.

g) THE "B" FILTER.—The "B" filter is a 4 × 4 in. sheet of

lead ½ in. thick, placed over the neck so as to eclipse the thyroid gland. It could, thus, aptly be called the "eclipse shield." A ½ in. layer will eliminate approximately 90 per cent of the primary thyroid radiation. A larger shield cuts off too much background; a smaller shield does not cover the source. If the filter is moved about a bit, the edges of the gland can be ascertained, or the filter can be shifted about until there is a minimum count. A count taken with the shield in place represents soft-tissue radiation, some primary radiation from the thyroid gland and some scattered radiation. The "B" shield offers a means of measuring soft-tissue radiation; and although it is obviously not too accurate a means, it cannot help but be an improvement on a thigh reading. It corrects errors in hypothyroid patients in whom the soft-tissue background is high, but it is not so important in hyperthyroid patients in whom the soft tissue I^{131} is quite low. A thigh reading gives a rough estimation of soft-tissue distribution; but if the thigh reading is higher than usual, the patient could be asked to return the next day when it will be less. Some correction may be made by this procedure.

h) THE PHANTOM.—Dr. Brucer emphasizes that the phantom should simulate the neck as nearly as possible and that it should produce a similar spectrum. By trial and error, he found the ideal phantom to be a cylinder of lucite 12.5 cm. in diameter and 12.5 cm. in height, with an opening for a capsule 2 cm. from the surface and 7.5 cm. deep. Such a "shallow" phantom with the standard close to the surface most closely simulates the neck.

i) FORMULAS.—Two formulas were considered most useful. According to formula No. 1:

$$TU = \frac{P_a - RB_a}{S_a - RB_a} \times 100 \qquad \text{Formula \#1}$$

where TU = per cent thyroid uptake,
$\quad P_a$ = patient count with "A" filter,
$\quad RB_a$ = room background with "A" filter, and
$\quad S_a$ = standard "A" filter.

According to formula No. 2:

$$TU = \frac{P_a - P_{ab}}{S_a - S_{ab}} \times 100 \qquad \text{Formula \#2}$$

where P_{ab} = patient count with "A" and "B" filters, and
S_{ab} = standard with "A" and "B" filters.

Dr. Brucer recommends formula No. 2. Many laboratories use the formula:

$$TU = \frac{P_a - \text{Thigh}_a}{S_a - RB_a}$$

where thigh_a = thigh count with "A" filter. Actually, the thigh reading does not vary much from room background except in the hypothyroid patients.

j) SOURCES OF ERRORS.—The principal sources of error when the ordinary counter and scaler is used are:

1. The phantom (not comparable to neck)
2. The formula (wrong one)
3. The kind of standard (not comparable to gland)

When the spectrometer is used for counting, the chief errors are due to:

1. The spectrum (poor choice of spectrum covered)
2. The phantom
3. The formula

The "A" filter gives a better answer with a poor phantom and low background. The "B" filter is better with a good phantom, low thyroid uptake and low sensitivity.

B. RECOMMENDED PROCEDURE

1. THE TRACER DOSE

There are two methods of securing a tracer dose: (1) by preparing it from a stock solution diluted from a regular shipment either as it comes direct from Oak Ridge or from a secondary supplier,* and (2) by purchasing it in capsule form from a secondary supplier. The second, or capsule method is by far the most convenient and the most useful one in the ordinary outpatient clinic or office practice.

---

* See Section D (pp. 284-286) of Chapter 14.

a) STOCK SOLUTION FOR TRACER DOSES.—A stock solution may be made up by diluting an accurately measured quantity of radioactive material taken out of an original shipment from the secondary supplier. This method is the cheaper one, and it has an advantage in that suitable quantities are pipetted out each day, so that the tracer dose always contains the same minimum number of microcuries. The assay may be conveniently made in a 25 ml. flask in a phantom.

In measuring stock solutions, as well as in measuring therapeutic doses, it is safe to accept the values as stated on the accompanying invoice from the secondary supplier. Consignments from Oak Ridge are not intended for direct use but must be processed and assayed before administration. Large laboratories may prefer to make their own assays by means of a Lauritsen electroscope,* but with very few exceptions the assay methods of the secondary supplier are superior to those of the ultimate user. If the laboratory wishes to calibrate its instruments, using I^{131} from another source, it can make use of an accurately assayed sample furnished twice yearly by the Nuclear-Chicago Corporation.

b) CAPSULE DOSE.—The capsule dose is obtainable from the secondary supplier at regular or irregular intervals, in any number and in any specified microcurie size. The batches, usually delivered at weekly intervals, are distinguished also by a weekly change in color. They are easily stored and easily handled, and to a great extent they eliminate the hazard of accidental contamination inherent in the use of liquids. The capsule may be given to the patient to take home with him, to take on another, more convenient, day. It also may be mailed to him, and thus save him a trip to the laboratory. Shipping regulations (41) state that radioactive material must emit no more than 10 milliroentgens per 24 hours (or 0.4 mr./hr.) on contact with the container. This restriction can be met by placing the capsule, for doses of 25 μc. or less, in a small pillbox and packing the pillbox within a paper box container, size 10 cm³ (Fig. 1). For a 50 μc. dose, the capsule should be surrounded by 2 mm. of lead.

Although all the capsules in a batch will, in most instances, be of the same strength, it is well to assay each capsule rather than

---

* See Chapter 16, pp. 314-337, and Figures 62 and 63.

to use them indiscriminately. A convenient method of handling them is depicted in Figure 1. The capsule is assayed in a lucite phantom; the data are inscribed on a suitable sheet, the sheets being numbered consecutively; and the capsule is then placed in a small test tube (Wassermann tube), on which the same number is inscribed, and the tube is stored in a hole drilled into a lead

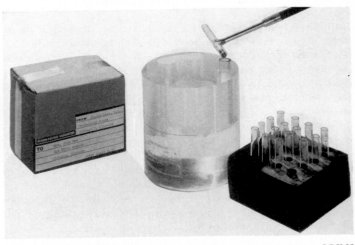

Fig. 1.—Mailing box for 25 μc. tracer dose, 4 × 4 × 4 in.; ORINS lucite phantom (Abbott Laboratories); and capsules stored in numbered test tubes in a lead brick.

brick. At the time of administration, the name of the patient and date are added to the sheet bearing the number on the test tube. The last-numbered capsule may be used as a reference source; it may be assayed again in the phantom at the time of the assay of the patient's neck and may be used to correct for decay and alterations in the counting mechanism. If one wishes, this step may be eliminated, without much loss in accuracy, by correcting the count of the delivered dose for decay by referring to decay charts.

c) SIZE OF DOSE.—To determine plasma[131] or PBI[131] with a well-type scintillation counter, the minimum dose should be 50 μc. Quantities as small as 10^{-5} μc./ml. or 10^{-2} μc./L. can be assayed in a well-type counter. This quantity is in the range found for the lowest level of PBI[131] following a 50 μc. dose.

For uptake studies the size of the dose will depend on the sensitivity of the counter, its background and the distance of the counter from the source. Let us assume that the preferred distance is 50 cm. from the center of radioactivity in the thyroid gland to the center of the crystal and that a scintillation counter is being used with a background of 300 counts per minute and sufficient sensitivity to give 400 cts./min./μc. at 50 cm. In most clinical work the period of counting is only 1–3 minutes. For this short time, statistical accuracy would necessitate a normal counting rate of 5 times background, or 1,500 cts./min., which, in this hypothetical instance, would be due to 4 μc. of I^{131} in the thyroid. A routine tracer dose should be chosen of such amount that it could be measured in the thyroid gland of a patient with a 10 per cent uptake or more. In this particular circumstance, a routine tracer dose of 40 μc. would permit an estimate of 10 per cent thyroid uptake at 50 cm. If a counting distance of only 10 cm. is chosen, the counting rate is increased 25 times, and a tracer dose of only 1 μc. would give a similar degree of efficiency, and one of 2 μc. would be ample. The shorter distance, however, would increase the error involved in estimating the depth of the center of radiation in the thyroid gland from the surface of the neck and would increase the error in the placement of the scintillation counter.

2. THE 24-HOUR THYROID IODINE-131 UPTAKE DETERMINATION

a) APPARATUS.—The following will be required:

A *scintillation counter* which has the following characteristics:
Crystal: NaI (Tl), 1½ in. O.D. × 1 in. thick.
Shielding: Should be 1 in. minimum about entire crystal and should overlap photomultiplier 1 in.
Collimation: Shield should extend 2 in. beyond crystal and should flare from 2 in. at proximal to 3 in. at distal end.
Filter: 1/16 in. of lead placed over crystal end (A filter).

A *scaler* having:
Discriminator: Variable from 0.1 to 3.0 volts.
Scaling factors: Binary or decade.
High voltage: 500–2,500 volts.

A *plastic phantom.**

A *lead shield,* 4 × 8 × 1 in. (one half of a standard lead
   brick), mounted on an adjustable stand (B filter).†

b) PROCEDURE.—The procedure is as follows:

1. Have the patient return to the radioisotope laboratory
   24 hours after he has received his tracer dose. He should
   sit in a cushioned armchair against a wall and be told to
   keep his head against the wall while readings are taken.

2. Place the scintillation counter at a distance (using a
   standard wood spacer) such that the center of the crystal
   is 47 cm. from the front of the neck (the thyroid is
   usually 3 cm. behind the front of the neck). The scaler
   and scintillation counter should have been "warmed up"
   before being used. Center the tube just below the cricoid
   cartilage.

3. Take a reading for 3 minutes at this position. This is
   called "reading P_a."

4. Center the lead filter (B) and place it 3 in. in front of
   the thyroid. The 8 in. dimension is on the horizontal
   plane and the 4 in. dimension on the vertical plane.

5. Take a reading for 3 minutes at this position (called
   "reading P_{ab}").

6. Remove the patient from the chair and place the phantom (and dose) so that its front is 47 cm. from the center
   of the crystal with only the "A" filter present. The doses
   used above must be prepared and assayed at the same
   time that the dose is administered to the patient—that
   is, 24 hours earlier. This will automatically compensate
   for physical decay corrections in the following calculation.

7. Take a reading for 3 minutes at this position (called
   "reading S_a").

8. Center the lead filter (B) and place it 3 in. in front
   of the phantom.

9. Take a reading for 3 minutes at this position (called
   "reading S_{ab}").

---

* Atomic Accessories, Bellerose, New York.
† Picker X-ray Corporation, White Plains, New York.

10. Then calculate the per cent uptake from the following formula:

$$\frac{P_a - P_{ab}}{S_a - S_{ab}} \times 100 = \text{Per cent uptake}$$

3. THE 24-HOUR URINARY IODINE-131 OUTPUT DETERMINATION

a) APPARATUS.—The following are required:

A scintillation counter identical to that described in Section 2, *a,* above.
A scaler identical to that described in Section 2, *a,* above.
Two 1,000 ml. polyethylene beakers.
One waterproof bowling ball bag.
Two 2 qt. Mason jars.

b) PROCEDURE.—The following procedure is used:

1. Give the patient the waterproof bowling ball bag containing the two jars, and tell him to collect in these containers all of his urine for 24 hours after his tracer dose and to return the following day.
2. After the tracer uptake measurement has been performed on the patient, dilute the standard dose into a 1 L. polyethylene beaker and bring it up to 1 L. of water.
3. Place the beaker so that its front is 47 cm. from the center of the crystal with only the "A" filter present. Take a 3-minute reading at this position (called "reading T_a").
4. Collect the urine from the patient and pour it into a large graduate or bottle. Determine its volume (V) (a dip stick is useful in this instance).
5. Put a 1,000 ml. aliquot of the urine into another polyethylene beaker and take a reading as in step 3. If less than 1,000 ml. is collected, add sufficient water to bring the quantity to 1,000 ml. in the beaker. This is called "reading V_a."
6. Remove the beaker and take a 3-minute background reading (called "RB_a").
7. Then calculate the per cent urinary I^{131} output from the

following formula if more than 1,000 ml. of urine is collected:

$$\frac{V_a - RB_a}{T_a - RB_a} \times \frac{V}{1,000} \times 100 = \text{Per cent urinary } I^{131} \text{ output}$$

8. Use the following formula if less than 1,000 ml. of urine is collected:

$$\frac{V_a - RB_a}{T_a - RB_a} \times 100 = \text{Per cent urinary } I^{131} \text{ output}$$

4. Blood Level: Protein-Bound Iodine-131 and Plasma Iodine-131

After the ingestion of the tracer dose of I^{131}, there is a rise in the level of total radioiodine in the plasma owing to absorption from the gastrointestinal tract. This is followed by a rapid disappearance from the plasma of inorganic I^{131} as a result of its removal by the kidneys and thyroid. After this decline, a slow rise is observed in the radioiodine in the plasma because of the incorporation of these atoms of I^{131} in the thyroxine or hormone fraction of the plasma. This effect reaches a maximum in 24–48 hours after the tracer dose has been taken and is a useful index, taken in conjunction with the thyroid-uptake study, in diagnosing thyroid function (42, 43, 44).

a) MATERIALS.—The following materials are required for the blood-level determinations:

Anion exchange resin (2 gm.).*
Trichloroacetic acid, 40 per cent, 1.5 ml.

b) APPARATUS.—The following apparatus will be required:

Scintillation well counter, 2 × 2 in. NaI (Tl).†
Thistle tube (No. 10–455): diameter, 45 mm.; diameter of stem, 6–7 mm.; length of stem, 300 mm.‡
Stirring rod, stainless steel, ¼ in. O.D. × 6½ in. length.

---

* Amberlite 1 RA-400 (C1), Analytical Grade, Rohm and Haas Company, Philadelphia, Pennsylvania.
† Picker X-ray Corporation, White Plains, New York.
‡ Fischer Scientific Company, Chicago, Illinois.

Plastic test tube.
5 ml. volumetric pipette.
Paraffin wax.
Test tube rack.
Ring stand.
Small beakers.

c) PROCEDURE.—Measurement of PBI[131] in microcuries per liter of plasma is determined in the following manner:

1. Prepare thistle tube by sealing tip of column (prior to its filling with resin) by dipping it in melted paraffin wax. After the paraffin hardens, use a 19 gauge needle to perforate the paraffin plug.
2. Fill thistle tube column section with approximately 2 gm. of the resin.
3. Pour 2 cc. of distilled water into column for uniform packing and wetting of the resin column before use. Use beaker under column to catch all excess water.
4. Five ml. of plasma is pipetted into reservoir portion of column. Effluent, free of inorganic iodide, is received in plastic tube containing 1.5 ml. of 40 per cent trichloroacetic acid. After the column is drained dry, it is washed free of any remaining plasma with 2 ml. of distilled water. Contents of receiving tube are then thoroughly mixed and centrifuged for 15 minutes. The supernatant liquid is carefully decanted, and the radioactivity of the PBI[131] precipitate is counted in a well scintillation counter for 15 minutes and a 15-minute background reading is taken.
5. From the total efficiency of the counter, it is possible to determine a conversion factor which may be used to calculate the amount of PBI[131] in microcuries per liter of plasma corrected for radioactive decay to the time of administration. The following relations apply:

PBI[131] (μc/L.) = Total counts in 15 min. × Conversion factor

where the conversion factor is

$$\frac{200 \times \text{Decay factor}}{15 \times \text{Efficiency} \times \text{disint./min./}\mu\text{c.}}$$

If a counter having 35 per cent efficiency (efficiency, 0.35) is used and if the counting is performed 24 hours after NaI^{131} administration (decay factor = 1.09), then the conversion factor is 1.89×10^{-5}. This factor is dependent on the efficiency of the counter and also depends on the scaler circuitry, pulse height selector setting and other factors.

d) SUMMARY AND RESULTS.—Table 1 gives the results obtained from 75 consecutive patients for whom the technique out-

TABLE 1.—RESULTS OBTAINED IN 75 CONSECUTIVE PATIENTS: PBI^{131} FOLLOWING 50 μc. DOSE

Class	Mean	S.D.	Range
Hyperthyroid...	0.135 μc./L.	±0.05	0.08 −0.23 μc./L.
Euthyroid......	0.028 μc./L.	±0.015	0.007−0.064 μc./L.
Hypothyroid....	0.029 μc./L.	±0.015	0.008−0.064 μc./L.

lined in this section was used. To obtain the percentage of dose per liter, multiply the figures in the table by 2. It is evident from the table that a clear separation can be made between hyperthyroid and euthyroid states. No such delineation can be seen between euthyroid and hypothyroid conditions. This inability to discriminate between the two states with PBI^{131} studies has been widely observed. This test performed in conjunction with the external thyroid pickup of I^{131} has been useful in the diagnostic evaluation of patients with thyroid disease.

5. CONVERSION RATIO OF IODINE-131 IN PLASMA

Some investigators (45) use as an index of thyroid function the conversion ratio of I^{131} in the plasma; that is, the ratio of protein-bound iodine to unbound or inorganic iodine at a specific time (usually 24 hours after administration of the dose). This figure is readily obtained in conjunction with the test described in Section A, 4, of this chapter.

a) MATERIALS AND METHOD.—All that is required is 50 μc. of NaI^{131}, in addition to a well-type scintillation NaI (T1) counter, and plastic test tubes, ½ in. O.D. by 4 in. length with metallic screw cap.*

---

* Source: Lusteroid Corporation, Maplewood, New Jersey.

b) PROCEDURE.—The method requires the following steps:

1. Pipette 1 ml. of whole plasma into the plastic test tube and count this in the scintillation well counter for 15 minutes.

2. The microcuries per liter of plasma are derived by multiplying the net counts per 15 minutes by the conversion factor, which is:

$$\frac{1 \times 1,000 \times \text{Decay factor}}{15 \times \text{Efficiency} \times \text{disint./min./}\mu c.}$$

3. The conversion ratio is obtained from

$$C_f = C_2/C_1$$

where C_2 is the PBI[131] level in microcuries per liter of plasma and C_1 is the total plasma I[131] level in microcuries per liter.

c) RESULTS.—It is generally accepted that a conversion ratio greater than 30 per cent at 24 hours after the dose indicates a thyrotoxic condition. This method does not yield results that can be used to indicate hypothyroidism.

d) COMMENT.—Some clinicians use the 72-hour plasma test as a screening test. Obviously, the total microcuries per liter herein derived is always greater than that derived from the PBI study; therefore, if the result obtained from step 2 above is below the level of 0.064 μc./L. of plasma, no useful purpose is served in processing the sample further for the PBI fraction. If the result obtained from step 2 is greater than 0.064 μc./L. of plasma, the steps outlined in the procedure for the determination of PBI may be carried out.

6. IN VITRO RED CELL TAGGING

a) MATERIALS:

10–120 $\times$ 10^{-4} μg. of I[131]-tri-iodothyronine.
Isotonic sodium chloride.

b) APPARATUS:

Scintillation well counter.
10 ml. Erlenmeyer flask.
Plastic 2 ml. syringe with needle.

c) PROCEDURE:

1. Add I^{131}-tri-iodothyronine to 3 ml. aliquot of whole blood in stoppered 10 ml. Erlenmeyer flask.
2. Incubate at 37° C. for 2 hours.
3. Determine radioactivity concentration of two 1 ml. aliquots of whole blood for 3 minutes.
4. Wash each blood sample 5 times in tenfold dilution of isotonic sodium chloride.
5. Determine radioactivity concentration of red blood cell (r.b.c.) mass in washed cells.
6. Calculate the following:

$$\text{Percentage uptake} = \frac{\text{Net counts in r.b.c.} \times 100}{\text{Net counts/ml. of whole blood}}$$

7. Correct percentage uptake to 100 hematocrit for comparison purposes.

d) RESULTS.—Average values of the 2-hour in vitro red blood cell uptake of I^{131}-tri-iodothyronine (TRI) are given in Table 2.

TABLE 2.—AVERAGE UPTAKE OF I^{131}-TRI-IODOTHYRONINE IN RED BLOOD CELLS IN 2 HOURS*

THYROID STATUS	%/100 HEMATOCRIT	
	Males	Females
Euthyroid............	15.2	13.9
Hyperthyroid.........	23.7	22.5
Hypothyroid..........	9.7	9.3

* After Hamolsky, M. W., *et al.*: Plasma protein-thyroid hormone complex in man: Further studies on use of in vitro red blood cell uptake of I^{131}-l-tri-iodothyronine as diagnostic test of thyroid function, J. Clin. Endocrinol. 19:103, 1959.

C. SOURCES OF ERROR DUE TO DRUGS

1. IODINE

If stable iodine (I^{127}) reaches the blood stream, it will diminish or inhibit the accumulation of I^{131} by the thyroid gland. Quantities of I^{127} above 1–2 mg. a day begin to interfere with this accumulation (46, 47). The amount of iodine contained in iodized salt and in some vitamin-mineral combinations is insufficient to inactivate uptake, but virtually all other types of iodine medication invalidate the results. The duration of the inactivation varies according to the type of goiter and the form of medication. Lugol's solution administered to a patient with a frank exophthalmic goiter may lose its inhibitory effect in a week; whereas, if given to a normal person, it may reduce uptake for many weeks, and to a person with a toxic nodular goiter, perhaps for many months.

From clinical observation it seems that, if a patient with toxic nodular goiter receives therapy with Lugol's solution, the thyroid I^{131} uptake never rises very much above normal. There is no uniform time lapse on which to rely in eliminating the adverse effect of iodine medication. If a patient has a frank exophthalmic goiter, however, an interval of 1 or 2 weeks will suffice for a I^{131} diagnostic test after medication with Lugol's solution has been discontinued. Desaturation can be hastened by the administration of thiocyanate and propylthiouracil (46). The effect of the dyes for gallbladder and kidney visualization lasts for many weeks. In one euthyroid patient who had been given gallbladder dye, the thyroid gland did not reach its maximum uptake for 4 months.

The depressing effect of Lipiodol® may last for many years. We have noted the effect 3 years after instillation of Lipiodol® for bronchiectasis and 8 years following a salpingogram to determine tubal patency.

2. ANTITHYROID DRUGS

The antithyroid drugs inhibit uptake for a few hours after ingestion, but the duration of the effect varies. Immediately following cessation of medication the uptake may be exaggerated, owing to iodine starvation. Most observers consider this compensatory effect to be of short duration, but it has been reported to continue for several weeks. Usually it can be assumed that a delay of 1 week is safe after the antithyroid compounds have been taken.

3. DESICCATED THYROID OR THYROXIN

Desiccated thyroid or thyroxin suppresses thyroid function in daily doses of 0.065 gm. or less. There are some rebound phenomena at 2 weeks; but after 3 or 4 weeks, in most instances, uptake is normal regardless of the duration of thyroid therapy. In a patient receiving desiccated thyroid, an intramuscular injection of 5 units of thyroid-stimulating hormone (TSH) vitiates the inhibitory effect (48).

4. OTHER INHIBITORS

Cortisone and ACTH diminish thyroid accumulation (49), as does desoxycorticosterone and progesterone (50). Para-amino-salicylic acid (PAS) retards uptake from 1 to 4 weeks after prolonged therapy (51). Thiocyanate medication prevents iodine trapping, washes out iodide and leaves the gland in an iodine-starved condition (52).

A complete résumé of the drugs that interfere with I^{131} uptake, written by Magalotti, Hummon and Hierschbiel, has been published in the January 1959 issue of the *American Journal of Roentgenology* (53), from which Tables 3 and 4 are reproduced.

TABLE 3.—CHEMICALS AND DRUGS THAT INTERFERE WITH
24-HOUR I^{131} THYROID UPTAKE*

A. IODINE CONTAINING COMPOUNDS:

These drugs all depress the 24-hour uptake but vary in degree depending on the type of thyroid. In general, the interference is usually longer with euthyroid patients and nodular goiters and much shorter with diffuse exophthalmic goiters. The average interval of depression is given.

General preparations (1–3 weeks):

Lugol's solution	Iodine suppositories
Iodides	Vitamin preparations (occasional)
Antitussives	Entero-Vioform
Iodine ointments (topical)	Diodoquin
Iodine tincture (topical)	Enterosept
Iodoform (topical)	Neo-Penil (penicillin)

Contrast media:

Aqueous solutions:

Diodrast (1–3 months)

Hypaque, Mediopaque, Neo-Iopax, Urokon, Miokon, Thixokon, Renographin (1–2 weeks)

Dionosil (British) (2–4 months)

Oily solutions (up to 1 year or more):

Lipiodol, Visciodol, Ethiodol, Iodochloral, Pantopaque

Cholecystopaques and cholangiopaques:

Cholografin (3 months), Telepaque (2 months), Priodax (1–3 months)

* From Magalotti, M. F., *et al.*: Effect of disease and drugs on twenty-four hour I^{131} thyroid uptake, Am. J. Roentgenol. 81:47, 1959.

TABLE 3. *(Continued)*

Uterosalpingopaques:
  Skiodan Acacia, Salpix (1 month)
B. OTHER CHEMICALS AND DRUGS:
  These preparations all depress the 24-hour I^{131} thyroid uptake, usually less and for a shorter time in hyperthyroidism. The average interval of depression is given when known.
  Antithyroid drugs (2–8 days):
    Thiouracil, propylthiouracil, methylthiouracil, iothiouracil (Itrumil), Muracil, methimazole (Tapazole), mercazole, Carbimazole
  Thyroid medication (1–2 weeks):
    Desiccated thyroid, thyronine, thyroxine, thyroglobuline
  Thiocyanates (1 week)
  Perchlorate (1 week)
  Nitrate
  Sulfonamides (1 week)
  Orinase
  Progesterone
  Adrenal cortical steroids (1 week or less):
    Cortisone, corticosterone, desoxycorticosterone, prednisone, prednisolone
  ACTH
  Resorcinol
  Cobalt (1 week or less)
  PAS and isoniazid (1 week after prolonged use)
  Butazolidin
  Amphenone (2–3 days)
  Antihistamines (1 week or less)
  Phenothiazine
  Pentothal (1 week)
C. COMPOUNDS THAT ENHANCE THE 24-HOUR I^{131} THYROID UPTAKE:
  Thyroid-stimulating hormone (TSH)
  Estrogens (not persistently)

TABLE 4.—VARIOUS IODINE PREPARATIONS WHOSE NAMES DO NOT REFER TO THE IODINE CONTENT*

Amend's solution	Child's Drikof	Organidin
Arocalcin	Endoarsan	Quin-O-Creme
Cal-A-Thesin	Entodon	Tamponets
Calcidin	Felsol	Thyractin
Ceradine	Limodin	

* From Magalotti, M. F.. *et al.*: Effect of disease and drugs on twenty-four hour I^{131} thyroid uptake, Am. J. Roentgenol. 81:47, 1959.

D. DIAGNOSTIC SIGNIFICANCE

1. THE 24-HOUR THYROID UPTAKE

Numerous comparative studies of the value of the various diagnostic tests for disturbance of thyroid function (54–62) show that all of the tests give reasonably accurate results, that no one of them is definitely superior to the others and that, above all, none of them, singly or in combination, is superior to the clinical history and examination. In 80–90 per cent of patients with hyperthyroidism, the physician will make the diagnosis with certainty on the clinical findings alone, and the laboratory findings merely confirm his opinion. In only about 10 per cent of cases is there any real diagnostic problem; but if there is a problem, the three laboratory tests in common use—the basal metabolic rate (BMR), the chemical protein-bound iodine (PBI) test and the 24-hour uptake of I^{131}—are of considerable help.

The 24-hour uptake test of I^{131} is not always reliable but it has some advantages. There are four basic errors in evaluating the results of uptake tests: (1) the patient has been taking iodine; (2) the test is not reliable in the group of patients with hyperthyroidism due to toxic nodular goiter; (3) the test is erratic in determining thyroid deficiency; and (4) in cases of toxic diffuse goiter, there is some overlapping of results between the euthyroids and the hyperthyroids. On the other hand, if there is a real diagnostic problem, it will usually be in a patient without thyroid enlargement. In this case, hyperthyroidism may be due to a diffusely hyperplastic gland, which will nearly always give a high uptake value even if the disease is of mild degree. The fact that the uptake study does not indicate the degree of hyperthyroidism but is, to a certain extent, an all-or-none reaction is of advantage from a purely diagnostic point of view but is useless, of course, if one is trying to estimate the severity of the disease. If the equipment is available, the tracer test is inexpensive and is subject to few unrecognizable technical errors—errors on the part of either the patient or the technician. If the equipment is purchased for the sole purpose of thyroid diagnosis, it is doubtful that the expense will justify the return, as measured by an improvement in diagnostic accuracy based on a combination of clinical judgment and the basal metabolic rate.

The 24-hour thyroid uptake of I^{131} is the most generally used determination and suffices for routine clinical purposes. However, as discussed previously, some other period (a 4-hour uptake) may be substituted with some increase in diagnostic accuracy. The difference, however, is so little that the convenience of the uptake time is the determining factor, rather than diagnostic accuracy. There is one disadvantage in all of the shorter periods, in that, if the patient is to be given a therapeutic dose, it is mandatory to know the maximum uptake, which is practically always reached in hyperthyroid patients by 24 hours. In fact, well within 24 hours the uptake curve reaches a flat plateau, or certainly one with

TABLE 5.—DIAGNOSTIC SIGNIFICANCE OF THYROID UPTAKE AND URINARY OUTPUT

Class	Thyroid Uptake (Mean Per Cent)	Urinary Output (Mean Per Cent)
Euthyroid	29	50
Exophthalmic goiter	75	16
Recurrent exophthalmic goiter ...	59	27
Toxic nodular goiter	51	29

very little slope, so that it matters little if the neck is assayed at any time between 18 and 30 hours. Of the other tracer tests that have been discussed or described, none increase clinical accuracy to such an extent as to warrant adoption in the ordinary laboratory. It is true that a battery of tests will better the statistical accuracy somewhat, but the betterment is unlikely to be worth the trouble and expense to obtain it. Neither hyperthyroidism nor hypothyroidism is such an obscure clinical entity as to require an expensive and complicated "thyroid profile" or an outline of all "the parameters of thyroid function."

A 24-hour uptake of more than 50 per cent indicates hyperthyroidism (see Table 5); one below 10 per cent (if there is no drug suppression) indicates hypothyroidism. The uptake test is not diagnostic in toxic nodular goiter, for it is possible for a patient to be very ill from a toxic nodular goiter and still yield normal results in the I^{131} thyroid uptake. Some of the discrepancy may be due to iodine medication. For example, if a nodular goiter is saturated with iodine, it does not rid itself of the element for many weeks or months, whereas an exophthalmic goiter turns the iodine over rapidly and recovers its avidity for iodine quickly. A high uptake is nearly always significant and is rarely found in a euthyroid individual without known disease. It does occur in a few cases of simple goiter due to iodine starvation, also in euthyroid patients who have recently discontinued antithyroid drugs, thyroid, thyroxine or tri-iodothyronine, and also in presumably cured Graves disease following either thyroidectomy or I[131] therapy. It is elevated only moderately and occasionally in congestive heart failure, in hepatic insufficiency, in nephrosis, in stool loss after ingestion of soybean flour, in pregnancy and in cold environment; and it has been reported high in patients with low concentration of serum chlorides. A low uptake demands a careful inquiry into the possibility of a drug suppression. If this can be ruled out, a low uptake is compatible with a diagnosis of hypothyroidism. Unfortunately, euthyroid subjects occasionally do have low uptakes, and hypothyroids occasionally have normal uptakes.

The uptake test is not decisively diagnostic in postoperative, recurrent toxic diffuse goiter, and much less so after treatment with I[131]. After such therapy the uptake is diminished long before the symptoms; it may drop to a very low level after 6–8 weeks, even though the patient still has symptoms, and then return to a normal or a high level; or it may continue at a low level if hypothyroidism ensues. If the uptake is high 2 or 3 months after therapy with I[131], most likely the patient still has symptoms or will have a recurrence of symptoms.

In hypothyroidism, either the PBI level or the basal metabolic rate is of greater diagnostic significance than I[131] accumulation.

Age has only moderate influence on the I[131] uptake. There is a tendency for the uptake to be depressed in persons over 60 years of age; but in children the uptake is in the normal adult range, although PBI[131] values up to the age of 4 years are significantly elevated (63–65).

Variations in the iodine avidity of the normal human thyroid as measured by the 24-hour I[131] uptake have been reported by Hare and Haigh (66) in repeated retest measurements in 28 euthyroid subjects. These investigators found a degree of variability outside the probable range of experimental error. They suggest that this normal fluctuation in iodine accumulation may be due to weather changes. Similar findings have been recorded by Francois and his associates (67) and by other investigators. In most instances, the variation is not enough to interfere with the validity of the test.

2. Use of Thyroid-Stimulating Hormone (TSH)

The following discussion is taken in large part from a recent review of the subject by Einhorn (68). The reader is referred to Einhorn's work for more detailed information and references.

The only thyrotropin available for clinical use is Thytropar® (Armour Laboratories, Kankakee, Illinois); it is furnished in ampules as a dry powder in 5- and 10-unit doses. When TSH is given by intramuscular injection, no effect on uptake occurs for 8 hours; thereafter there is a marked acceleration in uptake, which reaches a peak at the end of the first day, 18–24 hours after injection. During the second 24-hour period, the effect diminishes sharply but does not disappear entirely until 5 or 6 days have elapsed, after which there is a period of 1–2 weeks during which uptake is somewhat depressed. A dose response begins with 0.0031 USP units/kg. of body weight and rapidly reaches a maximum at 0.025 USP units/kg.; there is little or no increase beyond this point. There are a few adverse reactions beginning at a dose level of 0.05 units/kg. and reaching 10–15 per cent of cases at 0.3 units/kg. The symptoms, more common in females, consist of nausea and vomiting, cardiac embarrassment, fever and symptoms resembling those of hyperthyroidism. Although all of these calculations are based on a euthyroid status, personal observations indicate that they also hold at least for toxic nodular goiter.

Therefore, in administering TSH, it is very important to use a precise time-response. The tracer dose, or therapeutic dose, should be given 18–24 hours after the injection (24 hours is a satisfactory and more convenient time). An intramuscular injection of 5 USP units of Thytropar® is theoretically adequate and carries a low incidence of reactions. A 10-unit injection will occasionally lead to trouble.

The effect of TSH can be applied to advantage in many situations. It can be used to distinguish hypothyroidism in panpituitary deficiency from primary myxedema. In the former condition, there will be no uptake before the injection of TSH but a normal uptake after injection; in the latter condition, there will be no uptake either before or after. Uptake is inhibited in subacute thyroiditis, but this effect is overcome by TSH. If a patient is euthyroid and is taking thyroid medication, there will be an increase in uptake similar to that of a euthyroid person without medication. In this manner, one can establish the presence of a euthyroid state without awaiting the 3-week period after stopping medication. The test has also been applied in the diagnosis of strumolymphomatosa, since the uptake in this disease is usually not enhanced by TSH. In untreated cancer, however, there is enough normal thyroid present to give an increased uptake after TSH, as is the case also in simple nodular goiter.

The application of TSH to therapy is obvious and will be discussed later (Chapter 8). In toxic nodular goiter, where the uptake is frequently normal or low, the uptake can be increased to a level where therapy may become effective. Theoretically, TSH should be able to increase uptake in iodine-saturated diffusely hyperplastic glands. Unfortunately, in two patients with frank exophthalmic goiter with no uptake—one due to a Lipiodol® bronchogram for bronchiectasis performed 3 years previously, and the other to a Lipiodol® salpingogram to determine tubal patency 8 years previously—we were unable to obtain an uptake using a single injection of 10 units of TSH.

REFERENCES

1. Keating, J. R., Jr., and Albert, A.: Metabolism of iodine in man as disclosed with use of radioiodine, Recent Progr. Hormone Res. 4:429, 1949.
2. Crispell, K. R.; Parson, W., and Sprinkle, P.: Simplified technique for diagnosis of hyperthyroidism, utilizing one-hour uptake of orally administered I^{131}, J. Clin. Endocrinol. 13:221, 1953.
3. Morton, M. E.; Ottoman, R. E., and Peterson, R. E.: Thyroid uptake measured one hour after small oral doses of radioiodine, J. Clin. Endocrinol. 11:1572, 1951.
4. Kriss, J. P.: Uptake of radioactive iodine after intravenous administration of tracer doses, J. Clin. Endocrinol. 11:289, 1951.
5. Barrett, T. F., et al.: Practical application of scintillation counter in diagnosis of diseases of thyroid, J.A.M.A. 152:1414, 1953.
6. Greer, M. A.: Correlation of 24-hour radioiodine uptake of human

thyroid gland with 6-hour and 8-hour uptakes and accumulation gradient, J. Clin. Invest. 30:301, 1951.

7. Lowry, W. S. B.: Thyroid index factor, Acta radiol. 47:393, 1957.

8. Adams, D. D., and Purves, H. D.: Change in thyroidal I[131] content between 8 and 48 hours as an index of thyroid activity, J. Clin. Endocrinol. 17:126, 1957.

9. Meschan, I., et al.: Thyroid function assay with radioiodine; correlation of thyroidal clearance factor and percentage uptake, Am. J. Roentgenol. 81:74, 1959.

10. Friis, T., and Christensen, L. K.: Diagnostic use of radioactive iodine in thyroid disorders, Danish M. Bull. 6:1, 1959.

11. Schultz, A. L., and Zieve, L.: Thyroid clearance, uptake, and rate of uptake of radioiodine in hyperthyroidism, J. Lab. & Clin. Med. 50:335, 1957.

12. Larrson, L. G., and Jonsson, L.: Continuous registration of thyroid uptake after intravenous injection of radioactive iodine; rapid test of iodine concentrating function of thyroid, Acta radiol. 43:81, 1955.

13. Taplits, S.; Fine, A., and Rosenberg, L. S.: Immediate and continuous uptake studies of I[131] in diagnosis and treatment of hyperthyroidism, Radiology 67:544, 1956.

14. Astwood, E. B., and Stanley, M. M.: Use of radioactive iodine in study of thyroid function in man, West. J. Surg. 55:625, 1947.

15. Werner, S. C.: Diagnostic technics with radioiodine, M. Ann. District of Columbia 22:12, 1953.

16. Myant, N. B.; Pochin, E. E., and Goldie, E. A. G.: Plasma iodide clearance rate of human thyroid gland, Clin. Sc. 8:109, 1949.

17. Berson, S. A., et al.: Determination of thyroidal and renal plasma I[131] clearance rates as routine diagnostic test of thyroid dysfunction, J. Clin. Invest. 31:141, 1952.

18. Keating, F. R., Jr., et al.: Radioiodine-accumulating function of human thyroid gland as diagnostic test in clinical medicine, J. Clin. Endocrinol. 10:1425, 1950.

19. Nitowsky, H. M., and Puck, T. T.: Modified radioiodine test for thyroid function, J. Lab. & Clin. Med. 39:824, 1952.

20. McAdams, J. B., and Salter, W. T.: Comparative tests of thyroid function, Ann. Int. Med. 36:1198, 1952.

21. Foote, J. B., and MacLagan, N. F.: Thigh-neck clearance; simplified radioactive test of thyroid function, Lancet 1:868, 1951.

22. Ingbar, S. H.: Simultaneous measurement of iodide-concentrating and protein-binding capacities of normal and hyperfunctioning human thyroid gland, J. Clin. Endocrinol. 15:238, 1955.

23. Pochin, E. E.: Investigation of thyroid function and disease with radioactive iodine, Lancet 2:41 and 84, 1950.

24. Fraser, R.: Diagnostic procedures in thyroid disease, Postgrad. M. J. 33:312, 1957.

25. Mason, A. S., and Oliver, R.: Urinary excretion of radioactive iodine as diagnostic aid in thyroid disorders, Lancet 2:456, 1949.

26. Larsson, L. G.: Studies on radioiodine treatment of thyrotoxicosis; with special reference to behaviour of radioiodine tracer tests, Acta radiol. supp. 126, p. 5, 1955.

27. Morton, M. E.: Measurement of thyroxine synthesis with I^{131}; test for evaluation of thyroid function in equivocal states, California Med. 78:277, 1953.

28. Silver, S.; Fieber, M. H., and Yohalem, S. B.: Blood levels after tracer doses of radioactive iodine in diagnosis of thyroid disorders, Am. J. Med. 13:725, 1952.

29. Clark, D. E.; Trippel, O. H., and Sheline, G. E.: Diagnostic and therapeutic use of radioactive iodine, A.M.A. Arch. Int. Med. 87:17, 1951.

30. Barry, M. C., and Pugh, A. E.: Serum concentrations of radioiodine in diagnostic tracer studies, J. Clin. Endocrinol. 13:980, 1953.

31. Hanbury, E. M., Jr., et al.: Diagnostic use of I-132, J. Clin. Endocrinol. 14:1530, 1954.

32. Goolden, A. W. G., and Mallard, J. R.: Use of iodine 132 in studies of thyroid function, Brit. J. Radiol. 31:589, 1958.

33. Halnan, K. E., and Pochin, E. E.: Use of iodine 132 for thyroid function tests, Brit. J. Radiol. 31:581, 1958.

34. Berman, M.; Becker, D. V., and Benua, R.: Use of I^{131} in treatment of Graves' disease, J. Clin. Endocrinol. 17:1222, 1957.

35. Greer, M. A., and Smith, G. E.: Method for increasing accuracy of radioiodine uptake as test for thyroid function by use of desiccated thyroid, J. Clin. Endocrinol. 14:1374, 1954.

36. Werner, S. C., and Spooner, M.: New and simple test for hyperthyroidism employing L-triiodothyronine and twenty-four hour I^{131} uptake methods, Bull. New York Acad. Med. 31:137, 1955.

37. Smollar, L.: Hyperthyroidism: Diagnosis by failure of triiodothyronine to suppress uptake of iodine 131, California Med. 88:288, 1958.

38. Thode, H. G.; Jaimet, C. H., and Kirkwood, S.: Studies and diagnostic tests of salivary gland and thyroid gland function with radioiodine, New England J. Med. 251:129, 1954.

39. Burrell, C. D., and Fraser, R.: Iodide-repletion test, Quart. J. Med. 26:559, 1957.

40. Hamolsky, M. W.; Golodetz, A., and Freedberg, A. S.: Plasma protein-thyroid hormone complex in man: Further studies on use of in vitro red blood cell uptake of I^{131}-l-triiodothyronine as diagnostic test of thyroid function, J. Clin. Endocrinol. 19:103, 1959.

41. National Research Council: *Shipping Regulations: Problems Associated with Transportation of Radioactive Materials* (Nat. Acad. Series Pub. No. 205).

42. Freedberg, A. S.; Ureles, A., and Hertz, S.: Serum level of protein-bound radioactive iodine (I^{131}) in diagnosis of hyperthyroidism, Proc. Soc. Exper. Biol. & Med. 70:679, 1949.

43. Myant, N. B., and Pochin, E. E.: Thyroid clearance rate of plasma

iodine as measure of thyroid activity, Proc. Roy. Soc. Med. 42:959, 1949.

44. Williams, R. H.; Jaffe, H., and Bernstein, B.: Comparison of distribution of radioactive iodine in serum and urine in different levels of thyroid function, J. Clin. Invest. 28:1222, 1949.

45. Clark, D. E.; Moe, R. H., and Adams, E. E.: Rate of conversion of administered inorganic radioactive iodine into protein bound iodine of plasma as an aid in evaluation of thyroid function, Surgery 26:331, 1949.

46. Starr, P., and Liebhold-Schueck, R.: Theory of thyroid hormone action, A.M.A. Arch. Int. Med. 92:880, 1953.

47. Gordon, E. S., and Albright, E. S.: Treatment of thyrotoxicosis with radioactive iodine, J.A.M.A. 143:1129, 1950.

48. Levy, H. P.; Kelly, L. W., and Jeffries, W. McK.: Study of thyroid function by means of single injection of thyrotropin, Clin. Res. Proc. 1:94, 1953.

49. Kuhl, W. J., Jr., and Ziff, M.: Alterations of thyroid function by ACTH and cortisone, J. Clin. Endocrinol. 12:554, 1952.

50. Zingg, W., and Perry, W. F.: Influence of adrenal and gonadal steroids on uptake of iodine by thyroid gland, J. Clin. Endocrinol. 13:712, 1953.

51. Balint, J. A.; Fraser, R., and Hanno, M. G. W.: Radioiodine measurements of thyroid function during and after PAS treatment of tuberculosis, Brit. M. J. 1:1234, 1954.

52. Blackburn, J. A.; Keating, F. R., Jr., and Haines, S. F.: Radioiodine tracer studies in thiocyanate myxedema, J. Clin. Endocrinol. 11:1503, 1951.

53. Magalotti, M. F.; Hummon, I. F., and Hierschbiel, E.: Effect of disease and drugs on twenty-four hour I^{131} thyroid uptake, Am. J. Roentgenol. 81:47, 1959.

54. Schultz, A. L.: Interpretation of thyroid function tests in diagnosis of thyroid disease, Minnesota Med. 40:246 and 260, 1957.

55. Henkelmann, C. R.; Balbus, T. G., and King, E. R.: Evaluation of battery of thyroid function studies, M. Ann. District of Columbia 26:161, 1957.

56. Cassidy, C. E., and Vander Laan, W. P.: Laboratory aids to diagnosis in thyroid disease, New England J. Med. 258:828, 1958.

57. Goolden, A. W. G.: Comparison of radioiodine tests in diagnosis of hyperthyroidism, Brit. J. Radiol. 31:433, 1958.

58. Goldberg, I. J. L., and Fitzsimons, E. A.: Thyroidal accumulation of radioiodine as clinical test for hyperthyroidism, Brit. J. Radiol. 31:428, 1958.

59. Luddecke, H. F.: Basal metabolic rate, protein-bound iodine and radioactive iodine uptake: Comparative study, Ann. Int. Med. 49:305, 1958.

60. Rubenfeld, S., et al.: Radioiodine profile in diagnosis of thyroid disease, A.M.A. Arch. Int. Med. 100:266, 1957.

61. Perlmutter, M.: Practical application of thyroid function tests, New York J. Med. 58:3796, 1958.
62. Newburger, R. A., *et al.*: Uptake and blood level of radioactive iodine in hyperthyroidism, New England J. Med. 253:127, 1955.
63. Rosenberg, G.: Effect of age on 24 hour iodine 131 uptake in healthy males, Canad. Serv. M. J. 13:565, 1957.
64. Oliner, L., *et al.*: Thyroid function studies in children: Normal values for thyroidal I^{131} uptake and PBI^{131} levels up to age of 18, J. Clin. Endocrinol. 17:61, 1957.
65. Sheline, G. E.; Koulischer, N., and Pickering, D.: Thyroidal accumulation of radioiodine in children, A.M.A. J. Dis. Child. 93:391, 1957.
66. Hare, E. H., and Haigh, C. P.: Variations in iodine avidity of normal human thyroid as measured by 24-hour 131-I uptake, Clin. Sc. 14:441, 1955.
67. Francois, P. E., *et al.*: Variations in thyroid function in normal subjects, Clin. Sc. 17:545, 1958.
68. Einhorn, J.: Studies on effect of thyrotropic hormone on thyroid function in man, Acta radiol., supp. 160, p. 5, 1958.

CHAPTER 2

Isotope Dilution Techniques

QUANTITATION OF DILUTION may be precisely accomplished by labeling the substance in question with an isotope. Isotope dilution techniques have been widely employed in biologic systems for determining the volume of fluid compartments and studying the concentration and distribution of various foreign and physiologic components.

Of the dilution procedures used, several are considered of sufficient general clinical interest to be included below. Using radioiodine-labeled human serum albumin (I^{131}HSA), plasma volume may be determined and blood volume calculated by means of the peripheral hematocrit. Radioiodine-labeled human serum albumin is also adaptable for determination of ascitic fluid volumes. Chromium-51 as chromate is an acceptable labeling substance for red cells and, in the reduced state, for labeling plasma; and it can be used to determine the circulating volume of these components as well as the relative survival time of the erythrocyte. A variation of the dilution technique is employed in the determination of vitamin B_{12} absorption. In this test the vitamin is labeled with cobalt-60.

A. BLOOD VOLUME: RADIOIODINE-LABELED HUMAN SERUM ALBUMIN (I^{131}HSA)

1. INTRODUCTION

A simplified technique for determining blood volume is an extremely useful adjunct to the clinical evaluation of patients in any modern hospital. The use of labeled human serum albumin tagged with I^{131} ($I^{131}HSA$) has had widespread application. This substance is employed because it has several useful properties: it is not toxic; it mixes rapidly with the circulating blood; it remains in the vascular compartment for a reasonable period of time; and it may be quantitatively detected in very high dilution. The possible alteration of the albumin owing to the labeling process and the radioactivity has not demonstrably changed the conditions needed for isotope dilution studies.

Determination of the circulating blood volume with $I^{131}HSA$ by the above-described technique has another advantage. Using the well-type scintillation counter, the circulating blood volume may be determined by injecting only 2 μc. of I^{131}. Such low levels of radioactivity allow for serial determinations of blood volume to be made at daily intervals, or more often, without exposing the patient to significant amounts of radiation.

A critical appraisal of the technical source of error inherent in determining the circulating blood volume by dilution technique using $I^{131}HSA$ has been reported by Hlad and Tanz (15). These investigators have evaluated errors due to pipetting, geometry of sample containers, constant-delivery syringes, sedimentation of blood in sample containers, self-absorption and scatter in blood (as compared to water) and adsorption of radioalbumin to glassware. The largest errors are due to constant-delivery syringes and adsorption of albumin to glassware. The latter error may be corrected with carrier albumin.

Sources of error other than technical errors have been discussed by Reeve (22). The stability of the I^{131} to albumin bond is important. The principal factors influencing this bond are: the specific amount of I^{131} bound per molecule of albumin, the use of species-specific albumin and the age of the preparation. The presence of any appreciable quantity of free iodide will give false high-volume values. On the assumption that the I^{131} label remains bound to albumin, the rate of escape from the vascular compartment and the degradation rate would assume significance. If these values were constant, multiple sampling could be used to extrapolate the volume of the albumin space at zero time. One must further assume that the concentration of the injected serum albumin after intravascular mixing is homogeneous and, further, that the red cell space of distribution is equal to that of albumin. If whole blood volume is to be derived from dilution of albumin in the plasma, total red cell mass must be extrapolated from the venous hematocrit. Available evidence suggests that red cell concentration in venous blood is higher than the concentration in small vessels in various tissues and organs. The whole body hematocrit averages about 91 per cent of venous hematocrit (13). The relationship of venous hematocrit (H) to whole body hematocrit (H_o), is known as the F cells factor and is expressed as follows:

$$F_{cells} = \frac{H_o}{H}$$

This factor has become the subject of various recent studies (1, 11, 13, 14, 21, 28). The trapping of plasma in hematocrit determination is a further source of error in deriving red cell mass and whole blood volume from a labeled serum protein; this trapping introduces an error of about 2 per cent. For the laboratory concerned with practical clinical laboratory techniques, the factors discussed above become important in avoiding obvious pitfalls and sources of error.

2. TECHNIQUE OF ADMINISTRATION

With a tubular spacer, it is possible to attenuate geometrically the radiation impinging on the scintillation crystal. This attenuation may be quantitated (to avoid preparation of a dilute standard) by assaying the radioactivity in the dose of $I^{131}HSA$ before injecting it intravenously into the subject to be studied. This method is employed in the procedure described below. The preassembling of needles, syringes and test-tube counting containers will preclude last-minute assembling of small equipment. A mimeographed record form with simplified formulas will allow the technical personnel to calculate blood volume.

a) MATERIALS.—The following are required:

   3 μc. $I^{131}HSA$
   One 10 ml. vial of saline, physiologic

Syringes:
  One 2 ml. plastic
  One 10 ml. plastic, disposable
Needles, disposable:
  Two 20 gauge, 1½ in. long
Test tubes, two:
  One plastic, ⅝ in. O.D., 4 in. long, with metallic
    screw cap calibrated to 5 ml. (nonsterile)
  One, same as above, but sterile
  One Wintrobe tube

b) APPARATUS.—The following are required:

Scintillation well counter with 2×2 in. NaI (Tl)
    crystal
Scaler
Spacer—aluminum tubing ⅝ in. O.D., 8 in. long,
    ½ in. I.D.
  A shelf is provided 1 in. from the upper end
    of the spacer to assure uniform positioning
    of the test tube.

c) PROCEDURE.—The following procedure is used:

1. Transfer approximately 3 μc. of I^{131}HSA from dose vial
   to a sterile plastic test tube, using the 2 ml. plastic
   syringe. Dilute to approximately 2 ml. with sterile saline.
   Cap the tube with a sterile cotton plug.
2. Place the test tube and its contents in the aluminum
   spacer, 7 in. above the bottom of the well. Count the
   sample for 1 minute.
3. Aspirate the dose of I^{131}HSA from the plastic test tube
   with the same 2 ml. plastic syringe and needle used
   above.
4. Inject the dose into the patient's antecubital vein. The
   syringe should be flushed with blood several times.
5. Remove the needle from the syringe with forceps and
   place the hub end down in the test tube. Place the
   syringe into the tube with the delivery end down. Insert
   the test tube into the spacer as before, and obtain the net
   count for a 1-minute period.

6. In exactly 15 minutes, withdraw sufficient blood from the antecubital vein of the contralateral arm to obtain a 5 ml. aliquot of whole blood for assaying radioactivity plus a 1 ml. sample for determination of the hematocrit in a Wintrobe tube by centrifugation at 3,000 rpm for 15 minutes. Using a calibrated plastic test tube, count a 5 ml. aliquot of blood in the well counter for 1 minute (the spacer is not used). Should greater accuracy in the determination be necessary, similar aliquots can be withdrawn at 20 and 25 minutes, processed as above, and the values of counts per minute placed on a semilogarithmic graph. A straight line extrapolated to intersect the ordinate at zero time will give theoretical volume of distribution before loss from the vascular compartment.

7. Calculate the blood volume, using the following factors:

$$V_B = \frac{G \; (A_{1 \text{ ml.}} - A_{\text{Res.}})}{A_{5 \text{ ml.}}}$$

where V_B = whole blood volume,

$\quad G$ = attenuation factor of 2 ml. in spacer to 5 ml. in well,

$\quad A_{1 \text{ ml.}}$ = net counts/1 min. from 2 ml. dose in spacer,

$\quad A_{\text{Res.}}$ = net counts/1 min. from residual activity adhering to empty test tube, syringe and needle,

$\quad A_{5 \text{ ml.}}$ = net counts/1 min. from 5 ml. blood sample in well.

8. Calculate the volume of plasma (V_p) and the volume of the red cell mass (V_c) from the hematocrit (H):

$$V_c = V_B H$$
$$V_p = V_B - V_c$$

A correction factor for the hematocrit may be used. This correction applies to the discrepancy between venous and total body hematocrit and the trapping of plasma in determination of the hematocrit. The factor recommended is 0.915 times the hematocrit. The derivation of the attenuation factor (G) is obtained as follows: The spacer is placed in the well of the scintillation detector. A test tube containing 2 ml. (3 μc.) of NaI^{131} in NaI solution is placed in the spacer and a net count of activity obtained. The volume is brought up to 10 ml. with NaI solution. With a calibrated pipette, 100 λ (0.100 ml.) is transferred from the original test tube to a clean tube. The pipette is flushed twice with NaI solution, the activity is brought up to 5 ml. volume, and a net count is obtained in the well of the scintillation detector—without the spacer.

$$G = \frac{\text{Cts. well}}{\text{Cts. spacer}} \times 500$$

3. INTERPRETATION

The plasma volume value of 40.6 ± 4.4 ml./kg. as obtained with the $I^{131}HSA$ technique by Storaasli and his co-workers (27) compares favorably with a value of 43.08 ± 5.9 ml./kg. with Evans blue dye reported by Gibson and Evans (12), and with 39.3 ± 4.9 ml./kg. with chromic chloride by Frank and Gray (32). These values are essentially in agreement with values obtained in our laboratories. Employing a factor of 0.915 for correcting the hematocrit, the following so-called "normal" values have been found adequate:

> Whole blood volume = 73 ml./kg. (±5 ml.)
> Plasma volume   = 43 ml./kg. (±5 ml.)
> Red cell volume   = 30 ml./kg. (±5 ml.)

A substantial normal range exists with a decreased blood volume per unit weight in the obese patient, and a higher value in the asthenic person. This may indicate a correlation between blood volume and body surface area or, more likely, body density. In those who have recently lost weight, the blood volume may be better calculated on the basis of the usual weight rather than the weight at the time of determination. Alteration of blood volume in disease has been adequately discussed (5, 13, 16, 19, 27).

B. RED CELL VOLUME AND SURVIVAL
STUDIES: CHROMIUM-51

1. Introduction

A search for methods for determining the total mass of circulating erythrocytes has led investigators to use numerous substances to label these cells (13). Metabolic incorporation of radioactive iron, phosphate or potassium by the red cell are typical examples of isotopic labeling. Although extensively studied, these substances are not fully satisfactory because of limited physical half-life, biologic half-life in the erythrocyte, reutilization when released from destroyed cells or the necessity for the preparation of labeled compatible cells in donors who must receive relatively heavy doses of radioactivity. Combined studies using chromium with other isotopes have also been made (38).

For determining total red cell mass or cell survival time, the incorporation of the radioactive chromate ion in the erythrocyte offers several advantages over tagging with labeled physiologic red cell components. Under proper conditions of pH, temperature and duration of incubation, nearly 90 per cent or more of the tracer dose may be affixed to the cell content. In addition to this high specific affinity, the bond between cell and chromate is stable, the half-time of elution from the red cell being 75–80 days. During this period the activity may be readily counted, since the physical half-life of Cr^{51} is 26.5 days. Reincorporation of the isotope into new red cells apparently does not occur. Evaluation of the red cell survival technique has been discussed by Strumia and his associates (46).

2. Technique of Administration

Chromium-51-labeled chromate may be utilized to determine red cell survival, red cell mass and plasma volume. The labeling of erythrocytes with Cr^{51} chromate may be abruptly stopped by reduction with ascorbate. The reduced chromium will label to plasma proteins. Labeling to glassware as a source of error does not occur in the technique described below (43). This modification of the method described by Read (40) will label red cells and plasma with approximately equal concentrations of radioactivity.

a) MATERIALS.—The necessary materials are:

> Sodium chromate $(Na_2Cr^{51}O_4)$*
> Heparin solution, 1–1,000
> Sodium ascorbate, sterile solution

A sterile tray is prepared containing the following items:

> Two tuberculin syringes
> One 5 ml. syringe
> Three 10 ml. syringes
> One 50 ml. syringe
> Two 19 gauge needles, 3 in. long
> Three 19 gauge needles, 1½ in. long
> Two 25 gauge needles, 1½ in. long
> One syringe cap†
> One 1 ml. heparin cannula (needle adapter, capped at distal end with a rubber diaphragm for multiple puncture)
> Two 2 ml. centrifuge tubes

b) APPARATUS.—The following are required:

> Scintillation well counter, NaI (Tl)‡
> One scaler
> Plastic test tubes,§ ½ in. O.D., 4 in. long, with metal cap
> Centrifuge
> Two 100 ml. volumetric flasks

c) PROCEDURE.—The following procedure is used:

> (1) *Labeling of Erythrocytes with Chromium-51:*
>
> > (*a*) Withdraw approximately 45 ml. of venous blood from the antecubital vein, using a 50 ml. syringe wetted with 0.5 ml. of heparin. Fill a Wintrobe tube, using a sterile hematocrit needle, and deter-

---

* Source: Abbott Laboratories, Oak Ridge, Tennessee.
† Source: Becton, Dickinson & Co., Rutherford, New Jersey.
‡ Source: N. Wood Counter Laboratory, Chicago, Illinois.
§ Source: Lusteroid Corporation, Maplewood, New Jersey.

mine the hematocrit by centrifugation at 3,000 rpm for 30 minutes.

(b) Do not withdraw the needle from the vein; replace the syringe with a heparin cannula. Inject a drop of heparin through the diaphragm to fill the lumen of the needle.

(c) Using a 3 in. 19 gauge needle, aspirate the 50 μc. of $Na_2Cr^{51}O_4$ from the 2 ml. centrifuge tube with the 50 ml. syringe of blood. Flushing with a small amount of blood will wash the chromate solution from the tube. Replace the 19 gauge needle with a syringe cap, and agitate gently for 4 minutes. Mixing will be aided by including several milliliters of air in the syringe.

(2) *Determination of Labeled Red Cell Survival:*

(a) Obtain a 10 ml. aliquot of venous blood in a heparin-wetted syringe from the antecubital vein of the contralateral arm. After injection, allow an interval of 15 minutes for mixing. Obtain further venous blood at appropriate intervals (e.g., daily to 2 times per week).

(b) Determine the radioactivity of 3 ml. samples of whole blood and plasma. Determine the hematocrit of all samples but the initial 15-minute blood, for which the hematocrit obtained in "Labeling of Erythrocytes with Chromium-51" (1, *a*, above) may be used.

The apparent half-survival time of Cr^{51}-tagged erythrocytes may be defined as the interval during which half of the Cr^{51} disappears from the circulating erythrocytes. A correction is made for the physical half-life of the isotope but not for the elution rate of Cr^{51} from the red cells.

The radioactivity of the erythrocytes determined on the initial day of observation is considered to be 100 per cent of the Cr^{51} activity. Assay of whole blood and plasma radioactivity may be made at appropriate intervals, and the percentage of surviving labeled red cells ascertained.

$$\text{Percentage of surviving red cells} = \frac{\text{Cts./ml. of red cells day}_n}{\text{Cts./ml. of red cells day}_0} \times 100$$

A correction must be made for decay of Cr^{51} by using appropriate tables or by relating the decay to the decrease in radioactivity of the standard solution.

The determination of Cr^{51} activity per milliliter of erythrocytes is made by subtracting the plasma activity from whole blood activity and correcting for the hematocrit.

$$\text{Cts./ml. red cells} = \text{Cts./ml. whole blood} -$$
$$[(\text{Cts./ml. plasma}) (\text{plasmacrit})] \left(\frac{100}{\text{hematocrit}} \right)$$

The data may be plotted on a 2-cycle semilogarithmic graph with the ordinate indicating percentage and the linear abscissa time in days. In this manner, Cr^{51} half-survival may be obtained.

(3) *Determination of Circulating Red Cell Mass:*

The circulating mass of erythrocytes may be determined by relating the activity in the labeled injected red cells to the observed dilution in the circulating blood.

(a) Label the blood as described above ("Labeling of Erythrocytes with Chromium-51"). In addition, the volume and radioactivity of the injected cells and plasma must be determined. The following additional steps are necessary:

[1] After 8 minutes of agitating the blood with the sodium ascorbate, remove 5 ml. of the blood for standard preparation (see below).

[2] Weigh the 50 ml. syringe and contents on a triple-beam balance after removing the 5 ml. aliquot and following the reinjection of the blood, to determine the weight of injected blood. The volume of injected blood is then

obtained. Specific gravity of 1.050 is assumed for blood unless actually determined by the copper sulfate flotation method.

$$\text{Volume of injected blood} = \frac{\text{Wt. of injected blood}}{\text{Specific gravity of injected blood}}$$

Obtain a 10 ml. aliquot of blood from the contralateral arm in 15 minutes and assay the radioactivity in 3 ml. of whole blood and plasma in the scintillation well counter.

(4) *Preparation of Standard Solution:*

(*a*) Dilute a 1 ml. sample of the whole labeled blood and a 1 ml. sample of the labeled plasma used for injection to 100 ml. with distilled water in volumetric flasks.

(*b*) Assay for radioactivity 3 ml. aliquots of each standard solution in a plastic test tube, using the scintillation well counter. Calculate the cell mass, using the following formula:

Red cell mass =

$$\frac{(\text{Vol. injected blood} \times \text{hematocrit})\ [(\text{cts./3 ml. blood std.} - (\text{cts./3 ml. std.} \times \text{plasma})] \times 100}{(\text{Cts./3 ml. blood after 15 min.}) - (\text{cts./3 ml. plasma after 15 min.} \times \text{plasmacrit})}$$

(5) *Plasma Volume Determination:*

Since the Cr[51] activity bound to plasma has a much more rapid rate of elution than that from erythrocytes, the plasma volume is best determined by obtaining at least three aliquots of plasma; intervals of 15, 20 and 25 minutes following injection are appropriate, for during this time the radioactivity in the plasma diminishes at an exponential rate. Plot the activity on semilogarithmic graph paper, and extrapolate the curve to the zero-time intersection. Count 3 ml. samples in the scintillation well counter.

of the one which appears between the braces:

Red cell mass = (Vol. injected blood × hematocrit) [(cts./3 ml. blood std. —(cts./3 ml. plasma std. × plasmacrit)] × 100 / (Cts./3 ml. blood after 15 min.) —(cts./3 ml. plasma after 15 min. × plasmacrit)

Plasma volume =

$$\frac{\text{(Cts./3 ml. of plasma std.) (vol. injected blood) (plasmacrit)}}{\text{(Cts./3 ml. of plasma at zero time)}}$$

(6) *Whole Blood Volume:*

Whole blood volume is calculated by adding cell volume to plasma volume.

Whole blood volume = Red cell volume + Plasma volume

(7) *Whole Body Hematocrit:*

$$\text{Whole body hematocrit} = \frac{\text{Red cell mass}}{\text{Whole blood volume}}$$

3. RESULTS

a) SURVIVAL TIME STUDIES.—The apparent half-survival time of Cr^{51}-tagged erythrocytes may be defined as that interval of

TABLE 6.—APPARENT HALF-SURVIVAL TIME OF Cr^{51}-TAGGED ERYTHROCYTES IN THE NORMAL ADULT

Number of Cases	Half-Survival Time (Days)	Donor	Recipient	Author
3	25–29	Group 0	Group A	Necheles, Weinstein and LeRoy (39)
5	30–39	Genotype specific	Compatible	Necheles, Weinstein and LeRoy (39)
5	30–33	Self	Self	Necheles, Weinstein and LeRoy (39)
5	33–38	Heterotype	Compatible	Sutherland *et al.* (47)
5	28–35	Self	Self	Sutherland *et al.* (47)
5	Avg. 28	....	....	Read (40)

time during which half of the Cr^{51} activity disappears from the circulating erythrocytes. A correction is made for the physical half-life of the isotope but not for the elution rate of Cr^{51} from the red cells. This value in normal adults, as observed by several investigators, is recorded in Table 6. The values observed in various hematologic disorders are recorded in Table 7. Ebaugh, Emerson and Ross (30) reported 19 cases of erythrocyte survival studies employing donor cells of varying age; half-time of survival was not recorded, and many of the cases were followed for only several days.

TABLE 7.—APPARENT HALF-SURVIVAL TIME OF Cr^{51}-TAGGED ERYTHROCYTES IN VARIOUS HEMATOLOGIC DISORDERS

Diagnosis	Number of Cases	Half-Survival Time (Days)	Donor	Recipient	Author
Anemia:					
Congenital hemolytic....	4				
Presplenectomy.........	..	12, 11, 14, 15	Self	Self	Read et al. (41)
Postsplenectomy........	..	33, 27.5, 32, 27.5	Self	Self	Read et al. (41)
Acquired hemolytic.......	1				
Before cortisone........	..	7	Self	Self	Read et al. (41)
During cortisone........	..	10	Self	Self	Read et al. (41)
(Lymphatic leukemia).	1	2.5	Heterotype	Compatible	Read et al. (41)
Before cortisone........	1	1	Genotype specific	Compatible	Weinstein and LeRoy (48)
During cortisone........	..	7	Genotype specific	Compatible	Weinstein and LeRoy (48)
During cortisone........	..	28	Self	Self	Weinstein and LeRoy (48)
Secondary hemolytic......	1	4.5	Genotype specific	Compatible	Weinstein and LeRoy (48)
Hemolytic...............	4	18, 28	....	....	Sutherland et al. (47)
Hypoplastic.............	3	26, 25, 21.5	Self	Self	Read et al. (41)
Hypoplastic.............	1	25	Genotype specific	Compatible	Weinstein and LeRoy (48)
Thalassemia.............	1				
Presplenectomy.........	..	15.5	Self	Self	Read et al. (41)
Postsplenectomy........	..	25	Self	Self	Read et al. (41)
Myeloid metaplasia.......	3				
Presplenectomy.........	..	6, 12	Self	Self	Read et al. (41)
Postsplenectomy........	..	32, 30.5, 23	Self	Self	Read et al. (41)
Myeloid metaplasia.......	3	18, 37, 40	Genotype specific	Compatible	Weinstein and LeRoy (48)
Chronic lymphatic leukemia.	3	8, 23, 38	Genotype specific	Compatible	Weinstein and LeRoy (48)
Uremia.................	1	23	Self	Self	Read et al. (41)

The relationship between Cr^{51} half-survival time and actual red cell survival is a complex subject and not within the scope of a description of technique. It may be stated that elution of Cr^{51} from the red cell may be variable in disease. The shape of the survival curve is unquestionably influenced by the senescence of red cells. A change in red cell mass during the period of observation can markedly influence the interpretation of the Cr^{51} survival curve as related to actual red cell survival.

b) RED CELL MASS AND PLASMA VOLUME.—The normal

TABLE 8.—NORMAL VALUES OF ERYTHROCYTE VOLUME
IN NORMAL ADULTS

Total Red Cell Mass	Red Cell Volume (Ml./Kg.)	Liters of Red Cells per Sq. Mm. Body Surface	No. of Determinations	Subjects	Author
2351($\pm$290)	31.8 (3.5)	1.21 ($\pm$0.12)	25	Normal male	Sterling and Gray (45)
2081($\pm$508)	30.3 (5.6)	....	10	Normal adult	Gray and Frank (34)
....	29.5 (0.58)	....	8	Normal male	Read (41)

values observed by the authors, using this method, are as follows, as determined in 13 normal males:

> Red cell mass, 32.7 ml./kg.
> Plasma volume, 45.4 ml./kg.
> Whole blood volume, 78.1 ml./kg.
> Peripheral hematocrit, 46.0
> Whole body hematocrit, 42.1
> Whole body/peripheral hematocrit, 0.91

The normal red blood cell volume as determined by the chromate technique in the normal adult may be seen in Table 8, as determined by several other observers. Reilly and his co-workers (42) reported their findings in 89 hospital patients with conditions which they felt did not alter the blood volume. These findings were reported as whole blood volume; hematocrits were not given. The whole blood volume was 65.5 cc. ($\pm$ 5.95) per kilogram, or 2.49 L. ($\pm$0.28) per square meter of body surface. The whole blood volume of 56 cardiac patients was reported by the same investigators, who concluded that blood volume is increased in most cardiac patients with evidence of right ventricular failure but not in cases with left ventricular insufficiency or mitral stenosis alone. Several other reports have confirmed the presence of hypervolemia in congestive failure (29, 31, 33).

c) FACTORS AFFECTING LABELING ERYTHROCYTES WITH CHROMIUM-51:

1. *Chemical State.*—Red cells are selectively labeled by the chromate ion; the chromic ion is ineffective (36) but may be used to label plasma (32, 34).

2. *Concentration of Chromate.*—Between the range of 0.25 and 10.0 μg./ml. of blood, the per cent of binding of chromate ion does not vary appreciably (30). This per cent of binding decreases with increasing concentration of chromate (36). In concentrations above 37.5 μg. of chromate per cubic centimeter of red cells, the per cent of labeling drops off rapidly from 98 per cent until at 1,800 μg. only 10 per cent of the chromate is taken up by the cells (42). Increased chromate, from 20 to 30 times the amount of carrier chromate, increases red cell fragility (39) and in vivo survival (30).

3. *Time of Labeling.*—Labeling is rapid at higher temperatures. At 39° C., 90 per cent of the activity is incorporated in 5 minutes, compared to 50–75 per cent at 26° C. and 10–20 per cent at 1.8° C. The per cent of labeling at 26° and 39° C. does not increase over the 5-minute value when an assay is made at 30 minutes (30).

4. *Hydrogen Ion Concentration.*—Uptake of chromate by red cells increases in an acid pH, the uptake at pH 6.0 being 3 or 4 times more rapid than at pH 7.3 (30).

5. *Age of Erythrocytes.*—When the blood is stored at 4°–6° C. for periods up to 29 days, the ability to bind chromate is not reduced but is actually somewhat increased, which may be attributable to the decrease in the pH of the stored blood (30).

6. *The Suspending Media.*—The incorporation of chromate is more complete in saline suspension than in whole blood, the percentage bound being approximately 98 per cent in saline solution, compared to 85–90 per cent in whole blood (40).

7. *The Site of the Chromate-Erythrocyte Union.*—Fractionation studies have demonstrated that chromate is bound to the globin

portion of hemoglobin (36). Hemoglobin shows a higher affinity for the chromic ion than for chromate, implying impermeability of the red cell to the chromic ion (36).

8. *Stability of the Chromate-Erythrocyte Union.*—Chromate bound to the red cell does not exchange with chromate in the suspending media. Cation and anion exchange resins cannot remove the chromium bound to hemoglobin (36). In vitro the bond is so stable that the half-time of elution of the chromium from the red cell is 77 ± 12 days (39).

9. *The Reutilization of Chromium-51 from Destroyed Erythrocytes.*—Observers have been unable to demonstrate the reutilization of Cr^{51} from in vivo destroyed red cells to label new cells (36).

The foregoing information does not attempt to give a complete review of the problem of labeling erythrocytes with Cr^{51} but should serve adequately as a basis for instituting this procedure in the reasonably well-equipped radioisotope laboratory.

C. DIAGNOSTIC TESTS USING RADIOACTIVE CYANOCOBALAMINE (VITAMIN B_{12})

Vitamin B_{12} labeled with radioactive cobalt (Co^{60}, Co^{58} or Co^{56}) is a valuable tool for the diagnostic study of patients suspected of having pernicious anemia. It is also of aid in the study of patients with nervous system diseases simulating subacute combined degeneration of the cord and of patients with intestinal malabsorption. The following description of the normal physiology of vitamin B_{12} will lead to a better understanding of this tracer technique and the interpretation of the results.

The average diet contains about 10 μg. of vitamin B_{12} a day, particularly in meats and other animal protein foods. Of this amount, about 1–3 μg. are absorbed from the small intestine into the blood stream under normal conditions. Normal absorption will take place only when adequate amounts of intrinsic factor, a substance secreted in the stomach, is also present. Pernicious anemia results when the stomach fails to secrete adequate intrinsic factor. Disease of the small bowel may also prevent the absorption of vitamin B_{12}, even in the presence of adequate intrinsic factor.

The absorption of vitamin B_{12} occurs in the ileum (50, 54), and the maximal rate of absorption occurs 6–14 hours after oral administration (51). The newly absorbed vitamin B_{12} is present in the circulating blood in low concentration, largely bound to protein. Intermediate storage depots probably exist; however, over a period of 4–7 days most of the vitamin B_{12} is stored in the liver, remaining there for months or years. It is slowly released from this organ, maintaining a fairly constant blood level, which is essential for normal cellular metabolism. At the cellular level it is involved in methylation reactions necessary in the synthesis of nucleic acid precursors. A cellular vitamin B_{12} deficiency, such as occurs in pernicious anemia, leads to faulty maturation and function of many body tissues. This deficiency is manifested as megaloblastic anemia, sore and atrophic tongue, central nervous system dysfunction and gastrointestinal disorders.

The ultimate metabolic fate of vitamin B_{12} is unknown. Under normal circumstances, none is excreted in the urine. However, if the serum B_{12}–binding capacity is exceeded by large parenteral doses, more than half of the amount injected appears in the 24-hour urine collection (75).

1. Types of Tests

Four types of tests have been devised using radioactive cyanocobalamine (vitamin B_{12}) for the detection of pernicious anemia or intestinal malabsorption. The relationship of these tests to the normal physiology of vitamin B_{12} is illustrated in Figure 2, in which 2.0 μg. doses of vitamin $B_{12}Co^{60}$ are utilized as an example. Other isotopes of cobalt and a variety of dosages ranging from 0.05 to 3.0 μg. of B_{12} have been used. Smaller doses of B_{12} tend to result in greater percentages of absorption. The four methods are:

1. Detection of unabsorbed vitamin B_{12} in fecal samples collected over a 5–10-day period (67).
2. Detection of gamma rays emanating from the liver by a scintillation counter-type radiation detector 5–10 days after the oral dose (64).
3. Detection of the minute amounts of radioactivity appearing in the blood 8–12 hours after administration (60).

4. Use of a large parenteral dose of nonradioactive B_{12} to "flush" absorbed radioactive vitamin B_{12} into the urine, and measurement of radioactivity in a 24-hour urine collection (81).

For various practical reasons the fourth test has achieved the widest popularity and is the one discussed in detail here. The

$\underline{B_{12}Co^{60}}$ TESTS FOR INTRINSIC FACTOR ACTIVITY IN NORMAL SUBJECTS

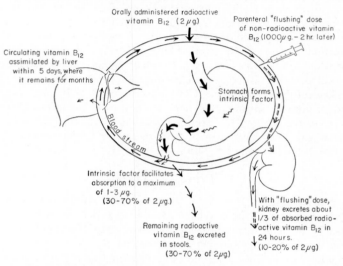

FIG. 2.—Relation of normal vitamin B_{12} physiology to various tests, using radioactive vitamin B_{12} as a tracer.

parenteral flushing dose has generally been administered 2 hours after the oral tracer, or at the same time. This variation has little effect on the amount of radioactive vitamin B_{12} excreted (79). Oral dosages of radioactive vitamin B_{12} most frequently employed have been 2.0 μg. (80), 1.0 μg. (81), 0.66 μg. (70), 0.5 μg. and 0.05 μg. (69). These varying doses give rise to differences in absolute and in percentage excretion, as will be discussed later. When a 2.0 μg. dose is given, most normal subjects will excrete

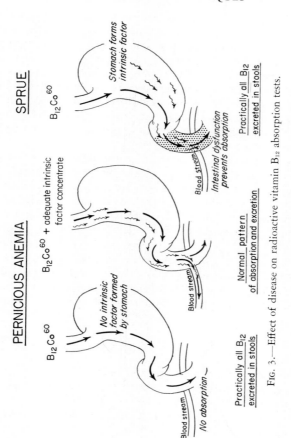

FIG. 3.—Effect of disease on radioactive vitamin B_{12} absorption tests.

10–20 per cent in the first 24 hours, an average of about one third of that absorbed (57).

Most of the early studies utilized Co^{60} as the radioactive label on the vitamin B_{12} molecule, inasmuch as this was the most readily available radioactive form of cobalt. This isotope emits hard gamma rays and has a half-life of 5.3 years. More recently, Co^{56} (62) and Co^{58} (68) have been used to tag the vitamin B_{12}.

These isotopes both emit hard gamma rays and have half-lives of about 72 days. Recently, $B_{12}Co^{58}$ has become generally available. Because of the long radioactive half-life of Co^{60}, and because the biologic half-life of vitamin B_{12} in the liver is ½–2 years (mean, about 1 year) (63), it has seemed prudent to limit the total $B_{12}Co^{60}$ to a minimum in any patient. The shorter half-life of Co^{58} makes this isotope theoretically more desirable than Co^{60}, although no untoward effects have been reported following the use of $B_{12}Co^{60}$. Even with Co^{58}, it is recommended that excessive total radioactivity be avoided.

Figure 3 illustrates vitamin B_{12} absorption in pathology related to B_{12} deficiency. In pernicious anemia, no intrinsic factor is excreted by the stomach. Therefore, only a negligible amount of radioactive vitamin B_{12} is absorbed and subsequently "flushed" into the urine (less than 3 per cent is recovered using a 2.0 μg. dose). If an adequate dose of a potent intrinsic-factor concentrate prepared from hog stomach is given orally with the radioactive B_{12}, the pattern of intestinal absorption and urinary excretion is the same as in normal persons. Where intestinal absorption is defective, as in sprue, only negligible absorption and excretion are evident, even with the addition of potent intrinsic-factor concentrates.

2. TECHNIQUE OF ADMINISTRATION

The isotopes Co^{60}, Co^{58} and Co^{56} emit similar types of radiations, and they may be detected by a number of methods. The simplest and most efficient method of detection utilizes a sodium iodide (NaI) scintillation crystal. Because of the relatively low concentration of radioactivity in urine specimens, various methods for increasing the ratio of sample counting rate to background counting rate have been employed. These include concentration of urine, denaturation of vitamin B_{12} with precipitation of cobalt (69), adsorption of labeled vitamin B_{12} on activated carbon (55), use of a large well counter (60), use of large urine volumes above or around the crystal (59) and attempts at reducing the background. The use of a large volume of urine above the crystal is simple and adequate and will be described here.

a) APPARATUS.—Required for the usual clinic load are:

One scintillation counter* 1½ in. O.D. × 1 in. thick NaI (Tl)

One dozen calibrated 1 L. polyethylene bottles with screw caps for collection of urine, to be used in counting

Six 4 in. diameter polyethylene funnels, to aid in urine collections

One jig or mount for containers, and a scintillation counter to provide for constant geometric relationship

Six 1 cc. Luer-Loc syringes, sterile

Six No. 23 needles, 1 in. long, sterile

One 1,000 ml. graduate

b) MATERIALS.—The following materials are needed:

(1) *Radioactive Vitamin B_{12}.*—For routine purposes, it is recommended that commercially available capsules containing dried vitamin B_{12} labeled with approximately 0.5 μc. Co^{58} be used. Vitamin B_{12} dosages are approximately 0.5 μg.† to 0.67 μg.‡ Similar dosage forms labeled with Co^{60} are also available.

(2) *Nonradioactive Vitamin B_{12}.*—This material, for parenteral use, may be obtained in 5 ml. vials containing 1,000 or 2,000 μg./ml. from a variety of sources.

(3) *Intrinsic-Factor Concentrate.*—This partially purified extract of hog stomach can be obtained in capsule form in dosage equivalent to approximately one USP unit from the same sources as the radioactive vitamin B_{12}. Kits are available containing all of the materials necessary for several tests. Only intrinsic factor preparations containing no vitamin B_{12} should be used; otherwise the test results may be markedly altered.

---

* Source: N. Wood Counter Laboratory, Chicago, Illinois (Model No. SC-2M); Nuclear-Chicago, Chicago, Illinois (Model No. DS-1); Tracerlab, Inc., Richmond, California (Model No. P20-M).

† Rubratope-58 Diagnostic Capsules, E. R. Squibb and Sons, Georges Road, New Brunswick, New Jersey.

‡ Radiocyanocobalamin (Co^{58}), Abbott Laboratories, Oak Ridge, Tennessee.

c) PROCEDURE.—The procedure is as follows:

(1) *Control Test:*

(*a*) Perform the test with the patient in the fasting state. The patient should not have received parenteral vitamin B_{12} during the preceding 2 days. Cognizance should be taken of other radioactive substances administered prior to the test, particularly I^{131} (53).

(*b*) Secure a large volume of pretest urine as a control. Generally, an overnight collection will prove adequate.

(*c*) Have the patient swallow a $B_{12}Co^{58}$ capsule with half a glass of water.

(*d*) Give 1,000 μg. nonradioactive vitamin B_{12} to the patient intramuscularly or subcutaneously.

(*e*) Give the patient two plastic bottles with screw caps and a plastic funnel for collecting urine. A shopping bag will be helpful to ambulatory patients. The patient should collect all urine from the time of $B_{12}Co^{58}$ administration until 24 hours later. If the volume is greater than 2 L., any household container may be used to collect the excess. If the patient fails to collect *all* urine during the 24 hours and if the $B_{12}Co^{58}$ content of that collected is less than the lower limits of normal, results should not be reported; the test should be repeated.

(*f*) Patient may eat a light breakfast 2 hours after the $B_{12}Co^{58}$ has been given.

(2) *Intrinsic Factor Test:*

Repeat the test with intrinsic factor concentrate if the control test is in the low range or if repeated tests are in the intermediate range (see section on Interpretation, p. 74). Do not repeat sooner than 4 days after a previous test. It has been recommended that patients receive no more than 3.0 μc. of $B_{12}Co^{60}$ (56), and the Atomic Energy Commission has set the permissible body burden of Co^{58} as 3 times that of Co^{60}. Thus, no more than 9.0 μc. of $B_{12}Co^{58}$ should be in the body at any time. For routine testing, it should rarely be necessary to approach these levels.

Intrinsic factor capsules are given simultaneously with $B_{12}Co^{58}$ capsules in the intrinsic factor test. All other details are identical to the control test (p. 72).

(3) *Measurement of Urinary Radioactivity:*
  (*a*) Measure the volume of the 24-hour urine collection. If it is less than the volume of the container used in counting, add water up to this volume and mix. If it is greater, mix and withdraw the necessary amount. It may be more feasible to measure proportional aliquots from separate collection bottles and to mix these aliquots for counting.
  (*b*) The total number of counts or total time of counting necessary will vary with the apparatus used. It is desirable to have a coefficient of variation of 5 per cent or less when radioactivity of 1 per cent appears in a liter of urine (± 2 standard deviations = 0.9–1.1 per cent). It is desirable to have a coefficient of variation of 1 per cent or less when radioactivity of 10 per cent appears in a liter of urine (± 2 std. dev. = 9.8–10.2 per cent). The time necessary to achieve these values, respectively t_1 and t_2, may be calculated according to the counts per minute of the various samples mentioned in the following formulas:

$$t_1 = 400 \times \frac{\dfrac{d - b}{10} + 2b}{\left(\dfrac{d - b}{10}\right)^2}$$

$$t_2 = 10,000 \times \frac{d + b}{(d - b)^2}$$

where b = counts per volume per minute for water used for background reading,

c = counts per volume per minute from 24-hour urine collection made preceding the start of the test (if significant amounts of radioactivity are detected, the test should be repeated at a future date),

d = counts per volume per minute for standard solution of radioactive B_{12}.

It is recommended that one oral dose be dissolved in 10 L. of water so that 1,000 ml. contains 10 per cent of the oral dose. An identical dilution used for a standard is also made by dissolving one oral dose in 1,000 ml. of solution and bringing 100 ml. of this up to 1,000 ml. with additional water.

Whichever time is longer should be used as the time for counting urine specimens.

(c) Calculate the per cent of excretion as follows:

$$\text{Per cent excretion} = \text{Liters/24-hr. urine*} \times 10 \times \frac{a-b}{d-b}$$

where a = counts per volume per minute for 24-hour urine collection.

Determine the values b and d each day a test is run, to compensate for differences in instrument response and for radioactive decay.

3. INTERPRETATION

The interpretation of the results is shown in Table 9. It is convenient to separate the percentages of excretion into *low, intermediate* and *normal* ranges. The intermediate range may be separated into *low intermediate* and *high intermediate* divisions midway between the extremes. Responses in the intermediate range are seldom observed, and when found, should be repeated for confirmation. When low intermediate responses occur, they are more suggestive of mechanisms producing low responses; and high intermediate responses may represent a low range of normal response. It is seen from Table 9 that limits of the three ranges vary, depending on the oral dose of radioactive

---

* If the 24-hour volume is less than that of the container used in counting, the volume of this container is used in the formula.

TABLE 9.—Classification and Interpretation of Urinary Excretion Tests Using Radioactive Vitamin B_{12} with and without Intrinsic-Factor Concentrates

Oral Dose	24-Hr. Excretion of Radioactive Vitamin B_{12}			Interpretation
	Low	Intermediate	Normal	
2.0 μg. 1.0 μg. 0.67 μg. 0.5 μg.	0–3% (60 mμg.) 0–4% (40 mμg.) 0–5% (33 mμg.) 0–5% (25 mμg.)	3– 6% (120 mμg.) 4– 8% (80 mμg.) 5–10% (67 mμg.) 5–10% (50 mμg.)	Over 6% Over 8% Over 10% Over 10%	
Pattern No.	Response Pattern			Interpretation
—	C*			Compatible with intrinsic-factor deficiency or intestinal malabsorption; test should be repeated with IFC.
I	C		IFC	Typical for intrinsic-factor deficiency (pernicious anemia).
II	C, IFC†			Typical for intestinal malabsorption (sprue, fistulas, etc.).
III	C	IFC		May indicate intestinal malabsorption with or without intrinsic-factor deficiency. Should repeat IFC test.
—		C		May be low normal or high abnormal. If repeat is consistent, retest with IFC.
IV		C	IFC	Mild intrinsic-factor deficiency.
V		C, IFC		Mild malabsorption or low normal.
VI			C	Normal; no need to repeat with IFC.

* C = Control test.
† IFC = Potent intrinsic-factor concentrate.

75

B_{12} both in percentage and in absolute excretions. It is unusual to obtain more than 25 per cent excretion of the administered dose with any of these doses. Representative data taken with doses of 2.0 μg. are shown in Figure 4.

A low or intermediate control response should always be followed by a test with intrinsic-factor concentrate. The great ma-

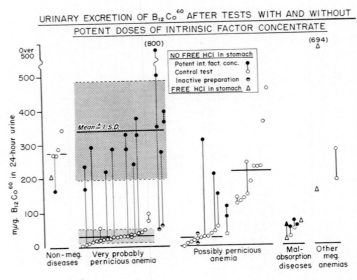

URINARY EXCRETION OF $B_{12}Co^{60}$ AFTER TESTS WITH AND WITHOUT POTENT DOSES OF INTRINSIC FACTOR CONCENTRATE

FIG. 4.—Representative data on 24-hour excretion of radioactive vitamin B_{12} (2.0 μg. $B_{12}Co^{60}$ orally, followed by 1.0 mg. of nonradioactive vitamin B_{12} parenterally).

jority of tests serve to clearly separate cases of intrinsic-factor deficiency, malabsorption defects and normal mechanisms of B_{12} absorption. Repeated tests may vary somewhat, owing to biologic or technical variation (58); but rarely do the subsequent interpretations change from one category to another.

Some patients may have all the typical clinical manifestations of pernicious anemia but show malabsorption or normal types of response to these tests. Some of these have free gastric acidity after histamine, and some may have evidences of poor nutrition or liver disease. In these cases the clinical abnormalities are due to a masked malabsorption syndrome, to dietary deficiency (77), to defective transport, storage or metabolism of vitamin B_{12}, or to an abnormality in some other biochemical system, such as that concerned with folic acid. Patients with true pernicious anemia who have been treated for some time with hog stomach intrinsic factor plus vitamin B_{12} orally may fail to show normal-range tests with intrinsic factor (82). This may represent an intraluminal reaction to foreign proteins, since the intrinsic factor of human gastric juice will still function normally.

An intestinal malabsorption pattern does not necessarily imply a mucosal block to vitamin B_{12} transport; it might also indicate utilization, adsorption, inactivation or destruction of either vitamin B_{12} or intrinsic factor in the intestinal lumen. One example is the megaloblastic anemia which sometimes accompanies the high intestinal infestation with certain Scandinavian strains of Diphyllobothrium latum, in which low-range tests are found both with and without intrinsic factor until the worm is eliminated or displaced to a lower portion of the intestine (76). Another example is found with intestinal blind loops or strictures, some cases of which have shown malabsorption type patterns which have been corrected by the administration of broad-spectrum antibiotics (65, 66). Presumably, these particular intestinal conditions predispose to growth of bacterial strains which inactivate vitamin B_{12} or intrinsic factor. It has been shown that intrinsic factor is inactivated in the normal upper intestine if it remains for too long a period (50). Some cases of hypothyroidism have demonstrated both a malabsorption type pattern and a lack of intrinsic-factor secretion (71). The exact mechanism in the condition is not clear. The lack of intrinsic-factor secretion may be documented by testing 25–50 ml. of the patient's gastric juice as an intrinsic-factor source in another patient with classic pernicious anemia. This amount is ordinarily equivalent to a potent dose of intrinsic-factor concentrate (81). It is interesting that many patients with malabsorption patterns (for example, due to nontropical sprue) will show an apparent lack of intrinsic-factor excretion as well as faulty absorption (74).

Occasionally, false positive tests have occurred. Temporary impairment has been noted in some acute infections (73). Renal impairment may give low 24-hour excretions (78) but apparently does not affect other types of tests using radioactive vitamin B_{12} (61).

Some elderly, achlorhydric patients with no other clinical or laboratory stigmata of pernicious anemia will show test results typical for pernicious anemia (72, 81). Presumably, these individuals are in a "pre-pernicious anemia" state. A poor diet plus the stress of intercurrent disease might be enough to bring an overt pernicious anemia.

This test has proved extremely valuable to the clinician. A diagnosis of pernicious anemia calls for lifelong therapy with vitamin B_{12} injections. Where this diagnosis has been well established on clinical grounds, tests with radioactive vitamin B_{12} have almost invariably confirmed it. Where the clinical evidence has been equivocal, these tests have shown that over half of such patients did not have pernicious anemia (52). The detection of masked pernicious anemia with subacute combined degeneration of the cord through the use of this test has been invaluable in the diagnosis of some patients with obscure neurologic disease (49).

4. REPORTING OF TEST RESULTS

It is suggested that the following examples of format be used for reporting results. The interpretations are paraphrased from Table 9 (p. 75).

PATIENT (1):

9-28-59. 0.5 μg. $B_{12}Co^{58}$ orally, followed by 1.0 mg. B_{12} parenterally. 24-hour urine contained 1.3% radioactivity. This is compatible with intrinsic-factor deficiency or intestinal malabsorption (usual range 0–5%). Test should be repeated with intrinsic factor for further diagnostic clarification.

PATIENT (1)—repeat:

Tests were made with 0.5 μg. $B_{12}Co^{58}$ orally, followed by 1.0 mg. B_{12} parenterally. 24-hr. urine radioactivity reported:

9-28-59. Control: 1.3%.

10-5-59. 30 mg. (about 1.0 USP unit) intrinsic factor: 14.2%.

This is typical for pernicious anemia (e.g., control 0–5%; intrinsic factor over 10%).

PATIENT (2):

10-15-59. 0.67 μg. $B_{12}Co^{58}$ orally, followed by 1.0 mg. B_{12} parenterally. 24-hr. urine contained 18.7% radioactivity. This is within the normal range (greater than 10%).

REFERENCES

BLOOD VOLUME: $I^{131}HSA$

1. Allen, T. H., et al.: Blood volume, bleeding volume and tolerance to hemorrhage in the splenectomized dog, Am. J. Physiol. 196:176, 1959.
2. Aust, J. B., et al.: A rapid method for clinical total blood volume determination using radioactive iodinated human serum albumin (RIHSA), Proc. Soc. Exper. Biol. & Med. 77:514, 1951.
3. Crispell, K. R.; Porter, B., and Nieset, R. T.: Studies of plasma volume using human serum albumin tagged with radioactive iodine, J. Clin. Invest. 29:513, 1950.
4. Erickson, J. R.; McCormick, J. B., and Seed, L.: Improved method for determination of blood volume using radioactive iodinated human serum albumin, Science 118:595, 1953.
5. Fields, T.; Kaplan, E., and Imperato, A. A.: Precision blood volume procedure using $I^{131}HSA$, Internat. J. Appl. Radiation 7:43, 1959.
6. ———, ———, and Terril, M.: Simplified technique for blood volume determinations using $I^{131}HSA$, J. Lab. & Clin. Med. 43:332, 1954.
7. Fine, J., and Seligman, A. M.: Traumatic shock: IV. A study of the problem of the "lost plasma" in hemorrhagic shock by use of radioactive plasma protein, J. Clin. Invest. 22:285, 1943.
8. Freinkel, N.; Schreiner, G., and Athens, J. W.: Comparison of late disappearance of T-1824 and iodinated albumin, Am. J. Physiol. 171:725, 1952 (abstr.).
9. ———; Schreiner, G. E., and Athens, J. W.: Simultaneous distribution of T-1824 and I^{131}-labelled human serum albumin in man, J. Clin. Invest. 32:138, 1953.
10. Friedell, M. T.: Effect of cigarette smoke on peripheral vascular system; radioactive iodinated albumin used as indicator of volumetric change, J.A.M.A. 152:897, 1953.
11. Muelheims, G.; Dellenback, R., and Rawson, R.: Red blood cell volume and distribution after bleed-out in the rat as determined by Cr^{51}-labelled red blood cells, Am. J. Physiol. 196:169, 1959.
12. Gibson, J. G., 2d, and Evans, W. A., Jr.: Clinical studies of the blood volume: II. The relation of plasma and total blood volume to

venous pressure, blood velocity rate, physical measurements, age and sex in ninety normal humans, J. Clin. Invest. 16:317, 1937.

13. Gregersen, M. I., and Rawson, R. A.: Blood volume, Physiol. Rev. 39:307, 1959.

14. ——— et al.: Cell volume, plasma volume, total blood volume and F_{cells} factor in the Rhesus monkey, Am. J. Physiol. 196:184, 1959.

15. Hlad, C. J., Jr., and Tanz, R.: An analysis of technical errors in radioalbumin blood volume methods and presentation of a modified method, J. Lab. & Clin. Med. 52:289, 1958.

16. Kaplan, E., et al.: Blood volume in congestive heart failure as determined with iodinated human serum albumin, Am. Heart J. 47:824, 1954.

17. Krieger, H.: Study of repeatability of plasma volume using I^{131} and T-1824 at two-week intervals, Clin. Res. Proc. 1:77, 1953.

18. ——— et al.: Appearance of protein tagged with radioactive iodine in thoracic duct lymph, Proc. Soc. Exper. Biol. & Med. 73:124, 1950.

19. ——— et al.: Use of radioactive iodinated human serum albumin in evaluating peripheral circulation, Ann. Surg. 136:357, 1952.

20. Levey, S.; Hower, J., and Loughridge, R. H.: Laboratory factors influencing determination of plasma volume using human albumin tagged with I^{131}, J. Lab. & Clin. Med. 41:316, 1953.

21. Rawson, R., et al.: Determination of residual blood volume required for survival in rapidly hemorrhaged splenectomized dogs, Am. J. Physiol. 196:179, 1959.

22. Reeve, E. B.: The contribution of I^{131} labeled proteins to measurements of blood volume, Ann. New York Acad. Sc. 70:137, 1957.

23. Roberts, L. N., et al.: Plasma volume, measured by iodinated albumin and T-1824 (Evans blue), Canad. M. A. J. 69:510, 1953.

24. Schultz, A. L., et al.: A critical comparison of the T-1824 dye and iodinated albumin methods for plasma volume measurement, J. Clin. Invest. 32:107, 1953.

25. Sear, H.; Allen, T. H., and Gregersen, M. I.: Simultaneous measurement in dogs of plasma volume with I^{131} human albumin and T-1824 (Evans blue) with comparisons of their long term disappearance from plasma, Am. J. Physiol. 175:240, 1953.

26. Sterling, K.: The turnover rate of serum albumin in man as measured by I^{131} tagged albumin, J. Clin. Invest. 30:1228, 1951.

27. Storaasli, J. P., et al.: The use of radioactive iodinated plasma protein in the study of blood volume, Surg., Gynec. & Obst. 91:458, 1950.

28. Wang, L.: Plasma volume, cell volume, total blood volume and F_{cells} factor in the normal and splenectomized Sherman rat, Am. J. Physiol. 196:188, 1959.

RED CELL VOLUME: Cr51

29. Brown, E., et al.: Blood volume and congestive heart failure studied by Cr^{51}, Co, and T-1824 methods, J. Clin. Invest. 33:919, 1954.

30. Ebaugh, F. G., Jr.; Emerson, C. P., and Ross, J. F.: The use of radioactive chromium[51] as an erythrocyte tagging agent for the determination of red cell survival in vivo, J. Clin. Invest. 32:1260, 1953.

31. Eisenberg, S.: The effect of congestive heart failure on total blood volume, red cell mass, and plasma volume as measured by radioactive chromium labeled red cells, J. Clin. Invest. 33:930, 1954.

32. Frank, H., and Gray, S. J.: The determination of plasma volume in man with radioactive chromic chloride, J. Clin. Invest. 32:991, 1953.

33. Funkhouser, R. K., and Pritchard, W. H.: A study of the blood volume in congestive heart failure, J. Clin. Invest. 33:934, 1954.

34. Gray, S. J., and Frank, H.: The simultaneous determination of red cell mass and plasma volume in man with radioactive chromic chloride, J. Clin. Invest. 32:1000, 1953.

35. ———— and Sterling, K.: The determination of the red cell volume by radioactive chromium, Science 112:179, 1950.

36. ———— and ————: The tagging of red cells and plasma proteins with radioactive chromium, J. Clin. Invest. 29:1604, 1950.

37. Kraintz, L., and Talmage, R. V.: Distribution of radioactivity following intravenous administration of trivalent chromium[51] in rat and rabbit, Proc. Soc. Exper. Biol. & Med. 81:490, 1952.

38. Mitchell, T. G.; Spencer, R. P., and King, E. R.: The use of radioisotopes in diagnostic hematologic procedures, Am. J. Clin. Path. 28:461, 1957.

39. Necheles, T. F.; Weinstein, I. M., and LeRoy, G. V.: Radioactive sodium chromate for the study of survival of red blood cells: I. The effect of radioactive sodium chromate on red cells, J. Lab. & Clin. Med. 42:358, 1953.

40. Read, R. C.: Studies of red cell volume and turnover using radiochromium, New England J. Med. 250:1021, 1954.

41. ————; Wilson, G. W., and Gardner, F. H.: The use of radioactive sodium chromate to evaluate the life-span of the red blood cell in health and certain hematological disorders, Am. J. M. Sc. 228:40, 1954.

42. Reilly, W. A., et al.: Whole blood volume determined by radiochromium-tagged red cells: Comparative study on normal and congestive heart failure patients, Circulation 9:571, 1954.

43. Small, W. J., and Verloop, M. C.: Determination of the blood volume using radioactive Cr[51]: Modification of the original technique, J. Lab. & Clin. Med. 47:255, 1956.

44. Spencer, R. P., et al.: Semimicromethod for blood volume and erythrokinetic determination, Acta haemat. 19:302, 1958.

45. Sterling, K., and Gray, S. J.: Determination of the circulating red cell volume in man by radioactive chromium, J. Clin. Invest. 29:1614, 1950.

46. Strumia, M. M., et al.: Uses and limitations of survival studies of erythrocytes tagged with Cr[51], Blood 10:429, 1955.

47. Sutherland, D. A., et al.: The survival of human erythrocytes esti-

mated by means of cells tagged with radioactive chromium, J. Lab. & Clin. Med. 43:717, 1954.

48. Weinstein, I. M., and LeRoy, G. V.: Radioactive sodium chromate for the study of survival of red blood cells: II. The rate of hemolysis in certain hematological disorders, J. Lab. & Clin. Med. 43:368, 1953.

DIAGNOSTIC TESTS USING RADIOACTIVE CYANOCOBALAMINE (VITAMIN B_{12})

49. Arias, I. M.; Apt, L., and Pollycove, M.: Absorption of radioactive vitamin B_{12} in nonanemic patients with combined-system disease, New England J. Med. 253:1005, 1955.

50. Best, W. R.; Frenster, J. H., and Zolot, M. M.: Observations on intrinsic factor and the intestinal absorption of vitamin B_{12}, J. Lab. & Clin. Med. 50:793, 1957.

51. ———; Landmann, W. A., and Limarzi, L. R.: Time pattern of vitamin $B_{12}Co^{60}$ urinary excretion in man after oral administration and parenteral "flushing," Blood 11:352, 1956.

52. ——— and Limarzi, L. R.: Diagnostic value of vitamin $B_{12}Co^{60}$ urinary excretion tests, Proceedings of the Sixth International Congress of the International Society of Hematology (New York: Grune & Stratton, Inc., 1958), p. 241.

53. ——— et al.: Studies on urinary excretion of vitamin $B_{12}Co^{60}$ in pernicious anemia for determining effective dosage of intrinsic factor concentrates, Blood 11:338, 1956.

54. Booth, C. C., and Mollin, D. L.: The site of absorption of vitamin B_{12} in man, Lancet 1:18, 1959.

55. Buchholz, C. H.: Concentration of vitamin B_{12} from urine by adsorption on carbon: A sensitive assay of radiocyanocobalamin in the Schilling test for pernicious anemia, J. Lab. & Clin. Med. 52:653, 1958.

56. Bull, F. E.; Campbell, D. C., and Owen, C. A., Jr.: The diagnosis and treatment of pernicious anemia, M. Clin. North America 40:1005, 1956.

57. Callender, S. T., and Evans, J. R.: The urinary excretion of labeled vitamin B_{12}, Clin. Sc. 14:295, 1955.

58. Chow, B. F., et al.: The urinary excretion test for absorption of vitamin B_{12}: I. Reproducibility of results and agewise variation, Am. J. Clin. Nutrition 4:142, 1956.

59. Corbus, H. F., and Nielson, H., Jr.: A simplified method for the urinary excretion test of absorption of cobalt[60]-labeled vitamin B_{12}, California Med. 89:400, 1958.

60. Doscherholmen, A., and Hagen, P. S.: Radioactive vitamin B_{12} absorption studies: Results of direct measurement of radioactivity in the blood, J. Clin. Invest. 35:699, 1956.

61. Dunn, A. L.; Walsh, J. R., and Holthaus, J. M.: Radioactive cyanocobalamin (vitamin B_{12}) in renal disease, A.M.A. Arch. Int. Med. 101:927, 1958.

62. Ellenbogen, L., and Williams, W. L.: Quantitative assay of intrinsic factor activity by urinary excretion of radioactive vitamin B_{12}, Blood 13:582, 1958.

63. Glass, G. B. J.: Radioactive vitamin B_{12} in the liver: III. Hepatic storage and discharge of $Co^{60}B_{12}$ in pernicious anemia, J. Lab. & Clin. Med. 52:875, 1958.

64. Glass, G. B. J., et al.: Uptake of radioactive vitamin B_{12} by the liver in humans: Test for measurement of intestinal absorption of vitamin B_{12} and intrinsic factor activity, Arch. Biochem. 51:251, 1954.

65. Halsted, J. A.; Lewis, P. M., and Gasster, M.: Absorption of radioactive vitamin B_{12} in the syndrome of megaloblastic anemia associated with intestinal stricture or anastomosis, Am. J. Med. 20:42, 1956.

66. Halsted, J. A., et al.: Mechanisms involved in the development of vitamin B_{12} deficiency, Gastroenterology 30:21, 1956.

67. Heinle, R. W., et al.: Studies of excretion (and absorption) of Co^{60}-labeled vitamin B_{12} in pernicious anemia, Tr. A. Am. Physicians 65:214, 1952.

68. Hutchison, J. S.; Townsend, S. R., and Cameron, D. G.: The advantages of cobalt[58]-tagged vitamin B_{12} in the study of vitamin B_{12} absorption, Canad. M. A. J. 78:685, 1958.

69. Kinnory, D. S., et al.: Determination of urinary excretion of radiocobalt-labeled vitamin B_{12} by cobalt sulfide precipitation, J. Lab. & Clin. Med. 50:913, 1957.

70. Klayman, M. I., and Brandborg, L.: Clinical application of cobalt[60]-labeled vitamin B_{12} urine test, New England J. Med. 253:808, 1955.

71. Leithold, S. L.; David, D., and Best, W. R.: Hypothyroidism with anemia demonstrating abnormal vitamin B_{12} absorption, Am. J. Med. 24:535, 1958.

72. MacLean, L. D.: The differentiation of achylia gastrica and achlorhydria by means of radioactive vitamin B_{12}, Gastroenterology 29:653, 1955.

73. Miller, A.; Corbus, H. F., and Sullivan, J. F.: A modified urinary excretion test for measuring oral cobalt[60]-labeled vitamin B_{12} absorption and its application in certain disease states, Blood 12:347, 1957.

74. Miller, O. N., and Unglaub, W. G.: A study of etiology of macrocytic anemia, J. Clin. Invest. 36:916, 1957.

75. Mollin, D. S., and Ross, G. I. M.: Vitamin B_{12} concentrations of serum and urine in the first 72 hours after intramuscular injection of the vitamin, J. Clin. Path. 6:54, 1953.

76. Nyberg, W.; Gräsbeck, R., and Sippola, U.: Urinary excretion of radiovitamin B_{12} in carriers of diphyllobothrium latum, New England J. Med. 259:216, 1958.

77. Pollycove, M.; Apt, L., and Colbert, M. J.: Pernicious anemia due to dietary deficiency of vitamin B_{12}, Clin. Res. Proc. 3:28, 1955.

78. Rath, C. E., et al.: Value and limitations of cobalt[60]B_{12} test, Am. J. Med. 20:954, 1956.

79. Reisner, E. J., Jr.; Rosenblum, C., and Morgan, M. C.: Urinary excretion of orally administered Co^{60}-labeled vitamin B_{12} in normal subjects and patients with pernicious anemia and sprue, Clin. Res. Proc. 2:56, 1954.

80. Schilling, R. F.: A new test for intrinsic factor activity, J. Lab. & Clin. Med. 42:946, 1953.

81. Schilling, R. F.; Clatanoff, D. V., and Korst, D. R.: Intrinsic factor studies: III. Further observations utilizing the urinary radioactivity test in subjects with achlorhydria, pernicious anemia, or a total gastrectomy, J. Lab. & Clin. Med. 45:926, 1955.

82. Schwartz, M.; Louis, P., and Meulengracht, E.: Reduced effect of heterologous intrinsic factor, Lancet 1:751, 1957.

CHAPTER 3

Localization of Tumors of the Brain and Eye

A. EXTERNAL MEASUREMENTS: IODINE-131

1. TECHNIQUE

INTRACRANIAL LESIONS MAY BE LOCALIZED by measurement of preferentially absorbed local concentrations of radioiodine (I^{131}). Approximately 0.35 mc. of sodium radioiodide (NaI^{131}) is orally administered under suitable radiation safeguards. Measurements of radioactivity at various areas of the skull are made from $\frac{1}{2}$ to 3 hours after the administration of the NaI^{131}. Brain-tumor tissue concentrates NaI^{131} to a greater extent than normal tissue. Increased amounts of I^{131} in tumors result in increased counting rates over tumor sites when the measurements are made external to the skull.

a) MATERIAL.—Radioiodine is available* in the form of a sterile solution of NaI^{131}, the specific activity of which is approximately 1.3–1.5 mc./cc. at the time of preparation. This radioactive substance emits two beta particles (0.3 and 0.6 Mev) and four gamma rays (0.8, 0.26, 0.36 and 0.6 Mev). The radiation detected by the Geiger counter† is primarily the 0.36 Mev gamma ray, for which the counter has an efficiency of 1.0 per cent. The half-life of I^{131} is 8.1 days.

b) EQUIPMENT.—The radiation detection equipment consists

---

* Source: Abbott Laboratories, Oak Ridge, Tennessee.
† See Chapter 16, esp. pp. 324–331.

of four major components: (1) a bismuth cathode Geiger counter of 4 cm. outside diameter; (2) a counter shield and allied mount; (3) an electronic indicator (scaler, or preferably a count-rate meter); and (4) a mechanical or graphic recorder.

The output socket of the Geiger counter is connected to a pre-amplifier, and the output socket of the preamplifier to a count-rate meter.*

A standard radium source is used in a reproducible geometri-

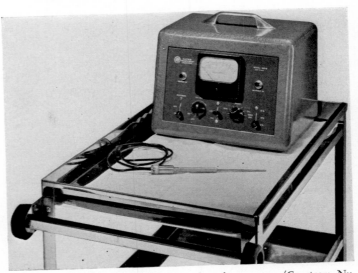

FIG. 5.—Typical count-rate meter and probe counter. (Courtesy: Nuclear-Chicago.)

cal arrangement for calibrating the counter before and after each test. Counters vary in sensitivity to gamma radiation, but the resulting differences in counting rates are within the range of variation of the readings obtained from normal patients. The

---

* Nuclear-Chicago count-rate meter, Model 1510 (source: Nuclear-Chicago, Chicago, Illinois), can be used. Style T-2 and D-34 counters were used (supplied by the N. Wood Counter Laboratory, Chicago, Illinois). Satisfactory count-rate meters and tubes of a similar nature are made by other manufacturers.

analysis of readings obtained from normal skulls is described in Table 10 on page 93.

The counter is mounted in a lead shield 1.2 cm. thick, a thickness which corresponds to four half-value layers for the gamma radiation of I^{131} (attenuation by factor of 16). The lead shield extends 1.2 cm. beyond the end of the counter.

After tests were made on shields of various designs, the rela-

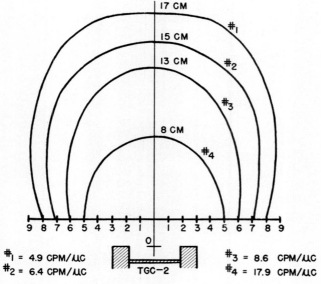

Fig. 6.—Isosensitivity curves of tube, T-2, used at Veterans Administration Hospital, Hines, Illinois.

tionship shown between the counter and the shield (see Fig. 5) was accepted as the one giving the best results. The shielded counter should be mounted on a device that will permit freedom of movement in all directions. A dental x-ray stand, yoke and swivel, or a camera tripod head, will serve.

The isosensitivity curves (Fig. 6) of the shielded counter (Fig. 7) used at the Veterans Administration Hospital at Hines, Illinois, demonstrate that the shielded counter is collimated only slightly. Actual practice has shown that counters with greater

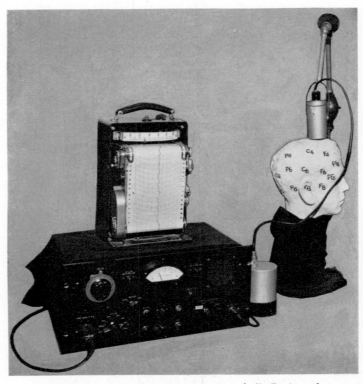

Fig. 7.—Placing of shielded counter against skull. Design of counter with only slight collimation gives best isosensitivity and solid-angle responses.

collimation are less satisfactory. The solid-angle response of the shielded counter is such that, even if the counter is moved by 30°, the readings are reproducible to within ± 5 per cent. This means that the placement of the counter against the skull is not particularly exacting, for variations in the positioning of the counter against the skull may, in practice, be as large as 15°. When the 30° limit is exceeded, there is a rapid decrease in the counting rate, which is reflected

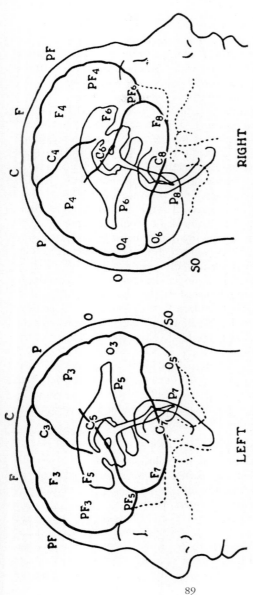

LEFT   RIGHT

Fig. 8.—F_7, center of counter is over zygoma; F_5, edge of counter is one finger width off the midline; PF_5, center of counter is above and behind the external canthus, with part of eye being covered by shield; PF_3, edge of counter is one finger width above eyebrow and the same distance off the midline; C_7, center of counter is over the external auditory meatus; C_5, edge of counter is just above the ear and one diameter above C_7; C_3, edge of counter is one finger width off the midline; P_7, center of counter covers the mastoid, just touching the back of the pinna and pointing forward and slightly upward; P_5, edge of counter is above and behind ear and one counter diameter above position P_7; P_3, edge of counter is one finger width off the midline; O_5, center of counter is just below the external occipital protuberance and a finger width off the midline; O_3, edge of counter shield is just above the external occipital protuberance and a finger width off the midline. Midline position: Center the counter over the glabella; adjacent positions are one shield diameter from the preceding position.

89

in the isosensitivity curves. The counting rates measured are dependent on the geometrical arrangements; thus, the counting rates reported here obtain only with a shielded counter of similar design, one which has the same isosensitivity and the same solid-angle response as the one described.

Measurements at Reid's base line, or even slightly below, are important in order to establish a reference point. The central part of the counter is centered on the malar bone, or external auditory meatus (Fig. 8, areas $F_{7, 8}$ and $C_{7, 8}$), in order to pick up radiations from the anterior temporal lobe, the hippocampus, the pituitary, the brain stem and the deep temporal lobe. If high concentrations are found here, the presence of midline lesions are indicated. The symmetrical site readings may here be equal because the counter will be equidistant from the center in such midline lesions. This finding may also be true in lateralizing lesions that are extensive enough to cross the midline. In lesions that are close to the midline in the middle cranial fossa, such as pituitary tumors extending out under the temporal lobe or hippo-campal tumors near the brain stem, the basilar readings will again be high, with slight differences of only 40–70 counts/minute to signify lateralization of the lesion. Placement over the mastoid (Fig. 8, $P_{7, 8}$) is made to detect posterior fossa or cere-bellopontine angle lesions.

The importance of the external occipital protuberance in the midline placements in order to differentiate supratentorial from infratentorial lesions is emphasized. To detect parasagittal lesions, particularly meningiomas, midline readings in addition to the symmetrical readings have proved valuable.

c) PROCEDURE.—The procedure follows:

1. Give the patient Lugol's solution orally 3 times, 10 drops each, the day before the test. On the day of the test, give an oral dose of 350 μc. of NaI^{131}, taking pre-cautions to prevent contamination.

2. After the material has been administered, place the counter in the inferior anterior temporal area (Fig. 8, left F_7) and keep it there until the counts reach a pla-teau. Before the plateau is reached, the counting rate drops with time. During this time (10–40 minutes),

differential measurements over the skull give fallacious results. As soon as the counting rate levels off and remains level for over 3 minutes, shift the counter to the symmetrical anterior temporal area on the opposite side of the skull (Fig. 8, right F_8).

3. Then place the counter directly on the scalp and keep it at "Normal," that is, at a right angle to the tangent at the particular position on the skull under study. Take readings of at least 3 minutes' duration over each site, and repeat over abnormal areas at frequent intervals of time from 20 minutes to 4 hours after ingestion of the NaI[131].

As seen in Figure 8, a minimum of 32 different positions are surveyed with the Geiger counter—positions which cover every area of the skull on and above Reid's base line, if the 2-in. diameter counter is used. These sites include 13 symmetrical positions on each side of the skull: 2 prefrontal (PF); 3 frontal (F); 3 central (C); 3 parietal (P); 1 occipital (O) and 1 suboccipital ($O_{5, 6}$). The even numbers represent the right half, the odd numbers the left half, of the skull. Six midline positions are also routinely surveyed: midprefrontal, midfrontal, midcentral, midparietal, midoccipital and midsuboccipital.

Within a minute or two after the ingestion of the material, the radioactivity at the surface of the head is at a maximum. This decreases rapidly over the next 10–40 minutes, until a plateau is observed. After this interval, and for the next 1½–2 hours, the decline in counts is gradual, so that symmetrical positions can be accurately studied, if care is taken to match areas properly on each side of the skull within 3–5 minutes. The most significant counting rates occur within 1–3 hours after the administration of the material; hence, suggestive areas of involvement must not only be rechecked several times during this period but must also be compared to the concentrations in adjacent areas, so as to delineate not only the main focus of the lesion but also its extent.

The counting rate during this significant period, with the equipment described, is of the order of magnitude of 1,000–2,000 cts./min.

It is essential to count at least all 32 sites. However, the limited significant time interval available for counting requires that the areas chosen for counting be randomly selected where possible and the suggestive areas be recounted several times for greater accuracy. At the end of 3 or 4 hours, the readings are only confirmatory, for the differential concentrations are no longer striking.

Because a large proportion of gliomas involve the temporal lobe, the routine procedure suggested is to move forward from the frontal (Fig. 8,* $F_{7, 8}$) positions to the prefrontal positions ($PF_{5, 6}$), and then backward to the central areas, $C_{7, 8}$. These positions are then compared to the parasagittal $PF_{3, 4}$ and $F_{3, 4}$ areas. The posterior fossa is examined ($P_{7, 8}$ and $O_{5, 6}$), and the remaining sites are covered with the counter. The scanning is completed with the 6 midline positions. The counting rate at the $F_{7, 8}$ position is used as the control reading; hence, this site is frequently remeasured throughout the test and is often compared consecutively with the $F_{3, 4}$ areas. This is especially true if midline or brain-stem lesions are suggested.

The standard error of a measurement is equal to $\pm$ 9 per cent, which is due to the standard error of counting of $\pm$ 3 per cent, the standard error of reading record of $\pm$ 3 per cent and the standard error in counting rate due to uncertainty in positioning detector of $\pm$ 7 per cent. The $\pm$ 7 per cent standard error results from the 30° solid angle of the shielded counter. The counting rates recorded on the chart are read to the nearest ten counts per minute. In normal subjects, readings over bilaterally symmetrical positions may vary by as much as $\pm$ 9 per cent. The most significant time for diagnostic purposes is the interval between 1 and 3 hours after the administration of the radioiodine. At this time, the counting rates in normal subjects lie in the range of 1,000–2,000 cts./min.; a variation of $\pm$ 9 per cent in these values amounts to 90–180 cts./min., respectively. In actual practice, differences between bilaterally symmetrical points seldom exceed 40 cts./min. Consistent differences of this amount or more are diagnostically suggestive.

---

* The numbering used in Figure 8 will be used throughout this section of the chapter.

2. ANALYSIS OF RECORDS AND RATES OF NORMAL SUBJECTS

In order to provide information on normal variations, a group of normal subjects was studied. The records and the counting rates at the 32 positions used were analyzed. It was found that the concentration of NaI^{131} decreases at a fairly constant rate

TABLE 10.—RADIOENCEPHALOGRAPH:* NaI^{131} MAXIMUM
READING (COUNTS/MINUTE)

POSITION	INTERVAL			
	$1–1\frac{1}{2}$	$1\frac{1}{2}–2$	$2–2\frac{1}{2}$	$2\frac{1}{2}–3$
$F_{7,\,8}$	2,070	2,300	2,300	2,300
$F_{5,\,6}$	1,150	1,150	1,265	1,265
$F_{3,\,4}$	....	....	1,265	1,265
F	....	....	1,265	1,265
$PF_{5,\,6}$	1,610	2,070	2,070	2,185
$PF_{3,\,4}$	....	....	1,380	1,380
PF	....	....	1,380	1,380
$C_{7,\,8}$	2,300	2,300	2,300	2,300
$C_{5,\,6}$	1,380	1,380	1,380	1,380
$C_{3,\,4}$	1,265	1,265	1,265	1,265
$P_{7,\,8}$	....	1,955	1,955	1,955
$P_{5,\,6}$	1,495	1,380	1,380	1,380
$P_{3,\,4}$	1,495	1,380	1,380	1,380
P	....	....	1,380	1,380
$O_{5,\,6}$	....	....	1,725	1,725
$O_{3,4}$	....	....	1,380	1,380
O	....	....	1,495	1,495
SO	....	....	1,840	1,840

* Bismuth cathode tube—sensitivity; 1,086 cts./min. for 10 μc. in 25 cc. volume, at 12.7 cm. distance (I^{131}).

between approximately ½ hour and 3 hours after ingestion. To simplify the analysis of the data, the following time intervals have been chosen: 1–1½, 1½–2, 2–2½ and 2½–3 hours (Table 10). The significant feature of the table is not the absolute values for counting rates at various positions; the important point is the relationship observed regularly between comparable positions used for measurement. Thus, the relationship between all the F points (Fig. 8) established a pattern which is typical in the normal and which will be disturbed in patients who have tumors underlying any one of these positions. Likewise, the midline positions, or the 3, 4, 5 and 6 positions (Fig. 8) are in constant relation to one another, as indicated in Table 10.

Just as the radiologist is acquainted with the normal variations in the ventricular system, or angiographic patterns of the brain, so the operator must be aware of the normal range of radioactive concentrations at specific time intervals and for the specific areas of the brain. Each of the 32 different locations in the skull normally vary in their radioactive concentrations at the same interval of time following the NaI^{131} administration.

If the observed concentrations in a presumed brain tumor are from 100 to 600 cts./min. greater than the statistically normal range at that particular time interval, then pathologic endothelial permeability must exist at that point. High concentrations are indicative of an organic lesion, whether strictly vascular or neoplastic in nature. If cerebral trauma is believed present—regardless of whether that trauma was due to an injury, to a recent epileptic seizure, to a recent air study or to a recent hematoma—the radioactivity concentrations will generally be high.

A repeat study performed from 10 to 14 days later will show a decreased radioactivity. This is consistent with the regressive vascular disturbances occurring in such lesions 2 weeks after the more acute episode. On the other hand, if the radioactive concentration still remains high, or becomes even higher, it is suggestive of a progressive vascular endothelial lesion, such as may be secondary to dedifferentiation changes in anaplastic neoplasms or to the effects of large doses of deep x-ray.

Recurrent tumors, regardless of their initial classification, show an increased uptake of I^{131} because of their increased cellularity, relative anaplasia and atypical, hyperplastic, relatively undifferentiated new capillary formations.

If there is a reversal of the normal basilar-parasagittal reading ratio (F_3 is greater than F_7 in a parasagittal meningioma) or if there is a difference in symmetrical readings greater than 60 cts./min., then the actual value of the I^{131} concentrations is not important, because focal disease must exist, although the lesion will probably be a relatively hypocellular or hypovascular one.

The I^{131} test does not differentiate an acute infection from an anaplastic tumor, because the disturbed capillary permeability in both types of lesions will result in an increased exudation of iodine. If the infection has gone beyond the stage of cellulitis, however, and a well-encapsulated abscess results, with central liquefaction necrosis and the absence of new blood vessels, then the I^{131} has no deranged blood vessels from which to escape; hence, normal concentrations are the result. This explanation is pertinent in differentiating an acute intracranial hemorrhage, with its resultant increased vascularity, from a chronic subdural or intracerebral hematoma, with its thickened relatively avascular highly fibrosed capsule and its large central chocolate cyst. The hematoma will yield readings depending on the amount of the cystic contents. In a cystic degenerative tumor, only the actively growing tumor tissue concentrates the I^{131}; whereas the cystic portions actually have a diminished uptake. When the preponderance of cyst fluid over tumor cells and tumor capillaries is too great, the I^{131} concentrations are not significantly increased. This gives rise to most of the expected errors in this method of diagnosis.

3. Normal Range of Concentration for Any Apparatus Ascertained

In order to ascertain the normal range of concentration for any particular apparatus, such as the counter described, it would be wise to administer 350 μc. of I^{131} to 10 or 20 "normal" patients. There should be clinical proof, as well as pneumographic and angiographic proof, that no space-occupying lesion exists. This applies to patients with and without neurologic signs and symptoms. A chart should then be made of the I^{131} concentrations for each of the 32 sites chosen to cover the topography of the skull.

These values can be recorded on the Esterline-Angus chart paper (4305—X) supplied with the Esterline-Angus automatic recorder.* The various ranges of counts-per-minute concentrations at each site at 30-minute intervals will be known for the first 3 or

---

* Source: Esterline-Angus Company, Inc., Indianapolis, Indiana.

4 hours after the injection in normal patients without tumor. The Esterline-Angus 5 milliampere recorder is connected to the direct-current output socket of the count-rate meter, and the scale of the meter is set so that 1,000 cts./min. gives full-scale deflection on the recorder. (Any commercially available recording milliammeter of comparable sensitivity may be used.) The chart speed of the recorder is 6 min./in.

It has been noticed that, after a plateau has been reached for any one position, the variation of the readings at that site are not greater than from 20 to 40 cts./min. regardless of whether the reading is 2 minutes or 12 minutes in duration. Each site is read for an average of 3 minutes. If differences of over 40–50 cts./min. occur at any two symmetrical sites, then these positions should be checked immediately. If the readings then show differences less than those expected (40 cts./min.), it is probable that the counter was not symmetrically placed, or that it was angulated and not flush with the skull, or that there was movement of the patient. In any event, every abnormality, whether pertinently high or not, must be rechecked immediately and again within a half hour at various half-hourly or hourly intervals thereafter. It is a persistent, and not a transitory, pertinent difference of I^{131} concentrations that indicates the presence of an organic lesion.

4. COMMENT

Ideally, the most accurate information would be obtained if the readings over symmetrically chosen areas occurred at the same instant of time. Readings should be made as consecutively as possible and, according to these standards, should be made within 3–5 minutes. In a restless patient it may be convenient to record two or three different positions on one side of the skull before contrasting these with their symmetrical mates on the opposite side. In that case, comparisons will be made after 15–30 minutes. It will then be observed that a gradual slope or decrease in the values at that site occurs with the passage of such an interval of time. This decrease would therefore permit discrepancies to appear; for the differences would then exceed the permitted 20–40 cts./min. expected between symmetrical sites in normal cases. Reference to the plotted concentrations on the proposed normal chart would help to clarify this feature, which is particularly important when the organic lesion is a relatively acellular or avascular one, such as an astrocytoma or calcified oligodendroglioma, or a cystic degenerative or necrotic lesion. In such instances, the differences are only between 40 and 90 cts./min., with the records as a whole being just above the highest expected normals at any particular interval of time.

If the lesion is highly anaplastic, a cellular one, or one with proliferative new blood-vessel formations as well, then the resultant increased permeability causes such high exudations of I^{131} that the readings are definitely pertinent because of their large values (80–200 cts./min. differences), and they persist even up to 4 hours following the intravenous administration of the NaI^{131}. This is especially true in the highly cellular meningiomas, glioblastomas, carcinomas and sarcomas when they do not show extensive cystic or necrotic changes.

A statistical analysis of 500 subject cases resulted in an accuracy of 61 per cent in those cases in which there were positively verified tumors (surgery, pathology, etc.). In the cases in which there was verification of the nonexistence of tumors, there was a test accuracy of 95 per cent. In other words, there is very little chance of obtaining a false-positive result (5 per cent), but there is a larger chance of getting a false-negative result (39 per cent). This degree of accuracy permits the use of this test as a convenient screening procedure.

B. INTERNAL MEASUREMENTS: PHOSPHORUS-32

1. Technique of Administration

It has been demonstrated that there is a high differential uptake of radiophosphorus (P^{32}) by most brain tumors following administration of this isotope. Some studies have indicated that tumor tissue will absorb from five to a hundred times the activity of similar specimens of normal brain tissue (10, 11, 12). Similar studies have indicated that gray matter has an activity ratio approximately twice that of normal white matter (13). Inasmuch as P^{32} emits only beta particles (practical range less than 0.5 cm.), it is possible, by means of a needle-sized Geiger counter, to probe into various areas of the brain during surgery and to determine the areas of highest concentration. When high differentials are observed on the recording meter, an abnormality is usually indicated, and so a surgeon may use this test as an aid in locating deep-seated lesions. The technique is simple. Relatively small quantities of radioactive materials and reliable electronic components are used.

a) EQUIPMENT.—Radioactive sodium phosphate* in the amount of 250 μc. will be needed, together with a cold sterilization solution, Zephiran® chloride, of 1:1,000 concentration.

A halogen-filled needle probe counter† is recommended. A count-rate meter with large indicating meter,‡ a plastic radioactive button with a ⅙ in. diameter hole, ¼ in. deep; a 4 × 10 × 2-in. sterilization tray; and a metal shield for the probe counter, ¼ in. deep by 8 in. long, comprise the apparatus required.

b) PREPARATORY STEPS.—Administer radio phosphorus, 250 μc. orally, to the patient 18 hours in advance of the surgical procedure. Give this in a paper cup under the usual radiation safeguards.

The needle counter with a counter shield and the radium button source may be cold sterilized. Place a rubber fingercot tightly over the connector end of the cable. Fasten the cot with a rubber band to prevent any fluid from coming in contact with the connector during sterilization. Place a metal tube shield over the probe end to protect it from mechanical shock. At least 12 hours before surgery, place the probe assembly, shield and button into a tray of Zephiran® chloride concentration of 1:1,000 containing antirust. At the end of the sterilization period, place the shield over the probe and place the probe and button on the operating table in the sterilization tray in preparation for the operation.

c) PROCEDURES:

(1) *Operating-Room Technique.*—Electronic: Note that the volume and high-voltage knobs on the count-rate

---

* Source: Oak Ridge National Laboratory, Oak Ridge, Tennessee, or Abbott Laboratories, Oak Ridge, Tennessee.

† Source: Anton Electronic Laboratory, Inc., Brooklyn, New York.

‡ Model 1615-B (manufactured by Nuclear-Chicago, Chicago, Illinois), or an equivalent.

meter are completely counterclockwise. Turn on the count-rate meter at least 15 minutes before it is to be used. Set the appropriate zero and calibration knobs to the correct positions. Set the operating switch to the "ON" position.

Take the connector end of the cable from the scrub nurse and, breaking through the fingercot, insert it into the coaxial connector on the rear of the count-rate meter. Have the nurse remove the protective shield and insert the probe into the radium button hole. Raise the high voltage until the first pulse is heard. Then raise the voltage an additional 35 volts. The button should now read a standard number of counts per minute as precalibrated. The instrument is then ready for use.

(2) *Operating Method:*

1. Choose an area in the brain considered to be normal.
2. Insert the probe at successive 1 cm. depths.
3. Record the readings at these positions on a record card in the form shown in Table 11.
4. After the normal readings have been noted, insert the probe in suggestive areas until a significant increase in counts occurs. The tumor areas will give an increase in counts over normal areas by at least

TABLE 11.—RECORD CARD FOR DATA COLLECTION DURING USE OF PROBE COUNTER AT SURGERY

Patient:	Serial No.:	Date:
Hours Dose:	Dose:	
Position: 1 cm. 2 cm. 3 cm. 4 cm. 5 cm. 6 cm.		

a factor of 5. In general, it has been found that, with the doses indicated, the normal counting rates will be below 50 cts./min., and abnormal counting areas will give a counting rate in excess of 250 cts./min.

5. After initial localization of the tumor area, insert the probe at adjacent areas in an attempt to demarcate the outline of the tumor area.

6. The sensitive area of the probe is at least 0.5 cm. from the tip of the needle. Beta radiation from P^{32} has a practical range in tissue of less than 5 mm.; therefore, after an initial high ratio has been obtained, insert the probe deeper to ascertain whether the probe is actually in the tumor or merely passing the outer edge of the tumor. If the probe is only passing the outer edge, the counts will *decrease* on slight increase in depth; if the probe is actually in the tumor, the counts will *increase,* in most instances, on slight increase in probe depth.

2. RESULTS

The technique described was studied at the Veterans Administration Hospital, Hines, Illinois. Confirmed localizations were made in at least 85 per cent of more than 30 cases. No untoward reactions were noticed with the material or the apparatus recommended.

C. IDENTIFICATION OF INTRAOCULAR TUMORS*

It has been well known for some time (14, 15, 16, 17) that certain radioactive materials (particularly P^{32}) are taken up selectively in rapidly growing neoplastic tissue; but this phenomenon has not been practically applied because, in most conditions,

* The research upon which this section (pp. 101–107) is based was performed by teams of investigators working under AEC Contract W31-109-eng-78 with Western Reserve University and was participated in by members of the Department of Surgery, Medicine and Radiology of the School of Medicine, Western Reserve University, Cleveland, Ohio.

the identification of malignant tissue can best be effected by histo-logic examination. It was realized, however, that the increased uptake of P^{32} in malignant tissue could be used to advantage in certain specific conditions. The one presently being considered is the identification of malignant tumors of the eye (18, 19, 20, 21, 22), for which histologic examination is only possible after enucleation of the eye; thus a radioactive material that will allow identification of malignant tissue in vivo is extremely useful. The major problem in the identification of intraocular tumors is that of differentiation between detachments of the retina caused by (1) underlying fluid, (2) benign inflammatory condition or (3) malignant growth. In most instances encountered, these three types of conditions are differentiable with the aid of the test to be described here. It should be stressed, however, that by itself this method does not provide a positive means of identifying any of the three conditions. The test should be considered only as an adjunct to available diagnostic procedures.

1. TECHNIQUE OF ADMINISTRATION

a) MATERIAL.—Because intraocular tumors can be accurately located by ophthalmoscopic examination and because these tu-mors lie close to the outside surface of the eye, it has been possi-ble and particularly advantageous to use a beta emitter for their identification. The advantage of using beta rays is that the meas-urement obtained by counting directly over the suggestive area is essentially unaffected by the radioactive material in the surround-ing normal tissue. This eliminates the masking effect of back-ground due to normal tissue, which complicates identification and localization measurements in which gamma emitters are used. The beta emitter chosen for the present study is P^{32}. The most important reason for the choice of P^{32} is that previous studies by other investigators (14, 15, 16, 17) have shown that P^{32} is selectively taken up by virtually all types of malignant tissue in concentrations from 2 to 500 times that found in normal tissue. Other reasons for the use of radioactive phosphorus are: (1) availability, (2) a half-life long enough to allow ease of use and (3) beta-particle energy such that most of the particles can penetrate less than 5 mm. of tissue. The average range is 3 mm., and this probably constitutes the maximum thickness of tissue through which increased concentrations can be easily identified.

b) APPARATUS.—The counting apparatus used consists of three types of special Geiger tubes,* along with usual scaling apparatus. The first tube is a small end-window tube with the end window mounted at right angles to the axis of the tube. This counter allows measurement over areas on the anterior hemi-

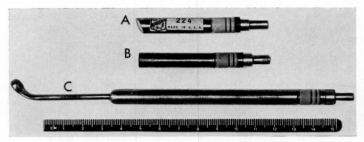

FIG. 9.—Geiger tubes for intraocular tumor localization. (Courtesy: Anton Electronic Laboratory, Inc., Brooklyn, New York.)

sphere of the eye and in some areas posterior to the equator when extreme rotation of the eye is used. The second type of tube is essentially the same as the first, with the exception that the window is mounted at an angle of 45° to the axis of the tube. This allows for measurement over more posterior portions of the eye. The third type (23) allows measurement at all posterior areas of the globe. The three special Geiger tubes are shown in Figure 9.

c) PROCEDURE:

1. Prepare the patient by instilling 1 per cent tetracaine hydrochloride or 4 per cent cocaine hydrochloride into the conjunctival sac.
2. Make a thorough ophthalmoscopic examination to determine the exact location and extent of tumor.
3. After making a check to determine that the counting apparatus is working properly, inject intravenously 500 μc. of P^{32} (or about 7 μc./kilo body weight) in sterile

---

* Source: Anton Electronic Laboratory, Inc., Brooklyn, New York.

isotonic saline solution. For a 70 kg. person, 500 μc. of P^{32} is far below the level of radioactivity that might produce manifest injurious effects; it is, however, greater than the generally accepted permissible dose. However,

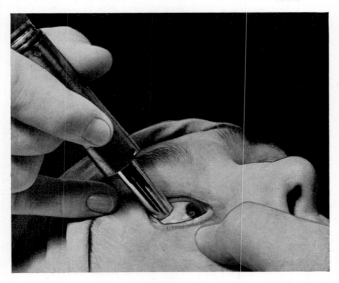

Fig. 10.—Window tube in use on eye. (From Thomas, C. I.; Krohmer, J. S., and Storaasli, J. P.: A.M.A. Arch. Ophth. 47:279, 1952.)

the exposure is less than that received during the course of most diagnostic radiologic procedures.

4. Immediately after injection, start the counting procedure by placing the counting tube directly in contact with the eye immediately over the suspected area (Fig. 10). Make a measurement for ½–1 minute in this location and record the count. Then move the counter to a normal portion of the same eye as far removed from the tumor site as possible and take a similar count. Continue this procedure by alternately counting over the area of the suspected tumor and the normal tissue for approximately 15 minutes. Then make additional series of

counts* over these areas at ½ hour and 1 hour after injection. Sometimes additional series of counts are made after 1, 2 or 3 days.

5. Plot on ordinary graph paper the variations in counting rate with time for the tumor and normal tissue. Determine the ratio of tumor to normal counts for various times and record it. The ratio that has proved most useful is the peak-to-peak ratio, that is, the ratio of the peak of the tumor curve to the peak of the normal curve.

d) ENUCLEATION.—In addition to the *in vivo* counting procedure, in all cases in which enucleation is thought necessary and performed, section the eye directly through the tumor. Use one half of the eye for preparation of histologic sections and radioautographs. From the other half of the eye, samples of tumor, sclera, retina, lens and other important sections may be obtained for assay of radioactivity. Place such samples in weighed porcelain counting dishes, dissolve them in concentrated nitric acid and then dry them; thin flat samples will result. After the samples have been dried and weighed, count them under identical conditions with a conventional laboratory Geiger-counter apparatus. Record the results in corrected counts per minute per gram of sample. The ratio of tumor to adjacent normal tissue in counts per minute per gram of sample are recorded.

2. RESULTS

The measurement of P^{32} uptake in suspected intraocular tumors is valuable in establishing the diagnosis: it is effective in determining whether retinal separations are produced by non-neoplastic or neoplastic disease. Because accurate diagnosis can often be made by ordinary clinical procedures and because the dose of P^{32} is somewhat above the recommended permissible dosage, it is suggested that cases be carefully screened and that positive diagnosis be made, when possible, by the usual clinical procedures. The test described should be limited to cases in which there is a question as to the diagnosis.

---

* Series of counts must be made. Because of low activity levels and the necessity for short counting times, single-count statistics are rather poor.

The success of the test depends largely on the determination of the exact location and extent of the suspected tumor. Ophthalmoscopic examination must be accomplished under the effect of a mydriatic in order to permit the most careful localization. Since the average range of the P^{32} beta particles is about 3 mm. in tissue, it is necessary to be certain that the counter is in as close proximity to the tumor as possible. For practical purposes, a distance of 5 mm. or more between the tumor and counter is unsatisfactory; therefore, when difficulty is experienced in placing the counter properly in apposition to the tumor, the significance of the result, particularly if it is a negative one, is doubtful. Because of this, it has been difficult in the past to study tumors situated in the posterior quadrant. The two early types of Geiger probes described (Fig. 9, *A* and *B*) could not be applied with any certainty in the posterior portion of the eye.

The newest type of probe design (Fig. 9, *C*) offers hope that posterior intraocular tumors may be properly measured by placing this counter directly over the area where the tumor lies. This will, in general, entail an operative procedure whereby Tenon's capsule must be opened and the counter placed immediately against the outside surface of the eye. It is believed that the best positioning of this counter will be obtained when a transilluminator (light pipe) (24) can be rigidly attached to the counter itself; then, by means of ophthalmoscopic examination, the light transmitted down the transilluminator can be used to position the counter properly.

It should be mentioned that the test described herein differs from tumor studies carried out by others in that measurements are made a short time after injection rather than after a period of 2–4 days. Studies (17, 19, 20, 21) made of superficial malignant tumors have indicated, for most subjects,* that in less than 15 minutes the ratio of tumor counts to normal counts reaches a maximum and that this ratio decreases for 1 or 2 hours after injection. After this decrease, a subsequent increase in ratio becomes evident and continues over the period studied, probably reaching a maximum in 4 or 5 days (Fig. 11).

---

* Patients with superficial malignant tumors were selected, so that a continuous recording of counts could be made. It has been subsequently borne out that intraocular tumors exhibit the same sort of curve.

The cause of increased activity in the tumor tissue in the early stages is uncertain, and is now under further investigation. It may be due to one or all of the following: (1) increased vascularity of the tumor, (2) more rapid transport of the inorganic phosphorus across the vascular membrane into extracellular space, (3) more rapid transport of P^{32} across cellular membrane into intracellular space and (4) more rapid incorporation of P^{32} into

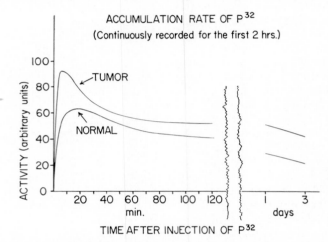

FIG. 11.—Typical P^{32} uptake curves for tumor and normal tissue. (From Krohmer, J. S., *et al.:* Radiology 61:920, 1953.)

nuclear and other cellular constituents. Whatever the mechanism may be for producing higher counts in neoplastic tissue after administration of P^{32}, it should be noted that measurements, as made by this method, have shown that neoplastic tissue may be identified at an early period. When the diagnosis has been questionable or borderline at early periods, further studies are made on the patients in 2 or 3 days.

It is fairly certain that the P^{32} measured later is actually incorporated in the nucleus and other cellular constituents. It is probably better procedure to make all measurements within 2 or 3 days. However, in actual practice it has been found that making the early measurement is advantageous because it can be done in a short time and patients need not be asked to return for later counts.

From experience with 68 cases of various intraocular lesions, the following data were obtained:

1. Tumors over which the counter can be placed show peak uptake ratios from 1.4 to 2.8, with an average of 1.8. The peak ratios usually occur within 15 minutes of injection and remain high for periods extending into days.

2. Retinoblastoma cases show inconclusive ratios, or the ratios vary considerably throughout the course of the measurements. Some of the difficulty may be attributable to the diffuseness of these conditions, so that a normal area is hard to find in the eye being studied.

3. Peak ratios in fluid detachments vary from 0.95 to 1.20, with an average of 1.05. The ratios remain low over all periods of measurement.

4. Peak ratios in inflammatory conditions range from 0.98 to 2.40, with an average of 1.33. In cases of inflammation, ratios often reach high levels early after injection and then rapidly decline to normal levels, generally at 1 hour and invariably within 3 days. Inflammatory conditions may thus be differentiated from tumors mainly through a decreasing ratio.

5. Benign tumors, hemorrhages and cysts yield normal or even subnormal ratios.

REFERENCES

1. Boyland, E., and McClean, D.: Factor in malignant tissues which increases permeability of dermis, J. Path. & Bact. 41:553, 1935.
2. Broman, T.: Cerebral vascular permeability in man: Supravital analysis of disorders of central nervous system, Acta med. scandinav. 118:79, 1944.
3. Brunschwig, A.; Schmidt, R. L., and Clark, T. H.: Intravital staining of malignant neoplasms in man by Evans blue, A.M.A. Arch. Path. 30:902, 1940.
4. Duran-Reynals, F.: Studies on localization of dyes and foreign proteins in normal and malignant tissues, Am. J. Cancer 35:98, 1939.
5. Gough, J.: The structure of the blood vessels in cerebral tumors, J. Path. & Bact. 31:23, 1940.
6. Ludford, R. J.: Vital staining of normal and malignant cells: Staining of malignant tumors with trypan blue, Proc. Roy. Soc., London, s. B, 194:493, 1929.

7. Sahs, A. L., and Alexander, L.: Vascular pattern of certain intra-cranial neoplasms: Studies with the benzidine stain, Arch. Neurol. & Psychiat. 42:44, 1939.

8. Seifter, J.; Bander, D. H., and Dervinis, A.: Alteration in permea-bility of some membranes by hyaluronidase, and inhibition of this effect by steroids, Proc. Soc. Exper. Biol. & Med. 72:136, 1949.

9. Virchow, R.: *Die krankhaften Geschwulste,* vol. 2, p. 141 (3 vols.; Berlin: A. Hirschwald, 1863-67).

10. Fields, T.: Mount, electronics, and indicator for probe counter, Nucleonics 10:60, 1952.

11. Selverstone, B.; Sweet, W. H., and Robinson, C. V.: The clinical use of radioactive phosphorus in the surgery of brain tumors, Ann. Surg. 130:643, 1949.

12. ————; Solomon, D. K., and Sweet, W. H.: Location of brain tumors by means of radioactive phosphorus, J.A.M.A. 140:277, May 21, 1949.

13. Erickson, T. C.; Larson, F., and Gordon, E. S.: The uptake of ra-dioactive phosphorus by malignant brain tumors, J. Lab. & Clin. Med. 34:587, 1949.

14. Kenney, J. M.; Marinelli, L. D., and Woodard, H. W.: Tracer studies with radioactive phosphorus in malignant neoplastic disease, Radiology 37:683, 1941.

15. Low-Beer, B. V. A.: Surface measurements of radioactive phosphorus in breast tumors as possible diagnostic method, Science 104:399, 1946.

16. Selverstone, B.; Solomon, A. K., and Sweet, W. H.: Location of brain tumors by means of radioactive phosphorus, J.A.M.A. 140:277, 1949.

17. Geffen, A.; Loevinger, R., and Wolf, B. S.: Surface activity fol-lowing administration of radioactive phosphorus, Radiology 56:857, 1951.

18. Thomas, C. I.; Krohmer, J. S., and Storaasli, J. P.: Detection of intraocular tumors with radioactive phosphorus: A preliminary re-port, Arch. Ophth. 47:276, 1952.

19. Krohmer, J. S., *et al.:* Detection of intraocular tumors with the use of radioactive phosphorus, Radiology 61:916, 1953.

20. ————, *et al.: The use of P^{32} in the Identification of Intraocular Tumors,* AEC Report NYO-4961 (July, 1954).

21. Thomas, C. I., *et al.:* Detection of intraocular tumors by the use of radioactive phosphorus, Am. J. Ophth. 38:93, 1954.

22. Dunphy, E. B., *et al.:* The uptake of radioactive phosphorus by intraocular neoplasms, Am. J. Ophth. 37:45, 1954.

23. Thomas, C. I.; Krohmer, J. S., and Storaasli, J. P.: Geiger counter probe for diagnosis and localization of posterior intraocular tumors, A.M.A. Arch. Ophth. 52:413, 1954.

24. ————, and Krohmer, J. S.: Transilluminator for use with the curved Geiger counter—an aid to localization of posterior intraocular neoplasms, A.M.A. Arch. Ophth. 55:413, 1956.

CHAPTER 4

Cardiovascular Studies*

A. PERIPHERAL VASCULAR STUDIES

ALTHOUGH THERE ARE MANY CLINICAL APPROACHES to the evaluation of the circulation in peripheral vascular disease, most of them are indirect methods and do not involve the direct measurement of blood flow in the extremities. Since Blumgart and his co-workers (1, 2) reported their measurements on circulation times by means of radium C in 1927, several methods for the evaluation of peripheral vascular circulation by means of radioisotopes have been investigated. Smith and Quimby (3, 4, 5, 6) utilized an intravenous injection of radiosodium (Na^{24}) and recorded *build-up curves* as the radioactive material was concentrated in the tissues of the foot. In this type of measurement a Geiger counter is placed against the sole of a foot, or other suitable site; and as the radioactive material comes into equilibrium with the site observed by the counter, the increased counting rate is recorded as a function of time. The concentration in the tissue depends on the amount of Na^{24} that has diffused from the vascular bed, and thus depends on the amount of blood containing the Na^{24} that is supplied to or flowing through the region per unit time.

A similar technique was used by Friedell and his associates (7, 8, 9), but with the substitution of radiophosphorus (P^{32}) for

* The research upon which this chapter is based was performed by teams of investigators working under AEC Contract W31-109-eng-78 with Western Reserve University and was participated in by members of the Department of Surgery, Medicine and Radiology of the School of Medicine, Western Reserve University, Cleveland, Ohio.

Na^{24}. In their technique the permeability of the capillaries to phosphate and the accumulation of P^{32} in the tissues is recorded. A reversal of this method was applied by Kety (10, 11) and, among others, by Elkin and his co-workers (12, 13), who measured the rate of disappearance of Na^{24} injected intramuscularly.

In all the methods utilizing a freely diffusible electrolyte, the effect measured is due not only to blood flow but also to the diffusion rate of the electrolyte across the capillary membrane to or from the extravascular space. Veall (14) has discussed the problem of separating counts from radioactivity in tissue space from that in intravascular space for such build-up curves.

With the foregoing investigations in mind, it appeared advantageous, in the study of peripheral vascular circulation, to separate experimentally the actual vascular flow from the effects of diffusion through the capillary walls and the equilibrium of the material in electrolyte space.

1. MATERIAL

In any circulation study, the primary requirement of a tagged material that is to be injected is its relatively slow disappearance from the circulating blood. Iodinated human serum albumin ($I^{131}HSA$) was selected for investigation because the material has only a minor loss from the vascular system for the period of measurement and can be used directly without the need of incubation. Since the primary information that is sought is how the injected material becomes mixed in the capillaries, there is perhaps some disadvantage in using a gamma emitter (e.g., I^{131}) as the tagging substance, because such a substance will allow the radioactive material in the blood in the larger vessels to contribute somewhat to the slope of the build-up curve that is obtained. However, the use of a gamma emitter is not a serious objection. In any mass of vascular tissue the blood in the capillary bed far surpasses that within the arterioles and venules, so that the tagged material in the arteries or veins is small compared to the capillary bed. Moreover, inasmuch as the detector is applied directly on the surface, the inverse square law becomes important. Thus, the contribution from the radioactivity within the deep vessels falls off rapidly because of the distance factor alone. It will therefore be noted that the measured radioactivity then arises primarily from the tagged albumin within the more superficial capillaries.

Some work was also done with red cells tagged with P^{32}, with the activity detected by means of a Geiger counter. This method restricts detection to the activity in vessels no more than 8 mm. from the surface and is useful where such restriction is desired.

2. Apparatus

The general experimental setup is shown schematically in Figure 12. Because most of the beta particles from I^{131} are ab-

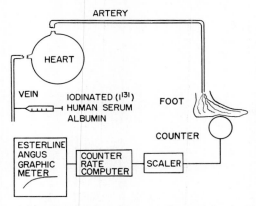

Fig. 12.—Schematic experimental setup for peripheral vascular flow measurements. (From MacIntyre, W. J., et al.: Radiology 59:852, 1952.)

sorbed in the first 1 or 2 mm. of tissue, these were filtered out and all curves were recorded by gamma detection by means of a scintillation counter.*

The Berkeley count-rate computer and scaler combination was used, but has no particular advantage over the conventional count-rate meters. It was felt originally that, if fast responses did occur, the computer would be better suited to reproduce these faithfully; however, such responses did not occur.

---

* See Chapter 16, pp. 331–335.

The counter was curved so that the palm of the hand or the sole of the foot could be comfortably placed in close apposition to the crystal itself. Lead shielding was used to prevent interference from radiation from the other extremities or other sites.

3. PROCEDURE

A room with constant temperature is preferred; but if this cannot be had, a quiet room, free from drafts and with a rela-

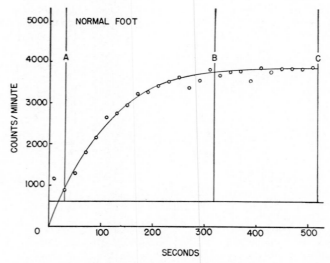

FIG. 13.—Typical equilibrium curve for peripheral vascular flow measurements. The latent period of the arm-to-foot circulation time (approximately 20 seconds) has been omitted. (From MacIntyre, W. J., et al.: Radiology 59:852, 1952.)

tively constant temperature is satisfactory. The method is mainly comparative: the patient's opposite extremity acts as control for the extremity under investigation. A scintillation counter is placed on the sole of each foot or the palm of each hand to obtain the characteristic build-up curve, which is recorded from each.

After an injection of 75–130 μc. of I¹³¹-labeled albumin in a volume of 1.5 ml. or less of physiologic saline solution is made into an antecubital vein, the counting rate, as obtained over the extremities, indicates the manner in which the radioactive albumin becomes mixed in the blood in the veins, arteries and capillaries. A typical curve is illustrated in Figure 13, and the section A–B shows a characteristic exponentially rising curve. This illustration shows the regular increase in activity that is a measure of the rate of mixing in the vascular bed. The curve indicates primarily the rate at which the tagged albumin is mixed with the normal plasma in the capillaries, and it therefore represents the manner in which the capillary beds may be cleared. The plateau B–C is indicative of the measured volume of the vascular bed. This plateau is reached when complete mixing has occurred between the injected and the normal plasma.

The curve may be mathematically approximated as follows: The capillary bed may be considered as a network of small-diameter pipes being fed by a large-diameter pipe (artery) and leading into a large-diameter exit pipe (vein). Radioactive measurement over this bed is then a measurement of activity (A) in the bed. This activity can be represented as the product of the volume of capillaries activated (V), that is, cleared of original blood and replaced with blood-containing iodinated (I^{131}) albumin, multiplied by the concentration (c) of the radioactive albumin in the blood in terms of microcuries per cubic centimeter. Then

$$A = Vc$$

The rate by which equilibrium is established is directly obtained by differentiating the quantity A with respect to time:

$$\frac{dA}{dt} = V \frac{dc}{dt} + c \frac{dV}{dt}$$

Since the mixing of iodinated (I^{131}) albumin is 90 per cent complete in about 1 minute and thereafter changes slowly, attaining complete mixing at about 10 minutes, as a first approximation the concentration (c) can be treated as a constant after 1 minute. Thus,

$$\frac{dc}{dt} = 0 \quad \text{and} \quad \frac{dA}{dt} = c \frac{dV}{dt}$$

This means that the uptake rate of the activity in the capillary bed is proportional to the rate at which the volume of blood within the capillaries is activated or cleared.

From a general point of view, the rate of activation of the capillary volume (dV/dt) will be directly proportional to the pressure (P) forcing the fluid through the tubes, and inversely proportional to the total resistance (R) which is acting to oppose the flow. It is also assumed that the rate of activation will be proportional to the volume of blood within the capillaries as yet unactivated $(V_f - V$, where V_f is the final volume activated). Inasmuch as the capillaries offer many paths of activation, the plasma will not necessarily follow the same paths each time, and the activation rate at any time must then be proportional to the paths that are still unactivated at that time. This expression of proportionality may then be represented as:

$$\frac{dV}{dt} \propto \frac{P\,(V_f - V)}{R}$$

or

$$\frac{dV}{dt} = \frac{kP}{R}\,(V_f - V)$$

where k is a constant of proportionality. This formula may be integrated to yield the equation:

$$V = V_f\,(1 - e^{-kPt/R})$$

This last equation describes the uptake curve as exponentially rising with respect to time. From this curve it is seen that the larger the value of the exponent kP/R, the higher the relative activity of the capillary bed will be at any time, and the faster the uptake curve will approach equilibrium. The foregoing examples illustrate the various factors which influence the uptake curve and which may be examined individually for their effect on the curve.

As the resistance (R) increases, the capillaries are activated at a slower rate, since a smaller volume of fluid will flow through the capillaries per unit time. If this resistance is due to the flow of viscous fluid, Poiseuille's law, which states that *the volume emerging from a pipe under a given pressure gradient is directly proportional to the square of the cross-section,* will apply. A decrease in the pressure *(P)* feeding the capillaries will also increase the time required for the curve to reach equilibrium.

The effects described can be tested by several methods: (1) dilation of peripheral arterioles and capillaries to reduce the resistance *(R);* (2) constriction of the artery or (3) constriction of the vein, both to reduce flow (increase resistance); and (4) increase of pressure *(P)* by increasing the heart rate by exercise or other stimulus.

4. RESULTS

Several experiments (15, 16) utilizing heat, cold and arterial and venous obstruction were performed in order to study the alterations in the clearance rate of the capillaries and in the volume of vascular bed as suggested by the mathematical approxi-

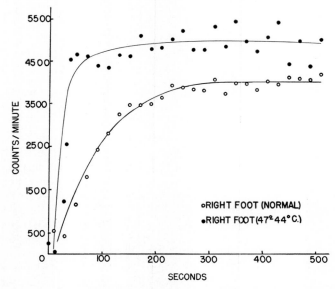

FIG. 14.—Effect of heat on peripheral vascular measurement. Note increased height of plateau and faster equilibrium time. (From MacIntyre, W. J., *et al.:* Radiology 59:853, 1952.)

mation for changes in peripheral resistance and pressure. Since heat causes vasodilation with a resultant increase in rate of mixing, a more rapid clearing or flushing of the capillary bed is obtained with decreased peripheral resistance. The volume of the vascular bed is increased with heat also, which is illustrated by a higher plateau. This effect, which may be due to dilation of arterioles, dilation of capillaries, or both, is illustrated in

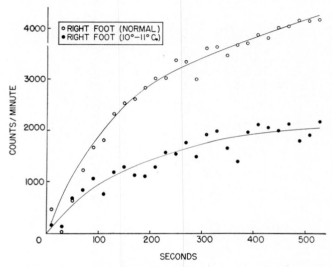

Fig. 15.—Effect of cold on peripheral vascular measurement. Note decreased height of plateau. (From MacIntyre, W. J., *et al.:* Radiology 59:853, 1952.)

Figure 14. Similar curves have been obtained (16) by the elimination of normal vasomotor tonus by blocking the posterior tibial nerves with procaine hydrochloride. Higher plateaus, reached in a short time, were noted consistently.

An increase in peripheral resistance, as caused by cold, would be expected to have the opposite effect of decreased rate of clearance and decreased height, as shown by Figure 15.

The effect of arterial obstruction, by digitally compressing the brachial artery, is shown in Figure 16. A prolonged gradual slope is noted until the compression is released, at which time an immediate rise is noted. As venous obstruction is applied, the plasma is pooled in the vascular bed (shown in Figure 17). No difference is noted in the slope, but a large increase in plateau due to increased entrapped volume of the capillary bed is observed.

This test has been applied (16) clinically for several different

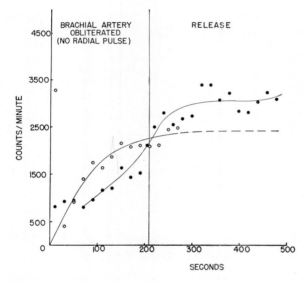

FIG. 16.—Effect of partial arterial obstruction on peripheral vascular measurements. o = right hand (normal); ● = right hand (obstructions). (Adapted from MacIntyre, W. J., *et al.*: Radiology 59:854, 1952.)

purposes: (1) to evaluate the state of peripheral circulation in such cases as arteriosclerosis; (2) to indicate possible benefits of surgical procedures by such means as observing the effect of a sympathetic nerve block before sympathectomy and (3) to evaluate the results of therapy, such as sympathectomies or the removal of obstructions or occlusions.

As stated, although this is still a comparative technique, greater control of the experiments may well lead to a quantiza-

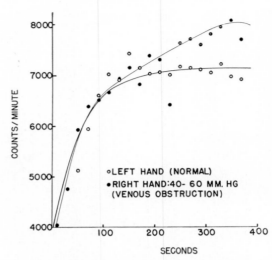

Fig. 17.—Effects of venous obstruction on peripheral vascular measurement. (Adapted from MacIntyre, W. J., *et al.:* Radiology 59:854, 1952.)

tion of the exponential factor and its actual relation to blood flow.

B. CARDIAC OUTPUT PROCEDURE WITH RADIOIODINE-LABELED HUMAN SERUM ALBUMIN (I¹³¹HSA)

The radioisotope procedure for determining cardiac output is similar to the dye-dilution techniques of measuring the capacities of a pump or of the heart. If a small volume of radioactive material is injected into the inflow tube of a pump, the fluid volume per stroke will be determined by the dilution of the material. This diluted volume can be summed or integrated over a prescribed period of time and the results quoted in terms of volume of flow per unit time or liters per minute (18–32).

Some investigators have used a scintillation counter placed over the aorta and made a continuous record of the radiation pickup. Adjunct electronic gear, such as count-rate meters, computers and tape recorders, have also been employed with the scintillation counter. The experience of most laboratories has been

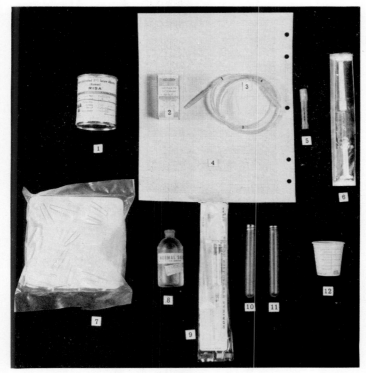

FIG. 18.—Materials for cardiac output test.

that these procedures were less accurate than the counting of individual blood samples collected over a 1-minute period. By using disposable plastic materials and very small radioisotope doses, the procedure described below allows for a maximum of accuracy and reproducibility and a minimum of complications and expense.

1. METHOD

a) MATERIALS (Fig. 18):

3 μc. radioiodine-labeled human serum albumin (I^{131}HSA) (Fig. 18, item *1*)

Heparin (*2*)

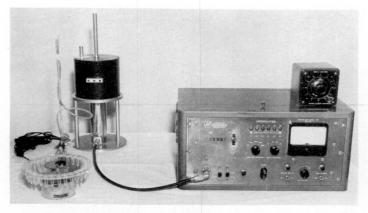

FIG. 19.—Counting and collection equipment for cardiac output test.

One plastic tube, 27 in. long, with 1½ in. needle
adapter (3)
One sheet of 3-cycle semilogarithmic graph paper (4)
One 20 gauge disposable needle (5)
One 2 cc. disposable syringe with 1½ in. needle (6)
Thirty 1 ml. microcentrifuge tubes (7)
10 ml. sterile saline solution (8)
One 5 cc. disposable syringe (9)
One sterile plastic test tube, 5 × ½ in. (10)
One nonsterile plastic test tube, 5 × ½ in. (11)
One 1 oz. paper cup (12)

b) EQUIPMENT (Fig. 19):

One scintillation well counter, 2 × 2 in.
One scaler
One ring stand
One aluminum well spacer, 10¼ in. long, ½ in. I.D.
One aluminum cup adapter
One 1 rpm motor
One plastic turntable with thirty ½ in. holes

c) PROCEDURE (Fig. 20):

1. Withdraw 3 μc. of I[131]HSA into the 2 ml. disposable
syringe and bring up to 2 ml. with sterile saline solution.

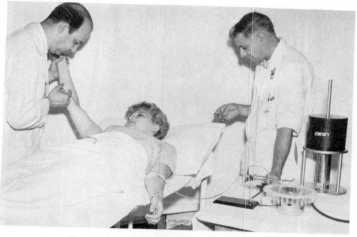

Fig. 20.—Injection and collection procedure.

2. Inject 2 ml. of the mixture into the sterile plastic test tube and count in 10¼ in. aluminum spacer above well counter.

3. Refill the 2 ml. syringe.

4. Place 30 microcentrifuge tubes into the turntable mounted on the 1 rpm motor.

5. Heparinize the 27 in. plastic tubing and adapter and set them in the ring stand directly over the centrifuge tubes (Fig. 20).

6. Connect the tubing to the Cournand needle which has been inserted into the brachial artery. After determining that the blood is flowing with no interference, permit the effluent of blood to continue to flow through the unfilled hole in the plastic disk into the paper cup.

7. Inject I^{131}HSA into a vein in the opposite extended arm. Raise the arm immediately after injection.

8. Start the turntable 6 seconds after the injection.

9. Stop the turntable after 30 tubes have been filled (1 minute).

10. Dilute the blood in each centrifuge tube to 1 ml. with a

measured and recorded number of drops of saline solution (20 drops/ml.).

11. Count each tube 1 minute in the aluminum cup in the well counter.

12. Withdraw 5 ml. of blood from the arm opposite the injected arm 15 minutes after the injection.

13. Count a 5 ml. sample for 1 minute in the plastic test tube in the well counter.

d) CALCULATIONS:

1. Record the volumes of each sample in column A of the Example on page 123.

2. Record the gross readings per minute in column B.

3. Subtract the background and record the net reading in column C.

4. Divide column C by column A to derive the net counts/min./1 ml. and record in column D.

5. Plot column D on the 3-cycle semilogarithmic paper as in Figure 21.

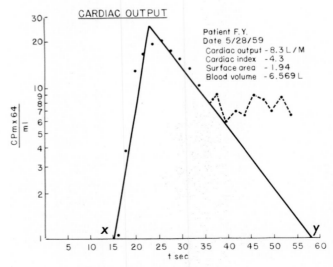

FIG. 21.—Typical cardiac output curve.

6. Extrapolate the curve at the end of the first cycle to abscissas (e.g., $t = x$ sec.).
7. Read the points from the curve between $t = x$ sec. (cts./min./1 ml. > 1.0) and $t = y$ (cts./min./1 ml. < 1.0) and record in column E.
8. Total column E.
9. The cardiac output is equal to:

$$\frac{\text{Cts. injected}}{\Sigma_{t=1 \text{ min.}} \text{ cts./min./1 ml.}} \times \frac{60 \text{ L.}}{1,000 \text{ min.}}$$

EXAMPLE

Patient: *F.Y.*

Date: *5/28/59*

Sample	Time	(A) Vol.	(B) CPM*	(C) CPM†	(D) CPM†/ml. (calculated)	(E) CPM†/ml. (plotted)
1	1			0		
	2			0		
	3			0		
2	4			0		
	5			0		
3	6			0		
	7			0		
4	8			0		
	9			0		
5	10			0		
	11			0		
6	12			0		
	13			0		
7	14			0		
	15			0		
8	16	0.60	5.9	0.5	0.8	1.5
	17					2.2
9	18	0.65	7.9	2.5	3.8	3.2
	19					5.0
10	20	0.65	13.6	8.2	12.6	7.4
	21					11.0
11	22	0.65	15.9	10.5	16.2	17.0
	23					25.0
12	24	0.60	16.8	11.4	19.0	23.0

* Gross counts × 64.   † Gross counts − background × 64.

EXAMPLE *(cont.)*

| | | | | | Patient: | *F.Y.* |
| | | | | | Date: | *5/28/59* |

Sample	Time	(A) Vol.	(B) CPM*	(C) CPM†	(D) CPM†/ml. (calculated)	(E) CPM†/ml. (plotted)
	25					21.0
13	26	0.60	17.4	12.0	20.0	19.0
	27					17.5
14	28	0.60	15.6	10.2	17.0	16.0
	29					14.5
15	30	0.60	14.5	9.1	15.2	13.5
	31					12.0
16	32	0.50	11.9	6.5	13.0	11.0
	33					10.0
17	34	0.55	10.9	5.5	10.0	9.2
	35					8.4
18	36	0.55	9.6	4.2	7.6	7.6
	37					7.0
19	38	0.55	10.2	4.8	8.7	6.4
	39					5.8
20	40	0.60	8.9	3.5	5.8	5.2
	41					4.8
21	42	0.50	8.8	3.4	6.8	4.4
	43					4.0
22	44	0.45	8.3	2.9	6.4	3.6
	45					3.3
23	46	0.50	9.7	4.3	8.6	3.0
	47					2.8
24	48	0.45	9.0	3.6	8.0	2.5
	49					2.3
25	50	0.45	8.5	3.1	6.9	2.1
	51					1.9
26	52	0.50	10.1	4.2	8.4	1.7
	53					1.6
27	54	0.45	8.3	2.9	6.4	1.5
	55					1.3
28	56	0.50	8.4	3.0	6.0	1.2
	57					1.1
29	58	0.45	8.2	2.8	6.2	<1.0
	59					<1.0
30	60	0.45	8.2	2.8	6.2	<1.0

* Gross counts × 64.
† Gross counts − background × 64.

Cts./2 μc. I^{131}HSA in aluminum spacer = 123.4

$$\text{Attenuation factor} = \frac{\text{Cts. spacer}}{\text{Cts. well}}$$

$$= 2,180$$

Therefore,

$$\text{Cardiac output} = \frac{(123.4) \times \text{attenuation factor}}{\Sigma \text{ col. E}} \times \frac{60}{1,000}$$

$$= \frac{123.4 \times 2,180}{323.5} \times \frac{60}{1,000}$$

$$= 8.3 \text{ L./min.}$$

REFERENCES

1. Blumgart, H. L., and Yens, O. C.: Studies on the velocity of blood flow: I, J. Clin. Invest. 4:1, 1927.
2. ———, and Weiss, S.: Studies on the velocity of blood flow: II, J. Clin. Invest. 4:15, 1927.
3. Quimby, E. H., and Smith, B. C.: Tracer studies with radioactive sodium on patients with peripheral vascular disease, Science 100:175, 1944.
4. Smith, B. C., and Quimby, E. H.: Use of radioactive sodium as tracer in study of peripheral vascular disease, Radiology 45:335, 1945.
5. ——— and ———: The use of radioactive sodium in studies of circulation in patients with peripheral vascular disease, Surg., Gynec. & Obst. 79:142, 1944.
6. ——— and ———: The use of radioactive sodium in the study of peripheral vascular disease, Ann. Surg. 125:360, 1947.
7. Friedell, M. T.; Drucker, E. F., and Pickett, W. J.: Histidine and ascorbic acid treatment of arteriosclerosis obliterans, with radioactive isotope estimations of circulatory effects, J.A.M.A. 138:1036, 1948.
8. Friedell, M. T., et al.: Radioactive isotopes in the study of peripheral vascular disease, Arch. Int. Med. 83:608, 620, 1949.
9. ———; Indeck, W., and Schaffner, F.: Radioactive isotopes in the study of peripheral vascular disease: III, Arch. Int. Med. 85:667, 1950.
10. Kety, S. S.: Quantitative measurement of regional circulation by the clearance of radioactive sodium, Am. J. M. Sc. 215:352, 1948.
11. ———: Measurement of regional circulation by the local clearance of radioactive sodium, Am. Heart J. 38:321, 1949.
12. Elkin, D. C., et al.: The study of peripheral vascular disease with radioactive isotopes: I, Surg., Gynec. & Obst. 87:1, 1948.
13. Cooper, F. W., Jr., et al.: The study of peripheral vascular disease with radioactive isotopes; II, Surg., Gynec. & Obst. 88:711, 1949.

14. Veall, N.: Some general problems in connection with the measurements of radioactivity in patients, Brit. J. Radiol. 23:527, 1950.

15. MacIntyre, W. J., *et al.:* I^{131}-labeled serum albumin: Its use in the study of cardiac output and peripheral vascular flow, Radiology 59: 849, 1952.

16. Krieger, H., *et al.:* The use of radioactive iodinated human serum albumin in evaluating the peripheral circulation, Ann. Surg. 136:357, 1952.

17. Stewart, G. N.: Researches of the circulation time and on the influences which affect it: IV. The output of the heart, J. Physiol. 22:159, 1897.

18. Kinsman, J. M.; Moore, J. W., and Hamilton, W. F.: Studies on the circulation: I. Injection method; physical and mathematical considerations, Am. J. Physiol. 89:322, 1929.

19. Moore, J. W., *et al.:* Studies on the circulation: II. Cardiac output determinations, Am. J. Physiol. 89:321, 1929.

20. Nylin, G., and Celander, H.: Determination of blood volume in the heart and lungs and the cardiac output through the injection of radiophosphorus, Circulation 1:76, 1950.

21. Pritchard, W. H., *et al.: The Measurement of the Early Disappearance of Iodinated (I^{131}) Serum Albumin from Circulating Blood by a Continuous Recording Method,* AEC Report NYO 4021 (Oct. 10, 1953).

22. Powers, S. R.; Rossi, H. H., and Papper, E. M.: An instrument for the measurement of cardiac output, Rev. Scient. Instruments 23:178, 1952.

23. MacIntyre, W. J.: A scintillation counter for measurement of I^{131} uptake in the thyroid gland, Proc. Soc. Exper. Biol. & Med. 75:561, 1950.

24. ————; Wirth, W. F., and Fessler, T. E.: *The Performance of Clinical Scintillation Counters,* AEC Report NYO 4018 (Aug. 17, 1953).

25. Kip, A., *et al.:* Design and operation of an improved counting rate meter, Rev. Scient. Instruments 17:323, 1946.

26. MacIntyre, W. J., *et al.:* The determination of cardiac output by a continuous recording system utilizing iodinated (I^{131}) human serum albumin: I. Animal studies, Circulation 4:552, 1951.

27. Pritchard, W. H., *et al.:* The determination of cardiac output by a continuous recording system utilizing iodinated (I^{131}) human serum albumin: II. Clinical studies, Circulation 6:572, 1952.

28. Hamilton, W. F., *et al.:* Comparison of the Fick and dye injection methods of measuring the cardiac output in man, Am. J. Physiol. 153:309, 1948.

29. Werkö, L., *et al.:* Comparison of the Fick and Hamilton methods for determination of cardiac output in man, Scandinav. J. Clin. & Lab. Invest. 1:109, 1949.

30. Kopelman, H., and Lee, G. D.: The intra-thoracic blood volume in mitral stenosis and left ventricular failure, Clin. Sc. 10:383, 1951.

31. Shipley, R. A., *et al.*: Analysis of the radiocardiogram in heart failure, Circulation Res. 1:428, 1953.
32. Huff, R. L.; Feller, D. D., and Bogardus, G.: Cardiac output by body surface counting of I[131] human serum albumin, J. Clin. Invest. 33:944 (A), 1954.

CHAPTER 5

Gastrointestinal Function Tests

A. FAT ABSORPTION WITH IODINE-131-LABELED TRIOLEIN AND OLEIC ACID

THE PATIENT WITH STEATORRHEA confronts the clinician with a very specific diagnostic problem. Steatorrhea is symptomatic of faulty digestion of neutral fat or malabsorption of fatty acids. Since faulty digestion and malabsorption have different etiologic connotations, it is important to differentiate between these two causes of fatty stools. The diagnosis of steatorrhea is largely clinical, but it may be verified by laboratory analysis of the stool for fat.

Triolein and oleic acid may be labeled with radioiodine (I^{131}). The stability of such a label has been confirmed by several means. Blood obtained after the ingestion of I^{131}-labeled triolein cannot be separated by dialysis; analysis of portal vein blood in such an instance shows that the I^{131} is carried by neutral fat and beta lipoprotein and that a direct proportionality exists between I^{131} blood assay and fat absorption in pancreatectomized dogs (8). It has been further demonstrated that in pancreatectomized patients, following a labeled fat meal, fecal I^{131} content is elevated and blood I^{131} has a low value (3). From the foregoing evidence and related studies, I^{131}-labeled triolein and oleic acid absorption is proportional to blood I^{131} levels (13). The I^{131} bond to triolein and oleic acid is more stable in the chloroiodo compound than in the di-iodo preparation.

By the use of a test meal of triolein labeled with I^{131} and another test meal of labeled oleic acid, three characteristic patterns are discernible in the blood levels of I^{131} activity. In the normal person, after the triolein or oleic acid meal the blood radio-activity levels are similar. The patient with a digestive defect (e.g., chronic pancreatitis) has a low I^{131} blood level following a triolein meal; but, since absorption of the products of digestion is unimpaired, I^{131} levels after an oleic acid meal are similar to those in the normal person. The patient with malabsorption cannot adequately absorb the product of digestion, and so blood levels of I^{131} are low following either the triolein or the oleic acid test meal (5). Normal and pathologic values are discussed below.

1. Technique of Measuring Fat Absorption

a) Materials.—The necessary materials are:

> 30 μc. I^{131}-labeled triolein or oleic acid
> 10 ml. carrier nonlabeled triolein or oleic acid
> 400 ml. fresh milk
> Vanilla extract or other flavoring extract
> Lugol's solution

b) Apparatus.—The following are required:

> Food blender, 1 qt. capacity
> Scaler
> Scintillation well counter
> 100 ml. volumetric flask
> Two volumetric pipettes:
>> One pipette, 10 ml. capacity
>> One pipette, 1 ml. capacity
> Cylindrical graduate, 500 ml.
> One 5 ml. syringe
> Two plastic test tubes

c) Procedure.—The procedure is as follows:

> (1) *Preparation of Patient.*—Patients selected for fat absorption studies are given Lugol's solution, 10 drops three times a day the day preceding the test. Oral feeding is suspended at 12.00 A.M. the day of testing. The test meal is administered at 8:00 A.M., and a 5 ml. venous blood sample is drawn at 12:00 noon. The patient may eat

lunch after this aliquot is drawn. Should more detailed studies be desired, blood samples may be drawn at intervals of 1–24 hours.

(2) *Preparation of the Test Meal.*—The test meal consists of 10 ml. of triolein or oleic acid labeled by the addition of 30 μc. of I^{131}-labeled triolein or oleic acid. The fat or fatty acid is suspended in 250 ml. of whole milk by mixing in a blender for 5 minutes. This uniform suspension of fat most closely approximates a physiologically stabilized fat emulsion. Palatability is improved by adding several drops of vanilla or other flavoring extract.

(3) *Preparation of the Standard Solution.*—The standard solution is prepared by diluting, in a volumetric flask, 1 ml. of the labeled milk to 100 ml., using nonlabeled milk as the diluent. This mixture is assayed for radioactivity in a scintillation well counter, 3 ml. of the milk standard in a plastic test tube being used for this purpose.

(4) *Determination of Percentage of Administered Dose in the Blood.*—By accepting the fundamental assumption that I^{131} activity in the blood represents absorbed labeled fat or fatty acid, the quantitation of this value is a relatively simple process. Preferentially, radioactivity in whole blood is determined rather than radioactivity in plasma, since the latter is a more variable and labile compartment than whole blood.

$$\text{Per cent ingested radioactivity/liter of blood} = \frac{\text{Activity/liter of blood} \times 100}{\text{Activity ingested}}$$

$$\text{Activity/liter of blood} = (\text{Cts./3 ml. sample/5 min.}) (333.3)$$

$$\text{Activity ingested} = (\text{Cts./3 ml. standard solution/5 min.}) (\text{Volume labeled milk}) (33.3)$$

A clinically adequate screening procedure in steatorrhea may be obtained if a single blood sample is drawn 4 hours after the triolein test meal and assayed for radioactivity, expressed as percentage of the administered dose per liter of blood. If the triolein test meal results in a normal blood level, no further testing is indicated. Should the triolein test be subnormal, an oleic acid test meal is given several days later. A blood sample is drawn preceding this second test meal, and the subsequent 4-hour level is corrected by this background level. Aliquots of blood obtained at various intervals may be assayed at the discretion of the observer.

2. INTERPRETATION

a) FAT ABSORPTION IN THE NORMAL INDIVIDUAL.—By the use of the method described above, the percentage of I^{131} activity measurable in the blood at varying intervals is found to be comparable with results obtained by other investigators (1–13).

The results furnish a criteria for the evaluation of blood radioactivity in normal and in pathologic fat absorption and digestion. Ingestion of the triolein test meal by 33 normal male subjects resulted in detectable blood levels in all instances in 30 minutes; then the radioactivity rapidly increased to a peak in 4 hours, slowly subsiding (Table 12). This pattern is graphically illustrated in Figure 22. The pattern of blood activity following ingestion of the oleic acid test meal closely parallels the results seen with triolein. The findings of an analysis made of the absorption of oleic acid in 11 normal males are shown in Table 13 and Figure 23. These findings indicate that the blood level of radioactivity following ingestion of the triolein or oleic acid test meal by the normal human male is confined within a narrow and characteristic range. The relatively wide scatter of observed radioactivity at ½ and 1 hours probably reflects variance in gastric emptying time and the possibility of rapid absorption of small amounts of free I^{131} (13). For the purpose of clinical evaluation, the levels observed at 4 hours are representative of peak levels and are found within the most reproducible range. The levels observed with triolein at 4 hours average 2.14 per cent, with an extreme normal range of 2.15 per cent, a standard deviation of ±0.50 per cent and a minimal coefficient of variation of 23.4 as compared to values at other time intervals. Average blood levels of 2.07 per cent of the ingested dose per liter of blood is seen 4 hours after

TABLE 12.—ABSORPTION OF INGESTED TRIOLEIN IN 33 NORMAL MALE SUBJECTS*

	No. of Hours after Ingestion							
	½	1	2	3	4	5	7	24
% activity/L. of blood, 4 ml. dose, 23 patients	0.23	0.64	1.28	1.83	2.18	2.18	1.77	0.59
% activity/L. of blood, 10 ml. dose, 10 patients	0.24	0.45	1.17	1.77	2.04	2.32	1.72	0.53
Av. % activity/L. of blood, 4 and 10 ml. dose, 33 patients	0.23	0.58	1.25	1.81	2.14	2.12	1.75	0.57
Max. range, 33 patients	0.08–0.56	0.23–1.20	0.55–2.64	0.94–2.79	1.37–3.52	1.24–3.31	1.05–3.07	0.28–1.09
Std. dev., 33 patients	±0.10	±0.26	±0.44	±0.48	±0.50	±0.57	±0.45	±0.20
Coefficient of variation	43.5	44.8	35.2	26.5	23.4	26.9	25.7	28.5

TABLE 13.—ABSORPTION OF INGESTED OLEIC ACID IN 11 NORMAL MALE SUBJECTS (4 ML. DOSE)*

	No. of Hours after Ingestion							
	½	1	2	3	4	5	7	24
Av. % activity/L. of blood	0.34	0.87	1.60	2.08	2.07	1.96	1.37	0.42
Range	0.02–0.58	0.11–1.77	0.87–2.77	1.24–3.41	1.41–3.28	1.15–2.62	0.92–1.99	0.15–0.94

* From Kaplan, E., *et al.*: Gastroenterology 34:901, 1958.

132

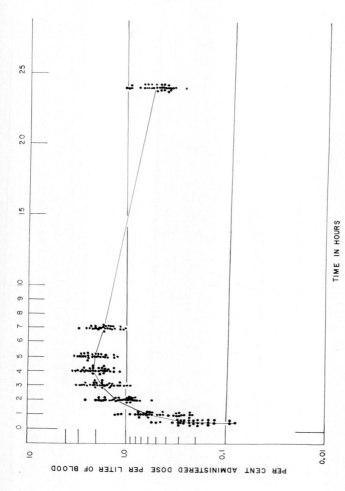

Fig. 22.—Absorption of ingested triolein in 33 normal subjects. Scattergram shows the mean and range of I131 blood levels after ingestion of labeled triolein by the normal male. (From Kaplan, E., *et al.*: Gastroenterology 34:901, 1958.)

TIME IN HOURS

PER CENT ADMINISTERED DOSE PER LITER OF BLOOD

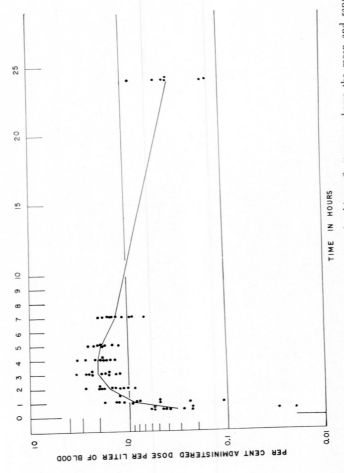

FIG. 23.—Absorption of ingested oleic acid in 11 normal subjects. Scattergram shows the mean and range of I^131 blood levels after ingestion of labeled oleic acid by the normal male. (From Kaplan, E., *et al.*: Gastroenterology 34:901, 1958.)

the oleic acid test meal. The normal values of radioactivity per liter of whole blood 4 hours after the triolein or oleic acid test meal is 1–4 per cent of the ingested dose.

A correction factor is unquestionably necessary when the subjects studied are of very large or very small size, because activity

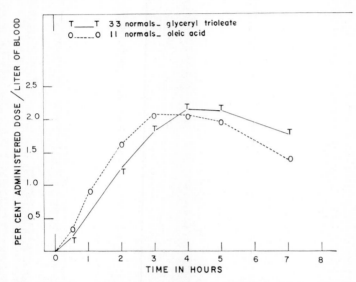

FIG. 24.—Comparative mean absorption of labeled triolein and oleic acid by the normal male. (From Kaplan, E., *et al.*: Gastroenterology 34:901, 1958.)

per unit volume of blood may be at variance with values reported.

Blood radioactivity following a test meal as compared to the triolein test meal reveals a peak level at 3, rather than at 4, hours; but no significant difference is observed in the peak levels obtained. The more rapid increase with oleic acid probably indicates that a period of time is necessary for the hydrolysis of triolein before absorption (Fig. 24). A similar lag is seen in the studies reported by Malm and his co-workers (7).

In the normal person, the quantity of oleic acid or triolein ingested makes little difference in the percentage of the admin-

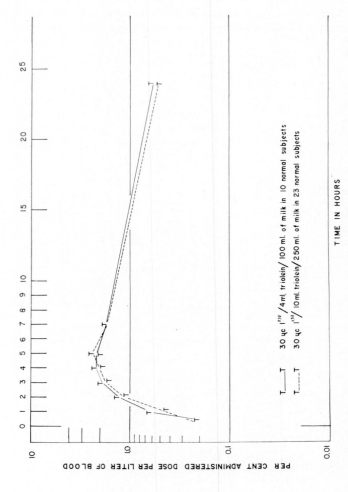

FIG. 25.—Comparative absorption of 4 and 10 ml. of labeled triolein by the normal male. (From Kaplan, E., *et al.*: Gastroenterology 34:901, 1958.)

136

istered dose observable in the blood. Malm and his associates
(7), using 5–10 ml. of oleic acid, and Isley and his co-workers
(4), using 0.5 ml., report levels comparable with the values we
have seen with 4 and 10 ml. Ruffin and his associates (8) gave
an emulsion of 50 per cent peanut oil with labeled triolein in a
dosage of 1 ml./kg. of body weight, while Grossman (2) used
60 ml. of vegetable oil as a vehicle for labeled triolein. The results which these investigators have reported in normals are comparable to those shown in Figure 25. This would suggest near
quantitative absorption of triolein and oleic acid by the normal
person over a relatively large range.

b) Fat Absorption in Digestive Defects with Steatorrhea.—In patients with digestive defects, particularly in those
with chronic pancreatitis with steatorrhea, the radioactivity in
the blood following the triolein test meal is consistently below
1.0 per cent; generally, it has been observed at 0.2–0.6 per cent
at 4 hours. These values show a slight increase at 7 hours but
remain below 1.0 per cent. In contrast, the blood level following
the oleic acid test meal is within normal limits. The triolein absorption may be slightly enhanced by treatment with pancreatin
(Fig. 26), although normal levels are not produced by this medication. The results obtained are compatible with suggestions by
Malm and his co-workers (7) and are also compatible with the
observation of Isley and his associates (4) in dogs with induced
pancreatitis. Turner (11) has also reported normal oleic acid absorption in steatorrhea of chronic pancreatitis. The depression of
triolein absorption in pancreatic insufficiency has been reported
repeatedly (1–4, 6, 8, 9, 11, 12). The conclusion is warranted
that physiologic absorption of triolein is dependent on adequate
pancreatic lipase, while oleic acid absorption is not influenced by
lack of this enzyme.

c) Fat Absorption in Absorptive Defects.—In patients
with malabsorption and steatorrhea, the blood level of radioactivity following either the triolein or oleic acid test meal is
decreased from that observed for the normal person. The expected
range is below 1 per cent of the administered dose per liter of
blood at 4 hours. Typical examples of triolein and oleic acid
absorption curves in malabsorption and the subsequent improvement with therapy may be seen in Figure 27.

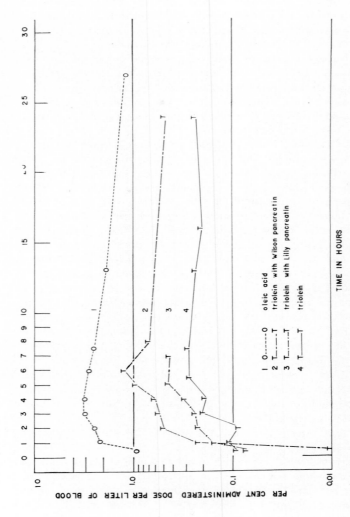

Fig. 26.—Characteristic absorption curves of labeled triolein and oleic acid in digestive defect (chronic pancreatitis). (From Kaplan, E., et al.: Gastroenterology 34:901, 1958.)

138

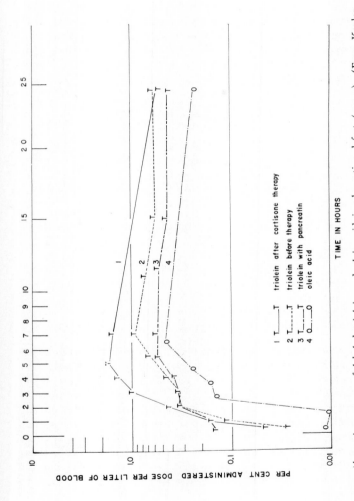

FIG. 27.—Absorption curves of labeled triolein and oleic acid in absorptive defect (sprue). (From Kaplan, E., *et al.*: Gastroenterology 34:901, 1958.)

It is well to reiterate the three categories of blood radioactivity observed using the combined triolein–oleic acid test meal procedure: In the normal person, a characteristic and similar level of activity is seen in the blood following either the triolein or oleic acid ingestion; in the patient with a digestive defect, oleic acid absorption is normal and triolein absorption is defective; and in the patient with an absorptive defect, both oleic acid and triolein absorption are subnormal.

B. ROSE BENGAL LIVER TESTS

1. INTRODUCTION

The liver is the metabolic center of the body; here a great number of chemical reactions are constantly taking place. Many tests reflecting specific aspects of liver function have been devised, namely:

1. The ability to store sugar, as in the galactose tolerance test.
2. The status of prothrombin production, a clotting factor related to vitamin K.
3. The level of an enzyme in the blood which under normal conditions is excreted into the biliary tract—e.g., alkaline phosphatase.
4. The conversion of benzoic acid to hippuric acid.
5. The elimination of an organic dye, such as bromsulfalein.

The foregoing are some of the tests which have been applied to determine the effects of various diseases on the liver. These tests are important because physical signs of liver disease are poor indicators of the degree of liver damage. There may, for example, be minimal evidence of liver cell damage with jaundice on an obstructive basis. Severe liver disease may not be suspected if the signs are minimal. These tests, however, all have their serious limitations, and the search for more sensitive and reliable tests of liver function is being carried on. A recent introduction of serum transaminase determination in the assessment of hepatic inflammation is an example of a new application. Undoubtedly, many more liver tests will be forthcoming in the not too distant future. At present, however, the accepted and most widely used test in diagnosing liver diseases is the bromsulfalein excretion test. This test is considered the more sensitive and reliable of the liver function tests, although it, too, has its serious limitations.

Radioisotope-labeled compounds have introduced and added several refinements to the established battery of tests used in diagnosing liver diseases (14, 15, 16). One of these compounds is radioiodine-labeled rose bengal, a dye taken up and excreted, essentially unchanged, by the liver cells into the bile. The determination of rose bengal, nonlabeled, depends on a colorimetric method; and this test, therefore, cannot be used in the presence of jaundice because of the color also produced by the bile. Labeled rose bengal circumvents this limitation and makes a more effective test. Also, the progress of patients with jaundice can be followed by serial determinations, using the radioactive test. In addition, some help in diagnosis is obtained in cases of obstruction, where bile does not flow into the intestine, by measuring the activity of the dye over the intestine.

Originally, there was a limitation to the labeled rose bengal test, since the counting was done over the liver and a great deal of overlap occurred among the values obtained for normal subjects and patients with hepatic disease. This limitation resulted from the fact that in the vicinity of the liver there are many structures which take up the dye, such as the gallbladder, the bile ducts and the intestines. Hence, the curves obtained in counting over the liver reflected, not the true liver uptake, but, instead, a number of events occurring simultaneously. This difficulty was overcome by Nordyke and Blahd (15), who found that counting over the patient's head, rather than over the liver, gave a declining curve of activity which was almost the same as the curve of extraction by the liver of the dye from the blood. Inasmuch as the liver is the only organ taking up significant amounts of the dye, the head-count curve is the reciprocal of the liver uptake of dye, and therefore a true reflection of the liver uptake.

The only liver function test utilizing radioisotopes that is of definite practical value at this time is this radioiodine rose bengal determination with the use of a probe placed on the head to determine the extraction of the dye from the blood by the liver. Also of some practical value is the count obtained by the use of a well-collimated scintillation detection probe held over the abdomen. Such counts determine the patency of the biliary flow into the intestine. This determination can be made at the same time as the head count is made. Other tests, including liver scanning, are still in the developmental stage. No crystallization of method and procedure has, as yet, occurred; nor has their clinical evaluation been extensive enough to warrant their routine adoption.

2. TECHNIQUE OF ADMINISTRATION

The radioiodine-labeled rose bengal determination is carried out as follows:

a) MATERIALS.—The materials needed are:

> One 5 cc. sterile plastic syringe
> One 22 gauge sterile needle, disposable
> Sterile radioiodine-labeled rose bengal, 25–30 μc. in 2–3 cc. of isotonic saline solution

b) APPARATUS.—The following are required:

> One detector probe, well collimated, containing a 1½ × 1 in. NaI (Th) scintillation crystal
> One count-rate meter
> One Esterline Angus recording graphic ammeter
> One standard scintillation probe, whose scintillation counter is ordinarily used for doing thyroid gland I[131] uptakes

c) PROCEDURE.—The fasting patient is placed in a comfortable position, lying on his back, and the probe is placed just touching, and perpendicular to the plane of, the right ear lobe. The count-rate meter is adjusted for minimum counts per minute, and the Esterline Angus recorder paper is placed at a speed of approximately 1 cm./min. Radioiodine-labeled rose bengal in the amount of 25–30 μc. in 5 cc. saline solution is then injected into the patient intravenously, and the curve of decline in blood activity is recorded.

By placing over the abdomen the well-shielded thyroid probe attached to a scintillation counter, directed inferiorly at 30° and with the opening of the probe below the liver, the arrival time of the dye into the intestine can be determined. Obviously, the dye will never arrive in the intestine during the period of observation if there is complete obstruction of the bile duct. Neostigmine, morphine, nitroglycerin and the presence of food will affect the bile flow and change the arrival time and the curve of intestinal accumulation of the dye. In patients with normal livers, the dye should begin to appear in the intestine within 15 minutes after injection. Giving the patient a glass of milk to drink during the procedure will stimulate the flow of bile into the intestine.

3. INTERPRETATION

The effects of toxic liver impairment on the test, as studied by Taplin and his associates (17), utilizing chronic carbon tetrachloride poisoning in rabbits, best illustrates the dynamics of the interpretation of the radioiodine-labeled rose bengal test. The simple recording of counts over the head and abdomen, *externally,* makes it possible to obtain the actual curves of disappearance of this substance from the blood stream and its arrival in the intestine. In the rabbits with liver poisoning, the dye took a longer time to reach low values in the blood stream when serial tests were performed as the poisoning progressed. On the 1st day, all of the dye was eliminated in 20 minutes; whereas, by the 73d day of poisoning, 50 per cent of the dye remained in the rabbit's blood stream 20 minutes after injection. The progressive increase in the degree of retention in the course of the 73-day period indicated a good correlation between the degree of damage to the liver cells and the dye retention. When a count was made over the abdomen below the liver before poisoning, the radioactive dye began to appear in the intestine 10 minutes after injection; as the disease progressed, less and less dye appeared in the intestine, reflecting the increased retention in the blood stream. Finally on the 73d day, when poisoning effects were at their maximum, no dye appeared in the intestine at all during the course of 20 minutes. The actual liver uptake diminished dramatically during the poisoning. Whereas before poisoning, 10,000 counts could be recorded over the liver 10 minutes after injection, on the 73d day only 3,000 cts./min. were recorded over the liver at the end of 20 minutes. The ability to follow the evolution of these functional liver changes with serial determinations (as was done) would have become impossible as soon as jaundice appeared if nonradioactive dye had been used. There is, however, no fundamental advantage to the use of labeled dye over the bromsulfalein

TABLE 14.—BLOOD DISAPPEARANCE RATES OF I[131]-LABELED ROSE
BENGAL BETWEEN 5 AND 20 MINUTES AFTER DOSE,
USING HEAD COUNTS*

Types of Cases	Blood Disappearance in Per Cent (Range of Values)	Average Percentage of Group	Comment
Normal subjects..	39–51	45	Based on fasting state.
Alcoholics.......	46–53	50	Above upper limits of normal in 50%.
Chronic hepatitis.	42–57	50	
Viral hepatitis...	45–90	55	Varies with stage of disease. With serial tests there is a progressive drop as jaundice appears.
Cirrhosis........	48–96	56	Short-interval serial determinations show no change.
Common bile duct stones........	53–87	....	Patients in the upper range had jaundice.
Common bile duct obstruction by tumor........	55–85	....	Serial testing shows no change.

* From Nordyke, R. A., and Blahd, W. H.: J.A.M.A. 170:1159, 1959.

test except in the presence of jaundice; also, labeling the dye makes it possible to use much smaller amounts of the dye itself.

When patients with viral hepatitis and jaundice are followed serially, their clinical improvement correlates well with the rate of disappearance of the dye as measured over the head. As reported by Nordyke and Blahd (15), patients with a retention in the blood stream of 39–51 per cent in the 20 minutes following an initial 5-minute equilibration period are in the normal range (Table 14). Patients with chronic alcoholism and Laennec cirrhosis show variable degrees of retention, ranging from 48 to 96 per cent in the 20-minute period following 5-minute equilibration. Patients with common duct stones show a range of 53–87 per cent, while complete common duct obstruction for several weeks seldom produces more than 85 per cent retention in 20 minutes following a 5-minute equilibration period.

The arrival time of the dye in the intestine detected by the probe over the abdomen is indicated by a sudden increase of counts over this area. If this increase is delayed by more than 17–20 minutes following the injection of the dye, the likelihood of extrahepatic biliary obstruction is greater. However, patients with both intrahepatic and extrahepatic obstructive jaundice of severe degree have prolongation of the time of arrival of the dye in the intestine for as long as 1 hour. Administration of a glass of milk may stimulate bile flow and help in the differentiation of extrahepatic from intrahepatic obstruction. A tumor blocking the common duct by external pressure may prevent any bile from passing, despite food stimulation. Neostigmine, nitroglycerin and amyl nitrate stimulate bile flow, while morphine depresses flow.

REFERENCES

FAT ABSORPTION WITH IODINE[131]-LABELED TRIOLEIN AND OLEIC ACID

1. Beres, P.; Wenger, J., and Kirsner, J. B.: The use of I[131] triolein in the study of absorptive disorders in man, Gastroenterology 32:1, 1957.
2. Grossman, M. I., and Jordan, P. H.: The radio-iodinated triolein test for steatorrhea, Gastroenterology 34:892, 1958.
3. ——— and ———: The use of I[131]-labeled triolein in the detection of steatorrhea, Clin. Res. Proc. 5:40, 1957.
4. Isley, J. K., et al.: Use of I[131]-labeled oleic acid in study of gastrointestinal function, Proc. Soc. Exper. Biol. & Med. 94:807, 1957.
5. Kaplan, E., et al.: Intestinal absorption of iodine[131]-labeled triolein and oleic acid in normal subjects and in steatorrhea, Gastroenterology 34:901, 1958.
6. McKenna, R. D.; Bourne, R. H., and Matzko, A.: The use of I[131]-labeled fat in the study of fat digestion and absorption in normal individuals and in patients with diseases of fat absorption, Gastroenterology 32:17, 1957.

7. Malm, J. R.; Reemtsma, K., and Barker, H. G.: Comparative fat and fatty acid intestinal absorption test utilizing radioiodine labeling; results in normal subjects, Proc. Soc. Exper. Biol. & Med. 92:471, 1956.
8. Ruffin, J. M., et al.: I^{131}-labeled fat in the study of intestinal absorption, New England J. Med. 255:594, 1956.
9. Shingleton, W. W., et al.: The evaluation of pancreatic function by use of I^{131}-labeled fat, Gastroenterology 32:28, 1957.
10. ———— et al.: A study of fat absorption after gastric surgery using I^{131}-labeled fat, Tr. Am. S. A. 76:145, 1956.
11. Turner, D. A.: The absorption, transport, and deposition of fat (thesis, Georgetown University School of Medicine, 1956).
12. Duffy, B. J., Jr., and Turner, D. A.: The differential diagnosis of intestinal malabsorption with I^{131} fat and fatty acid, Ann. Int. Med. 48:1, 1958.
13. Van Handel, E., and Zilversmit, D. B.: Validity of using I^{131} as a label for dietary and intravenous fat, Fed. Proc. 16:131, 1957.

ROSE BENGAL LIVER TESTS

14. Moertel, C. G., and Owen, C. A., Jr.: Evaluation of the radioactive (I-131 tagged) rose bengal liver function test in non-jaundiced patients, J. Lab. & Clin. Med. 52:902, 1958.
15. Nordyke, R. A., and Blahd, W. H.: The blood disappearance of radioactive rose bengal: Rapid simple test of liver function, J.A.M.A. 170:1159, 1959.
16. ———— and ————: The differential diagnosis of jaundice with radioactive rose bengal, Proceedings of the Second International Conference: Peaceful Uses of Atomic Energy, Geneva, 1958, Vol. 26 (New York: United Nations, 1958).
17. Taplin, G. V., et al.: New radiodiagnostic techniques for investigating parenchymal and obstructive liver and kidney diseases, Proceedings of the Second International Conference: Peaceful Uses of Atomic Energy, Geneva, 1958, Vol. 26 (New York: United Nations, 1958), p. 128.

CHAPTER 6

Radioautography

RECENT ADVANCES IN MEDICAL RESEARCH have pointed up the importance of cellular metabolism. In attempting to study the concentration, utilization and excretion of labeled compounds by organs or cell units, the ordinary biochemical or biophysical techniques use samples of tissue containing many types of cells. A milligram of liver will contain not only liver parenchymal cells but also bile-duct epithelial cells, blood vessels, connective tissue, reticuloendothelial cells and other cells. If an investigator were interested in the changes in the nucleic acid content of liver parenchymal cells in a regenerating liver, the analysis of a sample of the liver might reveal an increase of the nucleic acids. But before the investigator could ascribe this change to the parenchymal cell, he would be obliged to demonstrate that the increased concentration did not result from an increase in the number of nonparenchymal cells, from an increase in the concentration of nucleic acids in these cells or from increases in both the number and concentration of the substance in the nonparenchymal cells. It is, therefore, often necessary to obtain information about concentrations, rates and excretions at the cell level.

Radioautography, or autoradiography, is one of the simplest and cheapest techniques by which to discern differences in cell function. This method utilizes the fact that photographic emulsion may be darkened by radioactivity just as it is by visible light. If a piece of thyroid tissue taken from a patient who was given radioactive iodine (I^{131}) is placed on photographic emulsion, the beta particles given off by the I^{131} which concentrated in the patient's thyroid follicles will blacken the underlying emulsion.

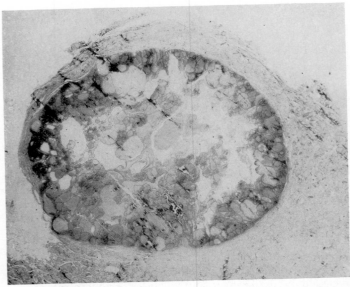

Fig. 28.—Radioautograph of human thyroid (nodular goiter) from patient who was given radioiodine (I^{131}). Isotope present in nodular goiter (large circumscribed dark areas), but none evident in surrounding normal thyroid. Tissue mounted directly on nuclear track emulsion. (Reduced from ×10.)

Histologic sections will often contain enough radioactive isotope to give an image on the emulsion. It is even possible to examine individual follicles of the thyroid and compare the darkening of the emulsion caused by the isotope in the follicles (Fig. 28). With the sensitive emulsions available today, single alpha or beta particles may even be recorded; for, as those particles leave cells or tissues, they may leave tracks in the emulsion and thus finger-print their tissue origin, course and termination (Figs. 29 and 30).

A. APPLICABILITY

Almost all types of biologic organisms have been studied by radioautography: human and animal tissues and excretions, pro-

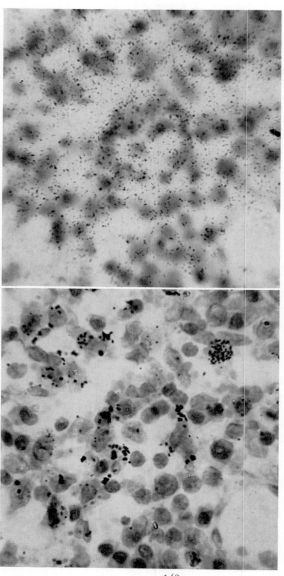

Fig. 29.—Tissue from mediastinal lymph node of a patient given radiogold (Au^{198}). Black granules are aggregates of colloidal gold in reticulum cells. (Reduced from ×900.)

Fig. 30.—Underlying nuclear track emulsion in focus. It supports tissue of Figure 29. Small random grains of reduced photographic emulsion and beta-particle tracks indicate radioactivity of the overlying aggregates of colloidal gold. (Reduced from ×900.)

tozoa, bacteria, fungi, viruses and tissue-culture cells (1). Minerals, solids, rocks, fluids and many industrial substances may also be examined by this method. In medical research the most extensive investigations have been those using radioactive iodine in thyroid disease, radiocalcium or radiostrontium in bone lesions and radioactive phosphorous in blood dyscrasias.

B. ISOTOPES

For the most part, radioactive isotopes giving off alpha or beta particles are used. Radioactive iodine (I^{131}), phosphorus (P^{32}), calcium (Ca^{45}), strontium (Sr^{90}), gold (Au^{198}), sulfur (S^{35}), carbon (C^{14}), tritium (H^3) and many other isotopes have been used (1). The last three may prove particularly useful because the corresponding nonradioactive element is such a common component of biologic tissues.

C. CONCENTRATION OF ISOTOPE REQUIRED

It is difficult to predict before experimentation the amount of isotope that must be given to organisms in order to obtain a radioautograph. Inasmuch as the physical characteristics of the isotope, the required ionization necessary to give a recognizable film density and the maximum limit of the exposure time period are known, it is possible immediately to set up rough limits of minimal activity which must be present in the specimen to give autographic images.

It has been shown (2) that, to obtain a density of 0.1 with a 15-day exposure on x-ray film, there must be a surface concentration in disintegrations per square centimeter per minute of 124 for C^{14}, 124 for Ca^{45}, 414 for I^{131}, 843 for P^{32} and 4,250 for Zn^{65}. These values indicate (3) that at least the following approximate tissue concentrations are required to obtain radioautographic activity from histologic sections under such circumstances: C^{14}, 0.05 μc./gm.; Ca^{45}, 0.05 μc./gm.; I^{131}, 0.2 μc./gm.; P^{32}, 0.4 μc./gm.; and Zn^{65}, 2.0 μc./gm.

The initial radioactivity required (4) to obtain a density of 0.6 on Eastman Kodak No Screen x-ray film with an exposure of 15 days is shown in Table 15. With Kodak Ltd. autoradiographic stripping film, the values required (4) to obtain a density of 0.5 above fog with an exposure of 10 days are given in Table 16. The figures in Table 16 could be considerably reduced if

TABLE 15.—AMOUNT OF RADIOACTIVITY REQUIRED TO OBTAIN DESIRED DENSITY

(Eastman Film X-ray)

Radioisotope	Radioactivity (μc./Cm.^{2})	Electrons per Cm.^{2}
C^{14}	3.6×10^{-4}	0.38×10^7
Ca^{45}	4.6×10^{-4}	2.0×10^7
I^{131}	9.8×10^{-4}	2.6×10^7
P^{32}	2.1×10^{-3}	7.2×10^7

TABLE 16.—VALUES REQUIRED WITH KODAK LTD. STRIPPING FILM

Radioisotope	Radioactivity (μc./Cm.^{2})	Electrons per Cm.^{2}
I^{131}	2.6×10^{-2}	0.56×10^9
P^{32}	5.5×10^{-2}	1.4×10^9

lower densities were used. Correspondingly, the required dose might be decreased by lengthening the exposure time in those isotopes with long half-lives.

D. PHOTOGRAPHIC EMULSIONS

The characteristics of the emulsions used in radioautography are listed in Table 17. The NTB emulsion requires about ten times as much radiation as does x-ray film. Stripping film (4) requires even more flux, about 10^7–10^9 particles/cm. About 1 μc./gm. of I^{131} is necessary for thyroid autographs with stripping film. The advantages of the sensitivity of the x-ray film and its poor resolution must be weighed against the better resolution and less sensitivity of the stripping film. The NTB emulsions are intermediate in sensitivity and resolution.

E. SENSITIVITY

The radioautographic method can detect small amounts of radioactivity in a minute sample, and it can record radioactivity

TABLE 17.—Photographic Emulsions Commonly Used in Radioautography of Biologic Tissues*

Type	Grain Size		Sensitivity	Resolution	Background	Remarks
	Microns	Uniformity				
Roentgen ray (No screen)	0.5–8.0	Very poor	Highest in nontrack autography	Poor	High	Good for gross localization or minimal concentrations
Medium lantern slide	0.5–1.0	Good	Medium	Good	Medium	Good for histologic localization of moderate concentrations
NTB	0.2–0.3	Best	Medium	Best	Low	Best for mounting methods
NTB₃	0.2–0.3	Best	Very high for beta particle tracks	Best	Increases very rapidly	Best for beta particle track autography
NTA	About 0.2–0.3	Best	High for alpha particle tracks	Best	Low; increases with time	Best for alpha particle autography
Liquid emulsion (Ilford G.5)	0.2–0.3	Best	High for beta particle tracks	Best	Low; increases rapidly	Very good for track autography
Kodak Ltd. stripping film	0.2–0.3	Best	Lowest	Best	Low	Best for cytologic localization

* From Fitzgerald and co-workers (3).

152

cumulatively over long periods of time at relatively little increase of background. In the small specimen, however, the isotope must be present in significant concentration; thus, if about 0.05 μc./gm. of C^{14} is required to produce evidence of radioactivity of a density of 0.1 on x-ray film after 15 days' exposure, this concentration of radioactivity would appear to be high in terms of the sensitivity of the efficient modern Geiger counters. However, such a concentration present in a tissue section 10 μ thick in an area of 10×10 μ (recognizable in the autograph by microscopy) represents (3) only about 1×10^{-9} gm., or 5×10^{-11} μc. With stripping film and P^{32}, the amount of isotope necessary (4) to produce a density of 0.5 with an exposure of 1 day is only 1.5×10^{-16} gm. of P^{32}. Track autography gives even more striking results.

F. SPECIMEN

A specimen of almost any size and shape may be used for autography, provided the radioactivity extends beyond a surface. Because of the absorption factors, specimens should be flat and thin.

a) GROSS SPECIMEN.—If localization of the isotope to small areas is not required, it is adequate to clean the specimen (e.g., a bone (5), or kidney) and place it on a piece of x-ray film in a darkroom (Fig. 32). The specimen is held against the film by weights, clips or tape to prevent displacement during exposure.

b) SMEARS.—Blood has been smeared directly onto the emulsion. Mouse and human leukocytes, normal and leukemic, intermittently give a pseudophotographic reduction superficially resembling radioactivity (3). Because Kodak Ltd. autoradiographic stripping film emulsion has been free of this artefact thus far, it has been used to cover either stained or unstained blood smears made on glass slides. Other emulsions may be used if covered with a thin protective coating.

c) MICRO-ORGANISMS.—Not infrequently, bacteria, yeast and other organisms are grown in media containing radioactive material, and this material must be removed from the surface of the organisms. Several investigators have reported techniques used with bacteria (6), fungi (6, 7, 8), yeast (Fig. 31) and paramoecia (1, 3).

d) Tissue Cultures.—Pelc and Spear (9) have used autography and tissue culture to demonstrate P^{32} in ovarian fibroblasts.

Fitzgerald and his co-workers (3) have shown the concentration of C^{14} in embryonic and mouse tumor cells, grown in a tissue-culture medium containing C^{14}-labeled nucleic acid pre-

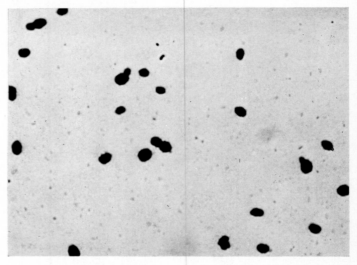

Fig. 31.—Radioautograph of yeast cells *(Torula utilis)* obtained by placing stripping film emulsion (Kodak Ltd.) over a smear of dry, unstained organisms. Yeast had been grown in a solution containing sodium acetate labeled with radiohydrogen (tritium, H^3). Average yeast cell is 5 μ long. (Reduced from ×2,000.) (From Fitzgerald, P. J., *et al.:* Science 114:495, November 9, 1951.)

cursors, by removing the central plasma clot, fixing the cells growing at a periphery of the preparation and covering them with stripping film.

e) Histologic Sections.—Formalin fixation is satisfactory for many autographic studies, although in rare instances tissues fixed in this solution give pseudophotographic effects, and occasionally some desensitize the emulsion. Tissues fixed in alcohol, acetone, or Carnoy's or Bouin's solution seem to be free of artefacts. Tissues fixed in Zenker's, Helly's or Schaudinn's solutions have given pseudophotographic effects if in direct contact with the emulsion (10).

f) Loss or Diffusion of Isotope.—In standard histologic processing, many isotopes or labeled substances may be wholly or partly dissolved out of the preparation; or there may be diffusion or translocation of the labeled substances. Some of the methods used to prove loss or diffusion of isotopes are: isotope-precipitating or non-isotope-dissolving fixatives, freezing, Carbowax and the other methods.

g) Freezing.—Ordinary freezing microtome and carbon dioxide may be used, and the sections may be transferred to photographic emulsion if the emulsion is covered by an impermeable coating. The freezing method of Linderstrøm-Lang and Mogensen may also be used. The freeze-drying techniques of the Altman-Gersh type have been used with some tissues (11).

h) Carbowax.—Fixation in cold propylene glycol and Carbowax embedding has cut down leaching of the isotopes and has shown greater retention of I^{131} and P^{32} in certain tissues fixed by this method than in those fixed by routine fixatives.

i) Isotope-Precipitating or Non-Isotope-Dissolving Fixatives (12).—Decalcification of bone often dissolves or, conceivably, causes translocation of isotopes. Attempts to precipitate isotopes in situ have been reported (3, 13, 14).

j) Bone.—Special embedding and sectioning techniques are necessary to prepare thin sections of undecalcified bones. Celloidin, Bioplastic (15) or other plastic media (13, 16) have been used for embedding. A rapid sectioning technique that cuts undecalcified sections 20–30 μ thick (15) and one in which the sections are only 5–8 μ thick have been described (13). Small pieces of undecalcified bone may be ground by hand down to a thickness of 20–50 μ (16).

Teeth and adjacent tissues have been embedded in methacrylate, cut with a saw and ground with a wheel. The embedding medium was then removed and the sections stained (16). Belanger (17) embedded specimens in paraffin, celloidin or in plastics, according to specimen hardness, and studied bone and soft tissues.

G. CONTACT BETWEEN SPECIMEN AND EMULSION (3, 18)

The type of contact between the specimen and the emulsion employed is governed by the detail desired in the autograph, the energy of the isotope, its concentration in the specimen, the size and shape of the object and other factors. If pseudophotographic effects caused by a chemical reaction between the specimen and the emulsion are a possibility (10, 19) and cannot be ruled out by the use of control material, a thin, inert, relatively impervious coating is interposed between specimen and emulsion. Parlodion, formvar and nylon films in 1 per cent solutions may be used. Three of the common techniques follow:

1. APPOSITION METHOD (3)

The apposition method (Figs. 32 and 33) is simple. It consists of placing a specimen with its radioactive surface against a

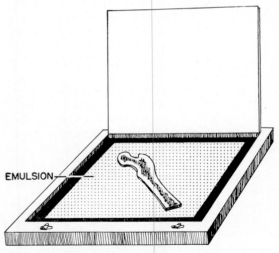

EMULSION

FIG. 32.—Gross specimens placed in contact with photographic emulsion. A thin sheet of impermeable nature may be placed between specimen and emulsion if isotopes of moderate or high energies are present. (From Fitzgerald, P. J., *et al.:* Lab. Invest. 2:122, 1953.)

photographic emulsion in the darkroom. Virtually all gross specimens are prepared in this manner (Fig. 32). The technique is outlined below in detail for use with histologic sections (Fig. 33):

1. If a protective layer is desired, the emulsion or the specimen is dipped in a 1 per cent solution of parlodion in amyl acetate, drained and dried for 8–10 hours.

2. Stained or unstained sections on a glass slide, paraffin

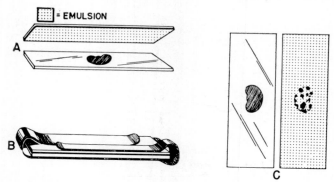

FIG. 33.—Histologic section on a glass slide covered with another glass slide which has a layer of photographic emulsion on one side. Emulsion and section are in contact. (From Fitzgerald, P. J., *et al.*: Lab. Invest. 2:122, 1953.)

embedded or deparaffinized, are placed against the emulsion surface of a 1 × 3 in. glass slide, so that the tissue and the emulsion are in contact (Fig. 33, *A*).

3. The respective short edges of the slide are aligned and fastened together with stainless-steel banker's clips (Fig. 33, *B*).

4. After exposure, the histologic section is separated from the emulsion (Fig. 33, *C*). Before photographic processing, the parlodion is removed from the emulsion by dipping the emulsion into amyl acetate for 5 minutes and then into decreasing concentrations of alcohol (95, 70 and 50 per cent), ending with water.

5. The radioautograph is developed, fixed, washed and dried (Table 18, p. 159). Embedded tissue on the apposed slide is deparaffinized. Unstained tissue may now be stained.

6. The autograph may be examined directly (Fig. 33, *C*) or realigned with the specimen. The histologic sections and the autograph may be mounted after proper alignment. The method is simple and shows that the gross localization of radioactive areas and the autograph may be used for densitometry. However, its resolution is poor and there is difficulty in realigning the object and the processed image.

2. MOUNTING METHOD

In this method the histologic sections (or other specimens) are mounted directly on the photographic emulsion (Fig. 34), and they remain bonded to the emulsion throughout photographic processing, tissue staining and mounting (3, 19).

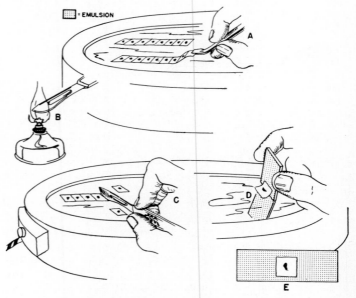

FIG. 34.—Histologic sections, or other specimens, mounted directly on photographic emulsion remain permanently bonded to the emulsion throughout the photographic processing and tissue staining. (From Fitzgerald, P. J., *et al.*: Lab. Invest. 2:122, 1953.)

1. Unstained paraffin-embedded tissue sections are floated in a water bath containing distilled water at 40° C. (Fig. 34, *A*). They are separated with a hot scalpel (Fig. 34, *B* and *C*). The flame and room lights are put out.

2. X-ray film or glass slides with lantern-slide emulsion or with nuclear-track emulsions are dipped into the water bath beneath

TABLE 18.—PHOTOGRAPHIC PROCESSING SCHEDULES*

EMULSIONS	DEVELOPER		STOP (H₂O) Sec.	FIX		WASH (H₂O) Min.
	Type	Min.		Type	Min.	
Roentgen ray	D-19	2	15	20% hypo	20	30+
Lantern slide	D-19	4	15	20% hypo	20	30+
Nuclear track (NTA, NTB, NTB₂, NTB₃)	D-19	5†	15	20% hypo	20	30+
Stripping film (Kodak Ltd.)	D-19	10	15	5% hypo	15‡	30+
Liquid (Ilford G.5)	D-19 (Ilford, dil. 1:3)	10–80	10 (min.) (2% acetic)	30% hypo	Twice clearing time	30+

* From Fitzgerald *et al.* (3).
† Development for 10–20 minutes is used for track work with NTB.
‡ Stripping films are rinsed briefly after fixing, immersed in a hardener (2 per cent potassium alum) for 5 minutes and then washed.

the tissue section, and the section is picked up on emulsion (Fig. 34, *D*), drained and air dried.

3. After drying, the section adheres to the emulsion (Fig. 34, *E*). It may be deparaffinized by immersing it in two changes of xylol (10 minutes in each) and allowing the xylol to evaporate. Deparaffinization may be done before or after exposure.

4. The preparation is exposed, developed, fixed, washed and dried. See Table 18 for the processing schedule.

5. The tissue is stained and mounted with a cover slip. The staining method is described later, on page 163.

The method described above permits easy correlation of tissue structure and radioactivity and has good resolution. Occasionally it desensitizes the emulsion or causes pseudophotographic effects.

3. COMBINED METHOD

A combination of the apposition and mounted methods may be used in which, in sandwich fashion, a glass slide containing emulsion is apposed to a specimen previously mounted on emulsion (3).

4. STRIPPING-FILM METHODS (3, 9, 21, 22)

Thin film emulsion flattened over histologic sections, organisms or cells (Fig. 35) smeared on a glass slide, with the emulsion in direct contact with the tissue or organisms, has been advocated by Pelc (9, 22). The specimen may be stained before covering it with the stripping film or through the permeable stripping-film base after exposure; or it may be left unstained and viewed by phase microscopy. Kodak Ltd. of London has provided the most satisfactory stripping film to date—5 μ of fine-grain emulsion on a gelatin base 10 μ thick, which is attached, emulsion side up, to a glass plate.

1. The glass slides to be used should be "subbed" so that the emulsion will adhere to the slides. Clean glass slides, 1 × 3 in., are dipped into a 0.5 per cent solution of gelatin containing 0.05 per cent chrome alum, and allowed to dry.

2. The sections are floated on a water bath, mounted on the "subbed" slides, drained and allowed to dry. They are deparaffinized in xylol and passed through decreasing concentrations of alcohol to water.

3. For some studies the specimen may be coated with parlodion by running the deparaffinized sections, stained or unstained, from xylol, through xylol–amyl acetate (1:1) and amyl acetate, for 2 minutes each and then dipping it into a 1 per cent solution of parlodion in amyl acetate. The preparation is dried for several hours and the parlodion layer is "subbed" and dried, so that film will adhere to it.

4. In the darkroom, a glass plate of stripping film, 4¾ × 6½ in., is cut with a razor blade ½ in. inside of and parallel to each

of its four edges. The central portion is divided into eight strips of approximately equal dimensions (Fig. 35, *A*).

5. Within a few minutes after the pieces are cut, they begin to separate from the glass support. By sliding a scalpel between the film and the glass, a piece of film may be freed from the glass

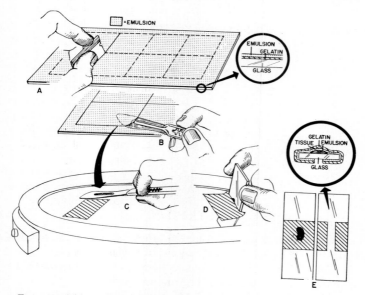

FIG. 35.—Thin strip of film emulsion placed over histologic sections, organisms or cells smeared on a glass slide. Emulsion is in direct contact with the radioactive object. (From Fitzgerald, P. J., *et al.:* Lab. Invest. 2:122, 1953.)

(Fig. 35, *B*), lifted off the plate, turned over and placed on the surface of clean, distilled water at 20° C., so that the film floats with the emulsion side down (Fig. 35, *C*).

6. The film is left on the water surface for 3 minutes, during which time it swells and expands.

7. The slide bearing the section is then immersed below the water surface, is brought close to the film and is withdrawn so that the film drapes itself about the slide (Fig. 35, *D*), covering

the section and overlapping the slides along the long edges (Fig. 35, *E*).

8. Excess water is allowed to drain off, and the preparation is dried in a desiccator.

9. The slides are exposed, developed, fixed and washed. (See Table 18 for the processing schedule.)

10. After photographic processing, prestained autographs should be dehydrated and mounted immediately.

11. Unstained specimens may be studied with phase contrast or stained through the stripping-film base after removing the parlodion, if present. Figure 35 illustrates the technique. Staining procedures may dissolve out some of the isotopes and should be postponed until after exposure (see p. 163).

This technique is best for cytologic studies because of its low background and high resolution. Its relatively low sensitivity and the difficulty of staining through the emulsion are disadvantages.

Many other techniques for special problems have been described in the literature (1, 3, 18).

H. EXPOSURE

Autographic slides, 1 × 3 in., are stored in black plastic, light-tight slide boxes sealed with photographic masking tape. Drierite ($CaSo_4$) is placed at one end of the box. Larger specimens are exposed in x-ray cassettes or in printing frames and are protected from light. All containers are labeled and stored in a dry refrigerator at 5°–10° C. After exposure, autographs are allowed to come to room temperature before processing.

I. PHOTOGRAPHIC PROCESSING

Procedures should be carried out with a scrupulously standardized technique regarding temperature, time and freshness of developing solutions. A Wratten 1 safelight is used. Small glass staining dishes (300 ml. capacity) accommodating glass trays, in which the 1 × 3 in. glass fit, may be filled with processing solutions and kept at constant temperature by immersion in running water kept at 19° C. Table 18 gives the processing periods.

J. STAINING

Because staining techniques may dissolve isotopes, they should be delayed, if possible, until after exposure. In the mounted and stripping-film methods, however, the specimen becomes bonded to the emulsion, and these methods require the use of special staining procedures.

Hematoxylin and eosin are heavily absorbed by the emulsion and they obscure autographic and histologic detail of mounted autographs. Thin 10 μ NTB plates are not so troublesome as the thicker emulsion. The following stains have been used fairly successfully: metaniline yellow and iron hematoxylin (10), cochineal (6), and celestine blue and hemalum (21). A Leishman-Giemsa stain has been suggested (24) for stripping film autographs of marrow cells.

K. MOUNTING

It is advisable to protect the autograph from dust by a cover slip as soon as possible after processing. The autographs may be dehydrated in increasing concentrations of alcohol, followed by xylol or toluol and mounting medium. Synthetic resin is used for some autographs, but glycerin jelly is used for stripping film (21).

L. INTERPRETATION

Visual observation of the radioautographic emulsion usually reveals whether radioactivity is present. Emulsion should be scanned with the high-dry objective of the visible-light microscope before it is considered negative for radioactivity. With stripping film, it may be necessary to do grain counts under oil immersion and apply statistical criteria to determine whether activity is present or absent. Phase contrast microscopy may be used with unstained objects, and it is helpful with the stripping-film methods (15).

Many artefacts occur in radioautography, but most of them can be readily recognized (3, 10, 18, 19). Morphologic experience or assistance is necessary in the proper interpretation of many autographs.

M. CONCLUSION

Radioautography is an advantageous adjunct to the standard counting technique. It is unique in its ability to indicate a possible correlation of isotope distribution and concentration with cellular structure and metabolism.

REFERENCES

1. Fitzgerald, P. J.: Radioautography in cancer, Cancer 5:166, 1952.
2. Steinberg, D., and Solomon, A. K.: The detection of Ca^{45}, I^{131}, P^{32}, and Zn^{65} by photographic film, Rev. Scient. Instruments 20:655, 1949.
3. Fitzgerald, P. J., et al.: Radioautography: Theory, technic and applications, Lab. Invest. 2:181, 1953.
4. Herz, R. H.: Photographic fundamentals of autoradiography, Nucleonics 9:24, 1951.
5. Lotz, W. E.; Gallimore, J. C., and Boyd, G. A.: Good gross autoradiograph of large undecalcified bone, Nucleonics 10:28, 1952.
6. Hammer, J. M., et al.: Use of radioactive isotopes in study of fungi and bacteria, Am. J. Clin. Path. 20:282, 1950.
7. Adams, A. M., and Miller, J. J.: Detection of radiophosphorus in cells and spores of fungi by radioautography, Nature 170:239, 1952.
8. Wheeler, H. E.: The use of radiocarbon for tagging fungi, Phytopathology 42:431, 1952.
9. Pelc, S. R., and Spear, F. G.: Autoradiographs of avian fibroblasts in tissue culture made with P^{32}, Brit. J. Radiol. 23:287, 1950.
10. Simmel, E. B.; Fitzgerald, P. J., and Godwin, J. T.: Staining of radioautographs with metanil yellow and iron hematoxylin, Stain Technol. 26:25, 1951.
11. Holt, M. W., and Warren, S.: Freeze-drying tissues for autoradiography, Lab. Invest. 2:1, 1953.
12. Blank, H.; McCarthy, P. L., and Delamater, E. D.: A non-vacuum freezing-dehydrating technic for histology, autoradiography and microbial cytology, Stain Technol. 26:193, 1951.
13. Arnold, J. S.: A method for embedding undecalcified bone for histologic sectioning, and its application to radioautography, Science 114:178, 1951.
14. Siffert, R. S.: The demonstration of P^{32} in bone by radioautography, Science 108:445, 1948.
15. Roofe, P. G.; Hoecker, F. E., and Voorhees, C. D.: A rapid bone sectioning technic, Proc. Soc. Exper. Biol. & Med. 72:619, 1949.
16. Sognnaes, R. F., et al.: A method for radioautography of specimens composed of both hard and soft structures, Anat. Rec. 104:319, 1949.
17. Belanger, L. F.: Improvements to the melted emulsion technique of autoradiography, Nature 170:626, 1952.
18. Fitzgerald, P. J., and Engstrom, A.: The use of ultraviolet micros-

copy, roentgen-ray-absorption, and radioautographic techniques in the study of neoplastic disease: A discussion of cytophysical techniques, Cancer 5:643, 1952.

19. Odeblad, E.: Artefacts in autoradiography, Acta radiol. 39:192, 1953.
20. Fitzgerald, P. J.; Foote, F. W., Jr., and Hill, R. F.: Concentration of I^{131} in thyroid cancer, shown by radioautography: A study of 100 consecutive cases showing relation of histological structure to the function of thyroid carcinoma, Cancer 3:86, 1950.
21. Doniach, I., and Pelc, S. R.: Autoradiograph technique, Brit. J. Radiol. 23:184, 1950.
22. Pelc, S. R., and Howard, A.: Techniques of autoradiography and the application of stripping film method to problems of nuclear metabolism, Brit. M. Bull. 8:132, 1952.
23. Diserens, H. W., and Hall, O.: A method for radioautographic localization of isotopes in tissues, Texas Rep. Biol. & Med. 10:286, 1952.
24. Lajtha, L. G.: Isotope uptake of individual cells, technic for stained autoradiographs and microphotographs for grain counting, Exper. Cell Res. 3:696, 1952.

CHAPTER 7

Scanning

THIS CHAPTER WILL BRIEFLY DISCUSS scanning apparatus and scanning techniques applicable in the clinical utilization of radioisotopes. A "scanning technique" is defined by Brucer (7, 8, 9) as "any method of detecting radiation inside the body from some point outside the body." To accurately interpret scans, a physician should possess basic knowledge regarding the following: the types of scanning, the component parts of the scanner, the variables of "resolution" and "contrast" (see p. 168), the factors essential for "quality scans," the selection of equipment, the procedures and the practical aspects for some uses of the scanner. For detailed and technical consideration of these phases, the references cited in the bibliography at the end of this chapter should be consulted.

A. INTRODUCTION

With the advent of the clinical utilization of radioisotopes, scanning techniques were devised to detect and record the localization, distribution and concentration of these materials in the living body. The early method of point-to-point scanning with a crude hand-held detector (usually a Geiger-Müller tube) of low sensitivity gave sketchy data concerning internally administered radioisotopes. The persistent desire to gain more information led to the mechanization of scanning. Advancing technology in electronics equipment and apparatus has transformed the original mechanical scanner of Cassen and Bauer (10) into a highly valuable diagnostic tool. It is now possible to purchase scanners which, with proper settings, can automatically scan body areas with a reasonable degree of efficiency. In fact, present-day scanners now produce scans which challenge the ability of the clinician to interpret them.

The ultimate result of scanning depends on the ability of the physician to interpret the scan accurately. Even with the best resolution and the proper factors of definition, the interpretation requires capabilities of the operator far beyond those built into the apparatus. However, the reverse also holds true, for, even with a complete knowledge of abnormal and normal physiology, it is impossible to interpret a scan when the resolution is poor or the factors of definition are improper.

The following factors must be included in any quality scan in order for it to provide useful data, according to *Radioisotope Scanning* (9):

The scan should be technically good, include some background area, and delineate clearly the outlines of the patient and some anatomical landmarks. The scanning mechanism should move equally fast in both directions, and the space between traversed lines should identify the approximate resolution of the scan. The legend on the scan should describe the patient by name or number, scanner used, dose and kind of isotope, time of administration of isotope, time elapsing from isotope administration to actual scanning, dot factor, scan speed in interpretable units, distance from collimator to the patient's skin, energy of radiation scanned, and interpretation sketch to assist the viewer. Lines should never be drawn on the actual scan (especially with a thick black marking pencil) as this is mutilation to important scientific data.

Even under ideal circumstances of scanning, it is possible to completely misread and misinterpret a scan. Errors can occur owing to malfunctioning of the machinery, to malfunctioning of the operator and to bias or human error of the interpreter. The adage "One tends to see and believe what those around him see and believe" is true in scanning. In *Radioisotope Scanning,* this is excellently illustrated by an original scan and five reproductions demonstrating reasonable interpretations of the scan when the interpreter used a thick black marking pencil, which distorts the data into making the viewer see what the interpreter did. The only marks that should ever be placed on the scan are those which will assist the physician in locating body landmarks, and even these marks should be made by an attachment of the machine on the scan.

The problem of interpreting the size and probable shape of unknown areas of activity is the crux of the area scan. Anyone who attempts to make interpretations of scans must study the resolution and definition of each piece of scanning equipment.

B. SCANNING APPARATUS

The present-day scanner usually consists of the following component parts: (1) detector, (2) collimator, (3) side shielding, (4) mechanical scanning mechanism, (5) pulse-height spectrometer and (6) scaler or rate meter. There are many variations of this basic system, each one being ardently advocated by its proponents.

Each part of the scanning apparatus has a significant effect on the "quality" of the scan. The measure of this quality is the *resolution* (ability to separate adjacent concentrations of radioisotopes) and the *contrast* (ability to differentiate between areas of slightly different activity) of the scan. All the parts also affect the sensitivity of the device, which determines how much radioactive material must be administered to obtain a scan of a given quality in a given length of time. The resolution of an area scan is determined by the detector, the collimator and the method of recording.

1. DETECTOR

In all scanning units now commercially available, the detector for gamma rays is a thallium-activated sodium iodide crystal ranging in size from 1×1 in. to 3×3 in. The commonly used size is 2×2 in. The sodium iodide crystal is optically matched to a photomultiplier tube, with the pulse from this unit being fed to a spectrometer.

2. COLLIMATOR

There is disagreement as to the type of collimator which will give the best definition for the scan. To a certain extent, the choice of collimator is dependent on the purpose for which it will be used. The open-bore collimator (a single ¾ in. bore about 6 in.

long) is used in various external tumor detection techniques, in the delineation of brain tumors, in dynamic circulation studies and in experimental procedures for liver uptake, excretion studies with radioiodine-tagged dyes, dynamic studies of kidney function and silicious-dust clearance of the lungs. Narrow single-hole collimators are inadequate for scanning purposes because the resolution is narrow in only two dimensions and can be increased only with a tremendous loss in sensitivity. This sensitivity loss can be compensated by widening the holes in the wide-angle collimator, but this causes complete loss of direction in the isoresponse lines. Wide-angle counters are used for tissue clearance studies to follow the rate of disappearance of the activity (usually only a fraction of a microcurie of radioiodine) injected interstitially. Focusing collimators varying from 12 holes, advocated by Shy and his associates (18) and by Meadows (16), to 61 holes, favored by Bell (2) and Bender (3), are usually best for mapping distribution of activity, such as thyroid scanning and brain-tumor scanning.

3. SIDE SHIELDING

For most uses, an adequate side shielding of the sodium iodide crystal should be a minimum of 2 in. of lead. This is necessary to reduce the count rate when the detector is away from the area of localization and to decrease the contribution of counts from the activity in other body areas to the scanned area. This is especially important when the ratio of concentration in the scanned area to that in other body areas is small and when the isotope used has gamma rays of high energy (example, the 0.637 value of I^{131}).

4. MECHANICAL SCANNING MECHANISM

The scanning mechanism is designed to move the detector automatically over a pre-set area. The size and shape of the scan can usually be varied with limiting switches. An electric motor powers the unit and may or may not have variable speeds for scanning. An electric drive moving the detector up and down is a useful feature found in most present-day machines. The primary functions of the mechanical portion of the scanner are to provide even and smooth movement of the detector system over an adequate area and to supply sturdy support for the detector and collimator. The size of the over-all unit is important in many cases, owing to the limited space usually provided for the isotope laboratory.

5. PULSE-HEIGHT SPECTROMETER

Formerly accepted merely as a useful accessory for the scanning unit but now recognized almost universally as an absolute neces-

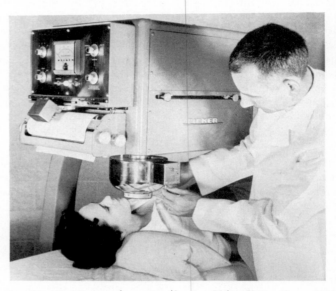

FIG. 36.—Positioning of scanner. (Source: Picker X-Ray Corp., White Plains, New York.)

sity for adequate scanning is the pulse-height spectrometer. The one exception to this is the application of positron scanning technique advocated by Brownell and Sweet (6, 19, 20). The spectrometer scans the height of the pulses coming to it from the detector and, through an upper and lower window, passes only those pulses which have values between the settings. Since the height of the pulse from the scintillating detector system is proportional to the photon energy striking the detector system, it is possible to reject background counts by selecting only the component desired.

For most scanning techniques, pulse-height spectrometry is essential because the scattered photons which have lost part of their energy can be discarded and only unscattered photons from the localized isotope are then recorded on the scan. This ideal condition is achieved only when the isotope used for scanning emits only a single-energy gamma (example, Cr^{51}). However, I^{131}, with a heterogenous emission pattern, is the most commonly used isotope for scanning. The spectrometer is usually set for the most abundant gamma ray, 0.364 Mev, to obtain the best counting statistics from the lowest possible dose of I^{131}. The higher-energy 0.722 and 0.637 Mev photons may be degraded (by scatter and insufficient shielding around the detector) to the point where their energies will be in the levels set for acceptance by the spectrometer. These photons may then be recorded as counts from one area when they originated from another area. The spectrometer does not completely eliminate the counts from gamma rays of higher energy than those for which it is set. The actual setting of the spectrometer may be a complex operation, as required by most units, or a simple turning of a knob to the correct isotope, as found on the Cliniscanner* (Fig. 36).

6. SCALER OR RATE METER

After the pulses pass through the spectrometer, they are fed to a scaler or rate meter unit, which is utilized to select the rate at which pulses are then fed to the data presentation system. Variation of the settings to match the activity level being scanned is essential for interpretable scans. Improvement of the data-recording unit systems, however, is making the settings less critical, since the newer ones have a wider dynamic range. Actual settings are too variable to be discussed in this text.

7. DATA PRESENTATION

a) MECHANICAL DOT RECORDER.—This system employs an electromagnet to move the stylus up and down and cause it to

---

* Picker X-Ray Corporation, White Plains, New York.

strike a piece of carbon paper and make an imprint on the paper below it. This type of recording unit, initially employed with the mechanization of the scanning techniques, is routinely available on most commercial scanners. The deficiencies of this type of recorder are a narrow dynamic range, easy jamming and difficult interpretation.

b) BACKGROUND CUTOFF OR BACKGROUND ERASE.—An improvement of the mechanical recording system through the use of a background cutoff system has been advocated by MacIntyre and Houser (14). In this system, a background level is established, below which no prints are produced by the recording system. When the background level is exceeded, all the information is recorded by the mechanical recording system. The main failing of this unit is the fact that it is difficult to set correctly the level of the background erase so that the wanted information will be obtained. These investigators have bypassed this problem by taking all of the information from the scaling unit on a tape recording and then replaying this information from the tape through the background cutoff system, with the cutoff level set at various levels. In this way, all of the information is recorded, and the scan which shows the areas of increased or decreased activity to the best advantage is then used for interpretation. The tape system is excellent but quite expensive and time consuming. Each level of replaying the taped information requires the same period of time as for the initial scan, or a multiple background erase and printing system must be utilized.

c) PHOTOGRAPHIC RECORDING SYSTEM.—A more promising method of recording information obtained from the scanning detector is the technique of photographically recording the data as advocated by Kuhl and his co-workers (12) and by Bender (3). This gives a permanent record which will not smudge or smear. In this photoscanning technique, the pulses from a scaler or rate meter are fed through an electrical or electromechanical system to a light bulb, which then shines on a photographic film to record the data obtained by the detector. In many cases the mechanical recording unit produces the desired information correctly, but the eye is not sufficiently acute to correctly interpret the increased or decreased count rate. It is much easier to detect a change in density on the film than it is to correctly gauge the distance between dots produced by the mechanical recording system. Other desirable features are the absence of the jamming difficulty and the non-linear recording, which takes a twofold increase in count rate and records it as a fourfold increase in density. The disadvantages of the photorecording system are that the scans cannot be observed during the time they are being produced and that it is quite ex-

TABLE 19.—Scan Recording Systems

Characteristic	Mechanical Dot Printer	Photographic	Teledeltos	Ideal
Reliability.............	Yes	Yes/no	Yes	Yes
Original information*..	No	No	Yes	Yes
Dynamic range†.......	Limited	Good	Good	Yes
Visible...............	Yes	No	Yes	Yes
Bias‡................	Yes	Yes	No	No
Filable..............	Yes	Yes	Yes	Yes
Compatible with present scanners.....	Yes	Yes	Yes	Yes
Noise level...........	Abominable	Nice	Low	Low
Cost.................	Moderate	High	Low	Low
Nonjam..............	No	Yes	Yes	Yes
Interpretable.........	Yes	Yes	Yes	Yes
Small change of activity level detectable......	No	Yes	Yes	Yes
Idiot-proof...........	No	No	Yes	Yes

* Original information: The recording system will print out the information as it is obtained without distortion.
† Dynamic range: Ability to accept and print out, in a usable manner, wide variations in concentrations.
‡ Bias: No time delay in recording accumulated information, so that information appears on the scan in the area that the detector picked it up.

pensive. The settings are fairly critical for the photorecording unit, but this also applies to the mechanical recording system, since incorrect scaling factors can completely obliterate the information that is desired.

d) Teledeltos Recording System.—Teledeltos is an electrosensitive paper on which an electric current will produce a density proportional to the applied current. This type of recording system was first utilized in scanning by Mueller and Myers (17) but proved unsatisfactory because the dots produced were not of uniform size or density. The problem of the use of Teledeltos has been overcome by Maxfield (15) through the use of a 60 cycle vibrating stylus to spread the resultant density in a straight line similar in appearance to that obtained with the mechanical stylus. The mark so produced, however, varies in density according to the activity detected, yielding a scan similar to that obtained with the photorecording system. Thus, the Teledeltos recording system has these advantages: the scan is visible during the time that it is being produced; and the system has a nonjamming factor, a wide dynamic range and an almost instantaneous response. In a session following the Symposium on Scintillating Scanning presented at the Naval Medical Center by the U. S. Naval Medical School in Bethesda, Maryland, in October 1958, advocates of the various scanning techniques concurred that the weakest section of the scanning apparatus at the present time is the recording system. The specifications of an ideal data presentation system were formulated by discussion after this symposium, and the existing systems were compared to the ideal system. Table 19 illustrates the specifications of this ideal system and compares the above-mentioned systems to the ideal one.

From the information in Table 19, it is evident that the mechanical recorder is the poorest of the recording systems. The photorecording system and the Teledeltos recording system with the vibrating stylus are closest to the ideal recording system.

C. RESULTS

1. THYROID SCANS

The most scanned organ of the body is the thyroid gland.

a) METHOD OF PROCEDURE:

1. Scans of the thyroid are made after an orally administered tracer dose of radioiodine (I^{131}), given 24 hours before the time of the scan. The dose of I^{131} for scanning ranges between 10 and 50 μc., depending on the sensitivity of the scanner to be used.

2. The scanner should be turned on for a warm-up of at least 1 hour, and the operation should be checked with a standard source. A focusing collimator is usually employed.

3. The scan is then carried out by positioning the patient under

the scanner. A small pillow or folded sheet placed between the patient's shoulder blades helps to extend the patient's neck and facilitates scanning of the thyroid gland. Explaining the procedure to the patient is essential.

4. An appropriate scale setting which has been determined by previous phantom work, by previous experience of the operator or by making trial passes over the thyroid is set and checked on the machine. The usual range is a scale of 4–32 for scalers or 1,000–3,000 range for rate meters.

5. The scan of the thyroid may be carried out from the superior

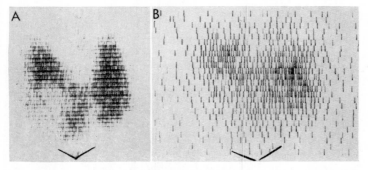

Fig. 37.—Scans of patient with multinodular goiter. *A,* Teledeltos recording. *B,* mechanical recording.

to the inferior, or vice versa. In either case, set the limiting switches so that the area scanned extends from the lower edge of the mandible to the junction of the upper and middle third of the sternum, including the lateral portions of the neck.

6. In a brief explanation of the procedure, the patient should be cautioned to swallow during the scan only when the detector is at one side of the scan area and is in the process of advancing to the next line of the scan. Swallowing at any other position may distort the thyroid pattern by producing areas of increased activity above the thyroid, which may be misinterpreted as abnormal areas of functioning thyroid.

7. Start the scanning mechanism.

8. Keep the lower surface of the collimator ½–1 in. closer to

the surface of the neck than is its focal distance. (Keep at distance of 1 in. for 1½ in. focusing collimator.) A motor-driven raising and lowering device for the detector is useful but should be operated only when the scanner is changing lines, since extraneous marks may be caused by the motor.

9. The anatomic positions usually marked are the cricoid cartilage and the suprasternal notch. Areas of thyroid abnormalities (e.g., scars, nodules) can also be marked. These positions are best designated at the beginning of the scan by the physician who interviewed the patient. A light localizer is essential to accurately indicate the anatomic positions. The points are marked as the scanner passes over them (Figs. 37–40).

b) INTERPRETATION.—The following factors must be considered to interpret the thyroid scan: the time following the tracer dose of I^{131}; the scale setting; the speed of the scanner; the spectrometer setting; the general outline of the thyroid gland (normal, absent section, additional areas of activity); and the activity within the thyroid gland (normal, increased activity, decreased activity). *Radioisotope Scanning* (9) discusses the details of these topics.

Evaluation of the question "Was the scale setting correct?" will influence the final interpretation of the scan, particularly if it was produced by a mechanical recorder. If the scale setting was too low, blank spots may be produced in the gland by jamming the recording stylus when the stylus is unable to move as rapidly as the rate at which it receives pulses from the scaler in the area of greatest activity. These false "cold areas" in the gland outline produced by this jamming of the stylus may cause the uninitiated interpreter to make a false diagnosis of a nonfunctioning nodule when, actually, the nodule was hyperfunctioning. Too high a scale setting will give poor visualization of the thyroid outline.

"Hot" nodules in the thyroid gland are usually detected with ease. "Cold" nodules, however, may show up as normally active areas if there is sufficient normally functioning thyroid tissue behind or in front of the cold nodule. Only when more than 50 per cent of the gland has been replaced with nonfunctioning tissue are areas of decreased activity in the thyroid gland usually demonstrated.

Discrete areas of decreased function within the thyroid gland

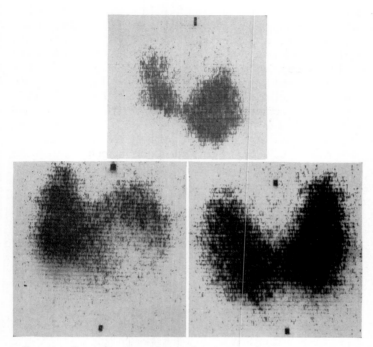

Fig. 38.—Scan of patient with nonfunctioning adenoma in right lower lobe of thyroid gland.

Fig. 39.—Scan of hyperthyroid patient with cyst in left lower pole of thyroid gland.

Fig. 40.—Scan of hyperthyroid patient with hyperfunctioning adenoma in left lower pole of thyroid gland.

may be caused by such conditions as hemorrhage into a nodule, nonfunctioning adenoma, cystic changes in the thyroid, colloid goiter and carcinoma. These must usually be more than 0.5 cm. in diameter before they can be identified by the scan.

There are also generalized areas of change identified by diminished concentration of the radioiodine in the thyroid gland. This state may be found in carcinoma; in suppression of the thyroid function by antithyroid drugs and previously administered iodine-containing materials; in acute thyroiditis; in chronic changes in the thyroid, such as Riedel's struma or Hashimoto's disease; and in degenerating colloid changes in the thyroid gland.

Areas of increased activity in the thyroid gland usually indicate a toxic nodule or a functioning nontoxic adenoma. Irregularity of the thickness of the gland, owing to variance in the size of the gland, may also produce areas of apparent increase in activity. Palpation of the gland and repeat scans on oblique planes will identify the variation in thickness as the cause of increased activity.

As a rule, it is not possible to make a positive diagnosis of a malignancy on the basis of a scan of the thyroid area alone. It is only possible to determine whether there is an increased, normal or decreased amount of activity in the area of the suspected nodularity. (The examiner should beware of the change in outline caused by swallowing and of normal areas of activity which may occur in the midline along the path of migration of the thyroid gland.) Occasionally, areas of metastasis can be definitely demonstrated; but, in the presence of a normally functioning thyroid gland, this is a fairly rare occurrence. If the thyroid gland has been surgically removed or ablated with the therapeutic doses of radioiodine, there may sometimes be demonstrated areas of thyroid metastasis which were not previously visualized.

In general, it can be said that scans of the thyroid gland are an aid in the estimation of the clinical potentialities of a nodule in the gland, the detection of marked irregularities in the gland size, the localization of substernal thyroid glands and, occasionally, the demonstration of areas of thyroid metastasis from carcinoma of the thyroid. Determination of the actual thyroid size from a scan, however, is very difficult, since the image presented by the recording unit will vary with the scale setting (especially with the mechanical dot recorder) and the amount of activity present in the thyroid gland. The final interpretation is dependent on the total clinical and laboratory findings plus the experience of the interpreter.

2. LIVER SCANS

In the use of scanning for large areas, such as the liver, there are certain obstacles, owing to the depth at which the radioisotope is deposited and the amount of intervening tissue. Therefore it is difficult to determine the exact structural changes which may have occurred, but gross changes are discernible. These are enhanced by the use of contrast variance, such as the closed-circuit television of Bender (5) or the background cutoff technique of MacIntyre and Houser (14). Initially, scans of the liver were tried, using RISA®. These scans were of poor quality, and the information obtained was not of diagnostic value. Recently, rose bengal tagged with I^{131} has been successfully utilized for liver scans. Rose bengal is concentrated by the polygonal cells of the liver and therefore gives an accurate outline of functioning liver tissue.

a) METHOD OF PROCEDURE:

1. The scanner should be checked for function and turned on for a warm-up for 1 hour.

2. Position the patient so that the area of the liver (as determined by palpation and percussion) will be covered. The limiting switches should be set accordingly.

3. A focusing collimator is commonly used, but a straight-bore collimator may be of greater value.

4. Inject intravenously 50–300 μc. (150 μc. ordinarily, depending on the sensitivity of the scanner) of rose bengal tagged with I^{131} (concentration of rose bengal between 0.2 and 5.0 mg.). (The rose bengal may be diluted with sterile isotonic saline solution to provide a dose of 1–2 cc. containing the previously listed concentrations.) If a prolonged period of time (above 60 minutes) is required for the scan, then a blocking dose of nonradioactive rose bengal, 50–100 mg., should be administered, to slow the rate of excretion of the rose bengal from the liver area.

5. Set the scale by making trial passes over the scan area.

6. The scan of the liver area is usually started 10 minutes after the injection, beginning the scan at the inferior border of the liver and setting the scanner to travel toward the superior portion of the body. By so doing, the amount of rose bengal which is excreted into the gallbladder and intestinal tract will not interfere with the delineation of the inferior margin of the liver. If the scan is started at the superior portion of the liver, by the

time the detector reaches the inferior border of the liver, activity in the duodenum and gallbladder will tend to obscure the actual inferior border of the liver.

7. The anatomic landmarks usually located are: the inferior costal margins; the outline of the liver, if it is palpable; and any palpable nodules. Again, the physician should mark the anatomic positions, using a light localizer.

8. If there is interest in the concentration of the rose bengal in the gallbladder, a scan of the gallbladder area may be carried out following the completion of the liver scan.

9. Following the scan, a laxative may be administered to the patient to speed the removal of the rose bengal I^{131} from the intestinal tract and decrease the radiation exposure. This is not an imperative procedure.

10. Colloidal radioactive gold (Au^{198}) has occasionally been employed for liver scans. The colloidal Au^{198} is picked up by the Kupffer cells of the liver. The dosage is usually 200–500 μc. of Au^{198} administered intravenously. Because of the large dose required, this isotope is usually relegated to scans for areas of metastasis in previously known carcinoma patients. Similar steps are taken as with the rose bengal I^{131}.

11. Radioactive manganese (Mn^{56}) is under experimental investigation for liver scans. The isotope Mn^{56}, with its half-life of 2.58 hours, is excellent for liver scanning if a nuclear reactor is in the vicinity. The Mn^{56} is administered either as manganese oxide or as manganese chloride in a colloidal form. The 0.8 Mev primary gamma of Mn^{56}, however, makes collimation a very difficult problem. The majority of the collimators available commercially appear as though they were nonexistant when they are exposed to gamma rays of such high energy.

b) INTERPRETATION.—The same factors utilized to produce the scan as outlined earlier, under "Interpretation of Thyroid Scans" (p. 176), must be determined here also.

Areas of abnormality in the liver will be shown as areas of decreased activity in the outline of the liver scan, when rose bengal I^{131}, Au^{198} or Mn^{56} are utilized for the scan. It is difficult to scan the liver adequately because of its configuration, with its convexity toward the detector, and because of the location of the greater mass of the liver in the right lobe. Therefore, small areas of decreased activity (less than 2 cm.) may be missed in the right lobe of the liver if they are seated fairly deeply. The mechanical recorder does not have a high-enough contrast enhancement adequately to delineate other than gross areas of decreased activity within the liver. For this reason, the photorecording or the Teledeltos recording unit is required for the best scans of the liver area. Because of the liver's unusual configuration, a special scanning unit was developed by Kuhl (13). This scanner rotates in a quarter arch around the circumference of the body, with the detector focused at the spine. This scanning procedure tends to spread the liver area out so that the mass of liver tissue which is "seen" by the detector at all times is essentially the same in depth. This facilitates detection of small areas of decreased activity which may be present in the right lobe of the liver.

Respiration, with its associated movement of the liver, may blur the margins of the liver, as does swallowing in thyroid scans. This movement may also hide small areas of decreased activity within the liver by smoothing out the pattern. Usually, areas of decreased density must be 2–2.5 cm. in diameter to be detected.

In interpreting liver scans, areas of decreased activity may be considered as due to areas of metastatic carcinoma to the liver, primary liver tumors, cirrhosis, liver failure, liver abscesses, incorrect setting of the scanning factors and rapid excretion of the tagged material from the liver. An exact tissue diagnosis cannot be made from the scan, but correlation with the clinical picture will often yield the correct answer.

3. GALLBLADDER SCANS

The visualization of the gallbladder by the use of a certain radioactive dye, di-iodophenolphthalein, is of importance in those patients in which the use of sufficient concentration to get an opacity for radiography is undesirable. Such visualization can be accomplished with a minimal amount of the dye and is an effective means of determining gallbladder function. As discussed above, a scan of the gallbladder can be immediately carried out following the rose bengal I^{131} liver scan and will demonstrate the concentration of the rose bengal in the gallbladder. The dose of radioactive material will vary from 50 to 300 μc.

4. Abdominal and Pleural Cavity Scans

The scanning of the abdomen after radioactive material has been injected into the abdominal or pleural areas is of importance. Radioactive gold (Au^{198}) is used. No additional administration other than the therapeutic dose is needed to carry out scanning for this purpose.

5. Vascular Structure Scans

Scanning of areas of the vascular system, such as the cardiac silhouette and the mediastinum, for the determination of tumor versus aneurysm is of importance. MacIntyre and Houser (14) have utilized scanning techniques to demonstrate blood pools within the body. This is very useful for delineation of areas of aneurysms and for the differentiation of an enlarged heart from a pericardial effusion. The radioactive material that is commonly used for this scanning technique is RISA® or chromium (Cr^{51}).

The scanning procedures and techniques will improve in the future as more of the interested clinicians apply their ingenuity and enthusiasm to the radioisotope field to aid them in solving the complex problems of their speciality. The hope for the coming years should be to obtain maximum information through the development of knowledgeable interpretations of the scanning possibilities.

REFERENCES

1. Allen, H. C.: A single bore collimator for brain tumor scanning (speech), Symposium on Scintillating Scanning at National Medical Center, U.S. Naval Medical School, Bethesda, Maryland, October, 1958.
2. Bell, P. R.: New developments in instrumentation for medicine, in *Radioisotopes in Medicine* (U.S. Atomic Energy Commission, September, 1953) pp. 170–185.
3. Bender, M. A.: Photoscanning detection of radioactive tracers in vivo, Science 125:443, Mar. 8, 1957.
4. Bender, M. A., and Blau, M.: A versatile, high contrast photoscanner for the localization of human tumours with radioisotopes, Internat. J. Appl. Radiation and Isotopes 4:154, 1959.
5. ———: Video contrast amplification applied to isotope scanning,

Society of Nuclear Medicine Meeting, June 17, 1959 (to be published).

6. Brownell, G. L., and Sweet, W. H.: Scanning of positron-emitting isotopes in diagnosis of intracranial and other lesions, *Peaceful Uses of Atomic Energy* (Geneva: United Nations Report, vol. 10, 1955), pp. 249–254.

7. Brucer, M.: Gamma ray absorption and radiation dosimetry, in *Radioisotopes in Medicine* (U.S. Atomic Energy Commission, September, 1953), pp. 103–158.

8. ————: The search for the hole, a study in scanning, *Medical Division Oak Ridge, Institute of Nuclear Studies* (U.S. Atomic Energy Commission).

9. ————: *Radioisotope Scanning—An Introduction to the Use of the Area Scan in Medical Diagnosis* (ORINS-20), (U.S. Atomic Energy Commission, January, 1958).

10. Cassen, B., and Bauer, F.: Possibilities and limitation of in vivo external counting techniques in biology and medicine, *Peaceful Uses of Atomic Energy: Radioactive Isotopes and Nuclear Radiations in Medicine* (Geneva: United Nations), vol. 10, (1956), pp. 244–248.

11. King, E. R., *et al.:* The production and medical application of short-half-life radioisotopes, *Radiology* 71:860, 1958.

12. Kuhl, D. E., *et al.:* A high contrast photographic recorder for scintillating counter scanning, *Radiology* 66:730, 1956.

13. ————: Rotational scanning of the liver, *Radiology* 71:875, 1958.

14. MacIntyre, W. J., and Houser, T. S.: A method for the visualization of the configuration and structure of the liver: Part B. A counting rate cut-off circuit for increased contrast in automatic scanning, *Am. J. Roentgenol.* 77:471, 1957.

15. Maxfield, J. R., Jr.: A small, compact and inexpensive scanner, *Symposium on Scintillating Scanning at Naval Medical Center of U.S. Naval Medical School at Bethesda, Maryland, October, 1958.*

16. Meadows, P.: Scanning—its value in medicine, *Symposium on Scintillating Scanning at Naval Medical Center of U.S. Naval Medical School at Bethesda, Maryland, October, 1958.*

17. Mueller, G. E., and Myers, W. G.: The Gremmicon, *News in Engineering,* November, 1955, p. 3.

18. Shy, G. M.; Bradley, R. B., and Matthews, W. B.: *External Collimation Detection of Intracranial Neoplasia with Unstable Nuclides* (Edinburgh: E. & S. Livingstone, Ltd., 1958).

19. Sweet, W. H., and Brownell, G. L.: The use of radioactive isotopes in the detection and localization of brain tumors, *Radioisotopes in Medicine* (ORO-125) (U.S. Atomic Energy Commission, 1953), pp. 211–223.

20. ———— and ————: Localization of intracranial lesions by scanning with positron-emitting arsenic, *J.A.M.A.* 157:1183, 1955.

PART II

ROUTINE CLINICAL THERAPY TECHNIQUE

CHAPTER 8

Treatment of Toxic Goiter
with Iodine-131

A. SELECTION OF PATIENTS

1. Exophthalmic or Toxic Diffuse Goiter

Therapy with radioiodine (I^{131}) in hyperthyroidism is primarily indicated in exophthalmic or toxic diffuse goiter rather than in toxic nodular goiter. The only major objection to the use of I^{131} is the possibility that this material is a carcinogen. Because of this danger, its application at first was selective, chiefly for poor-risk patients past 40 or 50 years of age, for those with relatively small goiters and for patients with postoperative recurrent exophthalmic goiter. As no tumors were observed, the threshold was gradually lowered to include virtually all patients with exophthalmic goiter who were over 40 years of age; and as each year passes with no evidence of carcinogenic effect, the limit is lowered by a year and sometimes more. At present it seems unlikely that the hypothetical danger of a future incurable cancer equals the 0.3–1.0 per cent mortality rate of a thyroidectomy.

There is evidence indicating that irradiation of the region of the neck in infants predisposes to cancer of the thyroid (1–9). The best evidence has been presented by Simpson and Hempelmann (1), who made follow-up studies on 1,502 infants who had been treated by x-ray for thymic enlargement. Of these, 11 developed thyroid cancer, while there were no instances of thyroid cancer in 1,933 untreated siblings. There has been one significant report, by Sheline, Lindsay and Bell (10), of the occurrence of thyroid nodules in children following therapy with I^{131} for hyperthyroidism: 5–10 years after therapy, thyroid nodules appeared in 3 of the 18 patients less than 20 years old. Two of these children with late nodules were among the 5 treated before age 10. One nodule showed invasion through its capsule and was classified as an invasive adenoma, a low-grade carcinoma. For the foregoing reasons, children should not be treated with I^{131}.

If the patient is very toxic, due to hyperthyroidism, some doubt may arise as to the advisability of administering I^{131} without preparation of the patient by means of one of the antithyroid drugs. Fortunately, the exophthalmic goiter patient tolerates I^{131} therapy very well; posttherapy reactions are not severe, but they do occur and can be fatal. A large weight loss, profound weakness or excessive nervousness is indication for a few weeks' preparation with propylthiouracil or Tapazole®. Itrumil® is not so satisfactory, in that it contains iodine and interferes with uptake during treatment. When sufficient improvement has been obtained, the medication is discontinued; 2 days later a tracer dose is administered; and, if the uptake on the following day is adequate, which it usually is, a therapeutic dose is administered. It is not advisable to wait too long, for the symptoms may recur.

For more detailed information on the use of I^{131} in the treatment of hyperthyroidism, the reader is referred to two excellent reviews, one by Chapman and Maloof (11) and the other by Lars-Gunnar Larsson (12).

2. Toxic Nodular Goiter

In toxic nodular goiter, thyroidectomy is still the preferred form of therapy. This operation is uniformly satisfactory; it removes the nodules; and it is followed by a low incidence of recurrence. In nodular goiter, therapy requires large doses of I^{131} and frequently several large doses.

The nodules are not completely destroyed by I^{131}; nevertheless, I^{131} therapy is effective as definitive treatment in this disease when the surgical risk is excessive, such as may frequently be the situation in patients over 70 years of age or in those with severe cardiac impairment. The therapeutic result depends on the percentage of thyroid uptake and the size of the goiter. If the thyroid accumulates less than 40 per cent of a tracer dose, the uptake should be enhanced by the use of thyroid-stimulating hormone (TSH) (see Chapter 1, under Use of Thyroid-Stimulating Hormone). Five units of TSH (Thytropar®*) is given intramuscularly; 24 hours later the tracer dose is administered, and it is assayed in the neck on the following day. If there is a substantial increase in uptake, a second 5 units is injected and the therapeutic dose given 24 hours later. By using TSH in this manner, the authors have been able to effectively treat a number of toxic nodular goiters heretofore not amenable to I^{131} therapy. A toxic nodular goiter with an uptake of more than 50 per cent will respond to therapy fairly satisfactorily. If a large nodular goiter accumulates less than 20 per cent of the tracer dose and the uptake cannot be increased by TSH, it is better to prepare the poor-risk patient with antithyroid drugs and arrange for a thyroidectomy, regardless of risk. Under no circumstances should Lugol's solution be administered if one contemplates using I^{131}, for, when this agent is used, the thyroid gland in nodular goiter does not recover its ability to accumulate iodine for many weeks. This effect does not occur in toxic diffuse goiter.

The patients in the category for treatment with I^{131} are usually very old and very ill, and it must be remembered that a reaction may be serious. There has been one known death during treatment and a number of sharp reactions have been recorded in the literature. If the situation is grim, preparation with large doses of propylthiouracil may be in order. Certainly, in most instances it is advisable to hospitalize the patient, get rid of any accumulated edema and quiet down the auricular fibrillation before administering internal radiation. A very ill patient, however, requires a definitive cure as quickly as possible; therefore, the severity of the illness should not induce one to give such small doses that they are relatively ineffective. In true toxic nodular goiter, little benefit is to be derived from doses under 20 mc.; and if the patient is in reasonably good condition, larger amounts are indicated.

---

* Armour Laboratories, Kankakee, Illinois.

B. CONTRAINDICATIONS

Iodine-131 is absolutely contraindicated in pregnancy 13 weeks after conception, at which time the fetal thyroid begins to function (13, 14). Russell, Rose and Starr (15) have reported on two women who received, at the thirteenth week of gestation, 225 mc. and 75 mc. of I^{131}, respectively, for thyroid cancer. The offspring of both women suffered from congenital hypothyroidism. Goldstein (16) reported on a pregnant woman receiving 71.7 mc. for carcinoma of the thyroid. Six days later an 18-week old fetus was delivered by abdominal hysterotomy, and the fetal thyroid was found to contain enough I^{131} to produce a radiation of at least 80,000 rads.

As stated above, I^{131} therapy is contraindicated in children.

C. ESTIMATION OF DOSAGE

An accurate method of determining dosage has not been devised. The dosage is usually estimated according to the weight of the gland and its ability to concentrate I^{131}. Actually, the size of the dose represents a compromise between a desire to produce an immediate and certain cure and an effort to prevent hypothyroidism. If positive control of hyperthyroidism is the prime factor, the dose should be high; but hypothyroidism will then be more frequent. If the dose is modified with a view to preventing hypothyroidism, control is less certain, and the necessity for repeated doses is likely. Regardless of the criteria for estimating dosage, most clinicians have arrived by trial and error at virtually the same dosage levels. It is generally accepted that the dose for an exophthalmic goiter should be approximately 70–100 μc. accumulated per gram of thyroid. If the thyroid uptake is 70 per cent and the effective half-life (EHL) is 5 days, which is the general average, then the dose is 7,000 roentgen-equivalents-physical (reps) or approximately the same number of rads.* As a crude estimate, then, one can figure that 70 μc. accumulated per gram of tissue equals 7,000 rep; 80 μc. equals 8,000 rep; 100 μc., 10,000 rep; and so forth.

* A rad equals 100 ergs/gm.

For an adult with a small diffuse goiter and high uptake, the minimal dose is roughly 4 mc. and the maximum 8 mc., the average being 6 mc. If the goiter is large, 1 mc. should be added for each estimated 10 gm. of weight. A first dose of 15 mc. is unusual, and one of 20 mc. is the upper limit. A toxic nodular goiter is nearly always larger than a toxic diffuse goiter; its percentage of uptake is usually less and it is not so radiosensitive as a diffusely hyperplastic gland. As a consequence, the dose required is larger, varying from 10 mc. to the maximum of 30 mc. permitted to an outpatient. Inasmuch as only poor-risk patients with toxic nodular goiter are treated in this way, the first dose is usually 20 mc. or more. Even this amount will usually need to be repeated at least once in toxic nodular goiter. If the patient has a large exophthalmic goiter (over 150 gm.), administration of more than one dose is routine. If the patient has a large toxic nodular goiter, repeated maximum doses of 20–30 mc. each are indicated.

Palpation is a very inaccurate method by which to estimate the weight of the thyroid gland. In most patients with exophthalmic goiter, there is a visible diffuse enlargement of the gland to about 1½ or 2 times normal size—that is, to 40–60 gm. If the gland is palpable but not visible, a 40 gm. estimate is reasonable; and if it is neither palpable nor visible, 30 gm. is sufficient. It is well to keep in mind that a small woman has a little goiter and that the estimate is likely to be too high. In a man, on the other hand, it is best to add 10 gm. to all the estimates; and if he has a thick muscular neck, to add another 10 gm.

The scan will permit a better estimation of the weight (17, 18). One may debate whether the increased accuracy is worth the expense and effort needed to utilize the gammagram, but one cannot deny that the scan will give a better estimation of weight than the fingers of the examiner. This is especially true if the examiner is not a surgeon and not accustomed to looking into the interior of the neck to see how wrong he can be. Allen has described the technique of the scan as follows: A tracer dose is given that will result in a concentration of 4–6 μc. of I^{131} per gram of tissue (many scintiscanners are effective with a smaller dosage). The dose is calculated by determining the uptake, estimating the weight of the gland by palpation and calculating the dose from the formula:

$$\frac{\text{Weight of gland} \times 4 \text{ or } 6 \ \mu\text{c.}}{\text{Maximum per cent thyroid uptake}} = \text{Oral scan dose } I^{131}$$

Twenty-four hours later an anteroposterior silhouette of the gland is obtained by scanning the neck. The area of each lobe is determined in centimeters by a planimeter, and the height of each lobe is measured. The weight of the lobe is calculated from the formula:

Weight of lobe = k (area thyroid lobe cm.^{2} × height of lobe cm.),

where the constant k equals 0.323 and is the coefficient of correlation of mean depth and height of a thyroid lobe determined experimentally only for normal or diffusely enlarged glands. The scan is not applicable to nodular goiter. Clode and his associates (19) have described a method of calculating weight by pneumo-thyroid laminagrams (roentgenograms following injection of air into the neck).

Theoretically, the most logical and most accurate units in which to estimate the dosage would be in equivalent roentgens or in rads. To make such calculation, it is necessary to know: (1) the percentage of uptake of I^{131}, (2) the effective half-life in the gland and (3) the size of the goiter.

The EHL is determined by administering a tracer dose and determining the thyroid I^{131} at 24-hour intervals, preferably every day for a week. Three or four determinations will permit calculation of the EHL but will not result in sufficient accuracy to be considered reliable. The EHL values usually average 5.2 days; but the spread is extreme (2–8 days), so that an average estimate is not of much value (20). The data are readily transferred to roentgen-equivalents-physical by assuming that 1 μc. of I^{131} uniformly distributed throughout 1 gm. of tissue will give 160 rep:

$$\text{Rep} = 160 \times \frac{\text{Dose } (\mu\text{c.})}{\text{Weight of thyroid (gm.)}} \times \text{Per cent uptake} \times \frac{\text{EHL}}{8}$$

This formula is not strictly accurate, in that it assumes that the dose is immediately accumulated by the thyroid gland. A correction can be made for this error, but the error affects the entire calculation only slightly.

The therapeutic dose behaves, to a large extent, as does the tracer dose (21, 22). A minimal estimated dose in radiation units should be about 7,000 rep/gm. Unfortunately, even if a predicted dose in roentgen-equivalents-physical could be accurately delivered, the clinical effect would not be reliably predictable. The inexplicable variations in the radiosensitivity of hyperplastic goiters are so great that it is doubtful whether the effort to calculate dosage in roentgens is worthwhile.

D. ADMINISTRATION OF THE DOSE

The technique of administration of I^{131} for toxic goiter is the same as that for large doses of I^{131} for cancer (see Chapter 10). Therapeutic doses can also be obtained in capsule form. The capsule dose is more expensive, but it is more convenient and reduces measurably the possibility of contamination and the health hazards to laboratory personnel. It is the method of choice if the laboratory treats only a few patients.

PRECAUTIONS.—Outpatients should be warned that their urine is radioactive and that they should be careful of it. They will be reassured if they are told that contamination is easily washed away. If a patient receives a large dose of I^{131}, it is best that he or she sleep alone for a few days, and probably not come into close juxtaposition with babies. Vomiting soon after the administration of the therapeutic dose is a distressing accident. This is likely to occur when the patient is exceedingly nervous and has not eaten. A small meal, such as coffee and toast, may obviate this difficulty.

E. RESULTS

1. USUAL EXPECTATIONS

For the first few days after the administration of I^{131}, the symptoms may be somewhat exaggerated. The increase of symptoms is not great; it is usually not noticeable to the patient but is sufficient to warn him to take life gently for a few days and to restrict his physical activities as the severity of the disease indicates. There may be some soreness about the neck, and often there is enough irritation to cause mucus and cough. The discomfort is usually so little that the physician learns of it only by direct questioning. Improvement of the symptoms begins at the end of the second week and is obvious in 3 weeks. The goiter begins to shrink at this time, and it disappears in 6–8 weeks. The improvement continues for 2–3, or 4, months, at which time the end result can be re-evaluated. At that time, having used an average initial dose of 6 or 7 mc. for exophthalmic goiters, about 65 per cent of the patients might be expected to be euthyroid, 25 per cent still to be hyperthyroid and 10 per cent to be hypothyroid. With the passage of months or years, there is a tendency to hypothyroidism. The effect on exophthalmos is the same as the usual surgical effect—diminution of stare, lending improvement to the appearance of the eyes, but little reduction in the actual proptosis.

A review of the literature (23) up to 1952 gave the results in 1,720 cases as follows: 80 per cent satisfactory results, 9 per cent incidence of hypothyroidism, 5 per cent unsatisfactory results and 6 per cent incomplete. Theoretically, in true toxic diffuse goiter, control is possible in virtually 100 per cent of the cases. Unsatisfactory results, other than hypothyroidism, are due in a large measure to errors in diagnosis and to discontinued treatment.

Sheline and Miller (24) have recently reported one of the largest, most carefully followed series of patients. Of 431 patients whom they treated, 29 had toxic nodular goiter, 78 had postoperative recurrent toxic goiter and 324 had toxic diffuse goiter. Toxicity was controlled in 95 per cent; hypothyroidism developed in 17 per cent; and there was recurrence in 3 per cent. Thyrotoxicosis was controlled in 59 per cent by one treatment. Death occurred in 3 patients with uncontrolled toxicity.

2. PERSISTENT HYPERTHYROIDISM AND THE SECOND DOSE

In prophesying the probability of a satisfactory outcome, laboratory findings are not so important as are the clinical findings. Taplits, Fine and Rosenberg (25) checked the 24-hour uptake in 107 patients 2 months after treatment with I^{131} and found a euthyroid uptake in 6 patients who were clinically hyperthyroid and 2 more patients who later developed hyperthyroidism. This discrepancy between the laboratory and clinical evidence can practically be eliminated by using curves of immediate uptake rather than the 24-hour uptake. Bauer (26) studied 60 patients treated with I^{131} and found that the rapid uptake of a tracer dose characteristic of toxic goiter persisted even though total uptake was reduced.

Schultz and Zieve (27) made an analysis of the value of the laboratory data in the early prediction of success or failure in

TABLE 20.—PROGNOSTIC VALUE OF TRACER TESTS PERFORMED
ABOUT 2 MONTHS (46–75 DAYS) AFTER TREATMENT*

Uptake	Number of Observations	Further Treatment Required	Euthyroid	Hypothyroid
Low to normal.	50	7	25	15
Borderline.....	106	15	79	12
High.........	146	110	36	0

* Adapted from Larsson, L.-G.: Acta radiol., supp. 126, p. 5, 1955.

I^{131} therapy in 66 patients. Of 25 patients who ultimately obtained a euthyroid state and had uptake studies in 6–9 weeks, 15 had 24-hour uptakes of 15 per cent or below; and of these, 3 were clinically hyperthyroid. Of 16 patients who did not obtain a remission and who had uptake studies in 6–9 weeks, 2 had a 9 per cent uptake and 1 a 24 per cent uptake. Both were clinically hyperthyroid. Of a similar group of 7 patients who became myxedematous, none had a normal uptake and 4 were still hyperthyroid clinically. These investigators concluded that at 6–9 weeks after therapy there are discrepancies between the clinical findings and the ultimate outcome, and between the clinical findings and the laboratory findings, but that there is sufficient correlation to set up the following criteria for handling the patient 6 or more weeks after I^{131} treatment:

1. If the patient is hyperthyroid clinically and the thyroid uptake and basal metabolic rate (BMR) are both either abnormally high or borderline, he will very probably fail to show improvement and should be re-treated.

2. If the patient is hyperthyroid clinically and his thyroid uptake or BMR is definitely normal, the course is uncertain and he should be observed further.

3. If the patient is euthyroid clinically, complete remission will very probably occur.

Lars-Gunnar Larsson (12) made an excellent investigation of the prognostic value of tracer doses after treatment. Table 20 is adapted from his article.

It must be recognized that soon after therapy there are discrepancies between the clinical findings and the ultimate outcome, and between the clinical findings and the laboratory findings. However, despite this, certain generalizations can be made, as follows:

1. If there is no clinical improvement whatever after 4 weeks, or if there is only slight to moderate improvement after 8 weeks, retreatment is indicated. This is especially true if there has been no reduction in the size of the goiter.

2. If there is well-marked clinical improvement at 2 months, one should await the course of events.

3. Soon after a therapeutic dose, the thyroid uptake is depressed to a greater extent than the symptoms would indicate. In 2 or 3 months the uptake rises to a higher level. A high uptake at 2 months usually means persistent hyperthyroidism. If there is a normal or low uptake, further treatment is much less probable and hypothyroidism is much more probable.

THE SECOND THERAPEUTIC DOSE.—If a patient shows no improvement whatever after 4 weeks and he is still quite ill, one will be forced either to give him another treatment or to place him on antithyroid therapy. There is much uncertainty as to the advisability of giving another therapeutic dose unless it is possible to do an uptake study; there have been too many examples of severely hyperthyroid patients whose thyroid, following I^{131} therapy, would not accumulate I^{131}. It is best to wait until enough I^{131} leaves the neck so that an uptake study can be made; this usually requires 6–8 weeks. At 4 weeks the better course of action is to place the patient on antithyroid therapy for 4–6 weeks, stop it, do an uptake study and, if it is elevated, give a second dose. The more common situation is to have a patient who at 2 or 3 months is better but far from well, or one who at 3–6 months still has persistent hyperthyroidism. In these cases the uptake is determined; and, if adequate, a second dose is administered. If the uptake is not adequate, the patient is placed on antithyroid therapy and the uptake is repeated. If a patient continues to be hyperthyroid, the gland will nearly always recover its avidity for iodine.

Estimation of the size of the second and the subsequent doses presents some additional factors to the already inaccurate criteria used in determining the size of the first dose. (1) It is obvious that the criteria used in estimating the first dose were in error. (2) The gland has probably decreased in size and may even be no longer palpable. (3) The uptake is at a lower level. One can use the same criteria as with the first dose, modified somewhat by the helpful evidence that the particular patient requires more I^{131} than the rules indicate. Usually the patient has had some improvement, the gland has shrunk to some extent and the uptake is lower. In this situation, a repeat dose of about the same size as the first one is in order. The dose, of course, can be varied up and down, according to the variability of the foregoing three factors.

3. HYPOTHYROIDISM

It is also important to recognize the onset of hypothyroidism. A patient with hypothyroidism is just as miserable, or perhaps more so, than one with hyperthyroidism. Hypothyroidism may occur early or late in the course of treatment. It can be suspected very early if the goiter and the symptoms disappear completely in 4 weeks, leaving the patient in a temporary euphoric state. It is recognized later by pains in the muscles, charleyhorses, tiredness, intolerance to cold, puffiness, a slow pulse rate and a mean disposition.

4. UNTOWARD EFFECTS

Severe reactions are not common. Large doses of I^{131} may be safely administered to very sick patients, but reactions do occur and must be taken into consideration. Two deaths have been reported following a therapeutic dose, and the cause of a third death is problematic. In exophthalmic goiter the reaction, or "storm," appears on the first or second day. There is nearly always some aggravation of symptoms during the first few days or the first week; but if the patient is in satisfactory condition after 48 hours, there is little cause for anxiety. If a possible reaction has been anticipated and the patient has been prepared for I^{131} treatment by antithyroid drugs, the dose should be administered soon after the withdrawal of medication. It may also be advisable to reinstitute antithyroid therapy or even administer Lugol's solution. If a severe reaction occurs in exophthalmic goiter, Lugol's solution or iodine medication will control it but will, at the same time, wash out most of the I^{131}. When the I^{131} is bound to the gland, the administration of stable iodine will not wash out the I^{131}; but in a very active gland, the hormonal secretion of I^{131} is high and this I^{131} is not reaccumulated. As a result, the EHL is sharply reduced. Although reactions in exophthalmic goiter can be easily controlled, this is not true of a reaction in a weak, elderly lady with a toxic nodular goiter and a bad heart. Such a patient is a much greater source of worry than one with a toxic diffuse goiter.

Radiation thyroiditis after the first few days is quite common but ordinarily is hardly noticeable to the patient. On direct questioning, the physician will usually find that the patient has had some vague soreness, cough and mucus. Very rarely will there be sufficient inflammation to cause a marked swelling and unbearable pain.

Kennedy and Fish (28) have reported the sixth case, and Vetter and Hofer (29) the seventh case, of leukemia following I^{131} therapy for thyrotoxicosis. The latter investigators called attention to the fact that in 5 patients the period between I^{131} therapy and the onset of acute leukemia was 18 months. These reports indicate that there may be more than a chance association between I^{131} therapy of thyrotoxicosis and the subsequent development of acute leukemia.

Genetic injury is possible but is not considered of enough moment to withhold radiation therapy. The total body dose and the gonadal dose is roughly 1 r./mc. of dosage. Thus, an average dose would about equal the radioactivity received by the average individual in a lifetime and would double the possibility of genetic injury due solely to radiation. The effect, of course, is enough to be considered along with radiation from other sources. The danger to the population as a whole, because of the small numbers involved, is exceedingly small, compared to the hazard produced by diagnostic roentgenography.

REFERENCES

1. Simpson, C. L., and Hempelmann, L. H.: The association of tumors and roentgen-ray treatment of the thorax in infancy, Cancer 10:42, 1957.
2. Duffy, B. J., Jr., and Fitzgerald, P. J.: Thyroid cancer in childhood and adolescence: Report on 28 cases, Cancer 3:1018, 1950.
3. Clark, D. E.: Association of irradiation with cancer of thyroid in children and adolescents, J.A.M.A. 159:1007, 1955.
4. Winship, T.: Carcinoma of thyroid in children, Pediatrics 18:459, 1956.
5. Majarakis, J. D.; Slaughter, D. P., and Cole, W. H.: Thyroid cancer in childhood and adolescence, Tr. Am. Goiter A. 1956, p. 412.
6. Fetterman, G. H.: Carcinoma of thyroid in children: Report of 10 cases, A.M.A. J. Dis. Child. 92:581, 1956.
7. Baron, S. H.: Does irradiation of infants and children cause cancer of thyroid? Laryngoscope 68:1267, 1958.
8. Petit, D. W.; Catz, B., and Starr, P.: Thyroid cancer in youth, California Med. 89:394, 1958.
9. Rooney, D. R., and Powell, R. W.: Carcinoma of thyroid in children after x-ray therapy in early childhood, J.A.M.A. 169:1, 1959.
10. Sheline, G. E.; Lindsay, S., and Bell, H. G.: Occurrence of thyroid nodules in children following therapy with radioiodine for hyperthyroidism, J. Clin. Endocrinol. 19:127, 1959.
11. Chapman, E. M., and Maloof, F.: Use of radioactive iodine in diagnosis and treatment of hyperthyroidism: 10 years' experience, Medicine 34:261, 1955.
12. Larsson, L.-G.: Studies on radioiodine treatment of thyrotoxicosis; with special reference to behavior of radioiodine tracer tests, Acta radiol., supp. 126, p. 5, 1955.
13. Chapman, E. M., et al.: Collection of radioactive iodine by human fetal thyroid, J. Clin. Endocrinol. 8:717, 1948.
14. Russell, L. B., and Russell, W. L.: Radiation hazards to embryo and fetus, Radiology 58:369, 1952.
15. Russell, K. P.; Rose, H., and Starr, P.: Effects of radioactive iodine on maternal and fetal thyroid function during pregnancy, Surg., Gynec. & Obst. 104:560, 1957.
16. Goldstein, D. J.: Uptake of iodine-131 by an 18-week human foetus, South African M. J. 32:239, 1958.
17. Allen, H. C., Jr.: Subtotal ablation of thyroid gland with single dose of radioactive iodine-131 for treatment of thyrotoxicosis, South. M. J. 49:1428, 1956.

18. Bauer, F. K., and Blahd, W. H.: Treatment of hyperthyroidism with individually calculated doses of I¹³¹, A.M.A. Arch. Int. Med. 99:194, 1957.
19. Clode, W., *et al.:* Importance of determination of weight of thyroid gland and clinical biologic factors in treatment of hyperthyroidism with I¹³¹, Am. J. Roentgenol. 81:65, 1959.
20. Seed, L., and Jaffe, B.: Comparison of tracer dose and therapeutic dose of I¹³¹ as to thyroid uptake, effective half-life and roentgen dosage, Radiology 63:541, 1954.
21. Friedberg, A. S.; Kurland, G. S., and Ureles, A. L.: Critical analyses of quantitative I¹³¹ therapy of thyrotoxicosis, J. Clin. Endocrinol. 12:86, 1952.
22. ———; Chamovitz, D. L., and Kurland, G. S.: Factors influencing uptake and turnover of I¹³¹ by thyroid gland, Metabolism 1:36, 1952.
23. Seed, L., and Fields, T.: *Treatment of Toxic Goiter with Radioactive Iodine* (Springfield, Ill.: Charles C Thomas, Publisher, 1953).
24. Sheline, G. E., and Miller, E. R.: Radioiodine therapy of hyperthyroidism, A.M.A. Arch. Int. Med. 103:924, 1959.
25. Taplits, S.; Fine, A., and Rosenberg, L. S.: Immediate and continuous uptake studies of I¹³¹ in diagnosis and treatment of hyperthyroidism, Radiology 67:544, 1956.
26. Bauer, F. K.: I¹³¹ uptake in treated hyperthyroidism, Am. J. M. Sc. 223:495, 1952.
27. Schultz, A. L., and Zieve, L.: Alterations in thyroid I¹³¹ uptake, basal metabolic rate, serum cholesterol following treatment of hyperthyroidism with radioactive iodine; value in early prediction of success or failure of therapy, Am. J. Med. 20:30, 1956.
28. Kennedy, W. M., and Fish, R. G.: Acute granulocytic leukemia after radioactive-iodine therapy for hyperthyroidism, New England J. Med. 260:76, 1959.
29. Vetter, H., and Hofer, R.: Acute leukaemia following radioiodine therapy of thyrotoxicosis, Brit. J. Radiol. 32:263, 1959.

CHAPTER 9

Therapy of Blood Diseases

THE ETIOLOGY OF POLYCYTHEMIA VERA and the leukemias remains obscure. No method of cure has yet been found. The present methods of therapy in leukemia at best prolong survival time and produce, in most instances, temporary symptomatic relief. At the moment, agents such as radiophosphorus (P^{32}) and triethylene malamine (TEM) have made the outlook for polycythemia vera more favorable than for leukemia.

A. ADMINISTRATION OF PHOSPHORUS-32

1. PHYSIOLOGY

During the first 4–6 days, approximately 20–40 per cent of an oral dose of P^{32} may be excreted in the stool. The amount of P^{32} excreted may be minimized if it is administered during a fasting state. Following intravenous administration, from 5–25 per cent of the dose is excreted in the urine during the first week. Subsequently the amount decreases to less than 1 per cent a day.

When P^{32} is administered, it is at first selectively concentrated to some degree in the nucleoprotein of cells in active mitosis in the marrow, liver, spleen and tumors. Apparently the marrow has the highest affinity for P^{32}, for studies in leukemic patients have shown a less favorable differential uptake of P^{32} in the liver, spleen and nodes, as compared with the marrow (15). Initially the P^{32} that localizes in leukemic white cells may be 4 or 5 times the amount in the red cells.

In tumor cells the concentration of P^{32} is greater in the nucleus than in the cytoplasm (12).

Eventually P^{32} is deposited in the bone as calcium phosphate. The interval required for this exchange depends on the turnover rate of the tissues. The effectiveness of a dose, therefore, depends on the total exchangeable phosphorus in the tissue, the rate of utilization of phosphorus and the rate of growth of new tissue. Because of this tissue exchange, P^{32} irradiates the marrow by two pathways: initially and internally, from within the cells; and later, externally, from without the cells, as it is deposited into the cortex of the bone.

2. DOSAGE

It has been repeatedly shown that there is no correlation between the dose of P^{32} and the equivalent amount of irradiation. Hypothetically, however, in a 70 kg. adult (presuming that no excretion occurs) 1 mc. of P^{32} would be equivalent to 0.6 r total body irradiation for the first day or 12 r during the complete decay of P^{32}.

Formulas for the estimation of dosage have been developed which take into consideration, among other factors, the area to be irradiated, the duration of irradiation and the rate of excretion (11). During the last 20 years sufficient experience with the use of P^{32} has been acquired to permit the establishment of predetermined dosage schedules which are as effective and safe as an individually calculated dose. Radiophosphorus may be given orally or intravenously. If given orally, food should not be given for 6 hours before and 3 hours after administration. No iron, phosphate or calcium should be administered within 24 hours of an oral dose.

Radiophosphorus is a pure beta emitter. Although protection against the beta radiation can be obtained by surrounding the material with a few millimeters of lead, there is secondary radiation ("Brehmstrahlung") of soft gamma rays in the vicinity. A solution of $Na_2HP^{32}O_4$ may be pipetted out of its container at a distance or withdrawn by hand into a shielded syringe and emptied directly into a waxed paper cup for consumption by the patient.

It is safe to accept the assay as stated by the distributor and to measure the intended number of millicuries according to the millicuries per milliliter stated on the invoice.

Fortunately, there is little health problem insofar as the patient is concerned. He is not sufficiently radioactive to injure anybody in close juxtaposition, and he does not excrete P^{32} in appreciable amounts.

B. TREATMENT OF POLYCYTHEMIA VERA

Polycythemia vera is a disease of insidious onset. The course is chronic and of long duration, provided that serious complications do not develop. The disease has a predilection for middle or late life. Numerous therapeutic agents have been tried with some

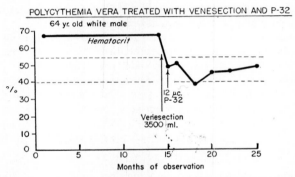

POLYCYTHEMIA VERA TREATED WITH VENESECTION AND P-32

FIG. 41.—A man, aged 64 years, had typical polycythemia vera. He declined treatment during a 14-month period of observation. Venesection of 3,500 ml. of blood over a period of about 2 weeks brought the hematocrit down from 68 to 49 per cent. He was then given 12.0 mc. of P^{32}. The hematocrit remained essentially within normal limits during the subsequent 10 months' observation. (From Best, W. R., and Limarzi, L. R.: Med. Clin. North America 31:220, 1955.)

success. One method of reducing the red cell count is to remove the peripheral blood either by venesection or by hemolysis. By another method, phenylhydrazine or acetylphenylhydrazine is used to produce hemolysis. However, the disadvantages of hyperbilirubinemia—secondary marrow stimulation, difficult dosage regulation and failure to control the platelet and white count—have limited the clinical use of phenylhydrazine or acetylphenylhydrazine. Depression of blood formation is another approach to lowering the blood count. Fowler's solution (potassium arsenite), nitrogen mustards and spray irradiation have been tried frequently. The use of Fowler's solution has been limited by the large dosage required, as well as the uncertain and difficult control of the cell levels. Nitrogen mustard also has several disadvantages: it requires hospitalization for administration; there are numerous side effects; and control of the cell counts is difficult. Roentgen irradiation, either locally to the spleen or diffusely as spray irradiation, has been effective. This procedure, however, requires considerable time, effort and expense. Radiation sickness is often severe.

Other treatments, such as the administration of benzol, ascorbic acid, choline, splenic extracts, iron-free diet, folic acid antagonists and splenectomy, are not generally adequate.

Venesection has the disadvantages of causing a hypochromic polycythemia, occasionally hypoproteinemia, and does not offer control of the white cell and platelet count. However, it is still the most effective means of giving immediate symptomatic relief to the patient. Venesection is now used concurrently with P^{32} (see Fig. 41) or triethylene melamine.

1. Phosphorus-32 Therapy

The use of radioisotopes affords a means of applying local radiation to diseased tissue with minimal irradiation of the surrounding normal tissue. The use of P^{32} in hematologic disorders was first reported by J. H. Lawrence (8) in 1940. Since then, P^{32} has been widely used by several investigators for various blood diseases (3, 4, 5, 6, 7, 14, 16, 17, 18).

2. Dosage

The dosage of P^{32} varies with the severity of the polycythemia and the weight and age of the patient. The severity can be determined by reviewing such essential data as symptomatology, hematocrit, the presence of complications and the ease with which the symptoms are controlled by simple venesection. In our experience, patients who require frequent venesections require larger doses of P^{32}. Relatively smaller doses are given to elderly patients. When there is doubt, smaller doses should be given.

It should always be remembered that, once the isotope has been given, there is, at present, no known method for counteracting its effects. In polycythemia vera, P^{32} may be given in small divided doses over a prolonged interval or in one total dose. A single total dose is preferred because less manipulation and fewer visits by the patient are required. This method also tends to hasten, as well as to prolong, the period of remission. The danger of

TABLE 21.—POLYCYTHEMIA VERA PATIENTS TREATED
WITH P^{32}: 55 CASES

Number of Patients	Number of Courses of Treatment	Total Dose* (Mc.)	Length of Each Remission (Months)
39. . . .	1	4.5– 8.5 (I) 3.0–12.0 (O)	6–42 (Av. 15)
12. . . .	2	8.0–15.0 (O-I)	3–15 (Av. 8)
4. . . .	3	13.0–23.0 (O-I)	6–10 (Av. 7)

* I = intravenous; O = oral; O-I = oral and intravenous.

marrow aplasia is theoretically greater but has not been observed by the authors.

A single oral dose of 6–12 mc. should be administered, after which the patient should be observed for from 3 to 10 months, initially at twice monthly intervals and subsequently at monthly intervals. A remission usually occurs within 3 months. In approximately 29 per cent of the patients a second course was required 6–10 months after the initial one. The second dose usually ranges from 3 to 10 mc. No side reactions were observed in 55 patients treated by this method (Table 21).

The administration of multiple small intravenous doses of P^{32} constitutes another method (9). Initially, 3 mc. of P^{32} are given intravenously. The patient is observed at first twice weekly and then at weekly intervals. At the end of 10–12 weeks the polycythemia is revaluated. If necessary, a second dose of 3–4 mc. is given intravenously. Again a 10- or 12-week observation period is maintained, at the end of which the patient's condition is evaluated. In Lawrence's group of 300 patients, 54 per cent required more than one course of therapy.

3. METHOD OF OBSERVATION

Frequent evaluation of the clinical and hematologic status should be made. This includes appraisement of the signs, symptoms and such laboratory data as hemoglobin and red cell count, hematocrit, white cell count, platelet count and peripheral

TABLE 22.—SYMPTOMATIC EFFECT OF P[32] IN 55 CASES OF
POLYCYTHEMIA VERA

	Relief (Per Cent)	Improvement (Per Cent)	No Improvement (Per Cent)
Fatigue	71	26	3
Heat tolerance	85	15	..
Dizziness and headache	90	10	..
Blurring of vision and excessive lacrimation	95	3	2
Pain in extremities	69	23	8
Paresthesia	73	27	..
Erythromelalgia	95	5	33
Pruritus	33	33	33

smear, before as well as after the initiation of therapy. The condition of the marrow may be evaluated before therapy is begun.

4. CRITERIA FOR REMISSION

Distinct symptomatic improvement usually occurs in those patients in whom satisfactory hematologic remission is induced. Hematologic remission constitutes a reduction of the hematocrit below 50, red cell count below 6 million, white count below 10,000. Theoretically, therapy cannot be considered adequate until the marrow reverts to a more nearly normal pattern. A remission should be evident within 3 months after therapy.

5. RESULTS OF TREATMENT

Table 22 summarizes the results of P[32] therapy in a series of 55 patients. Combined with the data from the literature in Table 23, these results give an over-all evaluation of the therapeutic effectiveness of P^{32}. Symptomatic improvement occurs in over 90 per cent of the patients treated. Some reports indicate that failure results from an inadequate dosage or the refusal of a patient to co-operate. Of the 55 patients observed by the authors, all showed some form of improvement. The greatest improvement was seen in the symptoms of headache, vertigo and erythromelalgia and in eye symptoms. Of the patients with anginal

TABLE 23.—EFFECTS OF P^{32} ON SYMPTOMATOLOGY AND PHYSICAL FINDINGS OF PATIENTS WITH POLYCYTHEMIA VERA*

Physical Findings and Symptoms	Number of Patients Treated	Increase	No Change	Decrease or Amelioration
Headache	294	. . .	4.8	95.2
Dyspnea	203	4.0	9.8	86.2
Vertigo	222	2.6	11.0	86.4
Eye symptoms	225	6.3	1.3	92.4
Gastrointestinal symptoms	139	12.9	12.9	74.2
Anginal pain	139	7.9	15.8	76.3
Fatigability	183	. . .	2.2	97.8
Heat intolerance	104	. . .	2.9	97.1
Erythromelalgia	63	. . .	. . .	100
Pruritis	115	. . .	23.5	76.5
Bone pain	97	. . .	6.2	93.8
Spleen	238	1.2	3.8	95.0
Liver	93	29.0	8.6	62.4
Hypertension	95	22.1	40.0	37.9
Cyanosis	89	. . .	59.5	40.5

* Summary from the literature and from a University of Illinois clinic series.

pain, 76 per cent were improved or completely relieved once remission was induced. If anginal attacks are frequent, phlebotomy may reduce the blood volume and viscosity; then the effect of P^{32} on the marrow may be manifested.

In 95 per cent of the patients, a significant reduction in the size of the spleen may be expected. In the series observed by the authors, two of the three patients with splenomegaly did not have palpable spleens following remission.

A significant reduction in the size of the liver occurred in more than half of the patients treated; however, 29 per cent developed hepatomegaly while being treated. The effects of a remission in lowering the blood pressure were variable. One fifth of the normotensive or hypertensive patients showed further elevation of blood pressure even though in a state of remission. A reduction in the degree of hypertension occurred in 38 per cent. A little more than half of the patients who were cyanotic remained so.

6. HEMATOLOGIC EFFECTS

Table 24 gives a summary of the results reported in the literature concerning the effects of P^{32} on the blood. Both the blood and the marrow reach normal values when a remission ensues.

TABLE 24.—EFFECTS OF P^{32} ON PERIPHERAL BLOOD OF PATIENTS WITH POLYCYTHEMIA VERA*

| | IN-CREASED | No CHANGE | DECREASED | | | NUMBER OF PATIENTS |
			Above Normal Range	Within Normal Range	Below Normal Range	
Red cell count......	0	3.7	3.7	92.6	6.1	378
Hematocrit........	0	...	8.7	91.3	...	160
White cell count...	0	5.7	8.24	86.1	18.2	352
Platelet count......	0	...	4.1	95.9	16.2	266

* Summary from the literature.

The red cell count becomes normal (less than 6 million) in 92 per cent of the cases. Anemia (less than 3.5 million red cells) may develop in 6 per cent. The white cell count also is reduced (less than 10,000) in 86 per cent of the patients with leukocytosis. A morphologic study of the blood shows normal distribution of the cellular elements. A right shift (disappearance of immature forms) in the granulocytic series occurs at the same time.

Blood volume studies in patients receiving P^{32} (9) show with equal frequency either a parallel fall in total red cell volume and plasma volume or a total fall in red cell volume with a reciprocal rise in plasma volume.

7. DURATION OF REMISSION

Remissions last from months to years. Approximately three fourths of the patients require further treatment by the end of the first year subsequent to initial therapy. Remissions as long as 4 years have been reported (9). Life expectancy has been increased so that most patients live from 5 to 20 years after onset of symptoms, with a median survival of 13.2 years (9).

8. COMPLICATIONS

Table 25 lists the causes of death, as reported in the literature, in polycythemic patients receiving P^{32}. Approximately 3 per cent

TABLE 25.—CAUSES OF DEATH IN PATIENTS WITH POLYCYTHEMIA VERA TREATED WITH P^{32}*

Total number of deaths	453
Acute granulocytic leukemia	2.7%
Carcinoma	0.9%
Aplastic anemia	0.5%
Thrombosis	1.6%
Miscellaneous	3.3%

* Adapted from Wiseman *et al.* (18).

eventually develop granulocytic leukemia. It has not yet been established whether or not this incidence is higher than occurs in untreated cases. However, the occurrence of fatal hemorrhagic and thrombotic complications (Table 26) is significantly reduced by proper P^{32} therapy, and this advantage outweighs the hazard of a slight increase in leukemia. Aplastic anemia after therapy is

TABLE 26.—THROMBOTIC COMPLICATIONS FROM POLYCYTHEMIA VERA*

Total number of patients	383
Percentage with thrombosis:	
Without P^{32} treatment	17.23
With P^{32} treatment	2.9

* Adapted from Wiseman *et al.* (18).

rare. Leukopenia (less than 4,500 leukocytes) may occur in 18 per cent. Thrombocytopenia (less than 100,000 platelets) is found in 16 per cent. Severe forms of thrombocytopenia are rare. These changes are presumably due to a suppression of granulopoiesis, megakaryopoiesis and erythropoiesis by the agent.

C. TREATMENT OF LEUKEMIA

Roentgen irradiation has long been the standard therapy in the chronic leukemias. In general, irradiation has had deleterious effects on the patient with acute or subacute leukemia, but newer developments in chemotherapy have been of value.

1. PHOSPHORUS-32 THERAPY

Radiophosphorus, like x-ray, is of little use in acute cases of leukemia. Roentgen irradiation is valuable in chronic leukemias for the management of localized leukemic infiltrates, such as in the spleen. In predominantly generalized involvement, however, P^{32} is of superior value.

2. DOSAGE

Several reports on the effect of P^{32} in chronic granulocytic leukemia have appeared in the literature. Dosage recommendations have varied with the investigators. In general, the regimen is similar to that used in polycythemia vera. Osgood and Seaman (14) recommend an initial dose of 2 mc., followed by similar or larger doses (maximum, about 6 mc.) at 1–3-week intervals, depending on the clinical and hematologic response. The dose is gradually reduced and the interval lengthened, depending on the course of the disease, until ultimately the patient receives a maintenance dose of 0.1–1 mc. every 1–3 months. Lawrence (10) advocates a course consisting of 1–3 mc.; thereafter doses of 0.5–2 mc. are given in weekly intervals until the desired effect is obtained. The end results are the same. Usually, larger doses are required in those patients previously treated by other means or who had had a previous remission. It is unnecessary and dangerous to attempt to reduce the white cell count to within normal limits when P^{32} is used for therapy. Leukemic patients with leukopenia must be treated cautiously, and they require frequent marrow evaluation.

3. RESULTS

Symptomatic improvement occurs in 50 per cent of the patients treated. The 5-year survival time, summarized from the literature, of 727 patients with chronic granulocytic leukemia treated with P^{32} is 20 per cent. As the white cell count decreases, the peripheral differential shifts to the right and the red cell count and hemoglobin rise. Although the blood findings may indicate a remission, the marrow may still be predominantly immature. This occurs in approximately 50 per cent of cases with blood remission (1). Other signs of improvement, such as a decrease in the size of the spleen, liver and lymph nodes usually accompany hematologic remission. However, complete remission cannot take place unless the marrow shows normal maturation.

Radiophosphorus has been less popular in the treatment of chronic lymphatic leukemia than in the treatment of chronic granulocytic leukemia. The dosage is similar in both conditions, but some investigators feel that a smaller amount of P^{32} is required in chronic lymphatic leukemia. The 5-year survival rate in 282 cases of chronic lymphatic leukemia reported in the literature is approximately 47 per cent. Lawrence (10) suggests that, of the patients surviving 5 years, 31 per cent will survive 10 years (approximately 14.5 per cent of the total). According to Reinhard and his associates (15), the drop in lymphocytes to below 50 per cent with reciprocal rise in granulocytes is not seen consistently. The anemia and thrombopenia are not improved so much in chronic lymphatic as in chronic granulocytic leukemia. The lymph nodes and spleen usually decrease in size after P^{32} therapy. The marrow condition is not altered, despite evidence of clinical and peripheral blood improvement (1).

D. RADIOPHOSPHORUS IN MISCELLANEOUS BLOOD DISEASES

Radiophosphorus has been used in the treatment of multiple myeloma, Hodgkin's disease, lymphosarcoma, reticulum cell sarcoma and giant follicular lymphoblastoma. The results have been disappointing. In general, P^{32} is not so effective in these conditions as are other forms of therapy.

E. THERAPEUTIC TRIALS OF OTHER RADIO-ISOTOPES

Radioactive stilbamidine has been produced in the hope of selectively irradiating myeloma cells. The compound is synthesized by building radioactive carbon into its structure. Apparently the uptake ratio between normal and myeloma cells is not great enough to warrant therapeutic use (16).

Radiosodium (Na^{24}) has been used in the treatment of the chronic leukemias, with results similar to those of P^{32}. Radiosodium has the advantage of having a half-life of only 14.9 hours and less variable excretion; thus regulation of the dosage to conform with the changing course of the disease is facilitated. Apparently, Na^{24} does not have a predilection for any tissue, and therefore the radiation administered is comparable to total body radiation.

Radiogold (Au^{198}) is administered intravenously in a colloidal state. It is localized in the reticuloendothelial system, such as liver, spleen and lymph nodes. With this isotope, favorable results have been reported in the treatment of the lymphoblastoma group.

Colloidal suspensions of radioactive chromic phosphate, yttrium and zirconium have been used in the treatment of blood disease. It is too early to predict which of these agents may have therapeutic value.

Radiostrontium seems to improve some of the symptoms of multiple myeloma.

F. CONCLUSION

Radiophosphorus (P^{32}) is the only isotope of practical effectiveness in the treatment of certain blood disorders, such as polycythemia vera, chronic granulocytic leukemia and chronic lymphatic leukemia. Other isotopes appear to be promising but require further clinical application before final assessment can be made.

REFERENCES

1. Berlin, N. I., and Lawrence, J. H.: Changes in the bone marrow differential in chronic leukemia treated with P^{32} and Y^{90}, Acta med. scandinav. 140:99, 1951.
2. Best, W. R., and Limarzi, L. R.: Newer agents in the management of leukemia, polycythemia vera and plasmocytic myeloma, M. Clin. North America 39:201, 1955.
3. Diamond, H. D.: Radiosotopes in medicine, J. M. Soc. New Jersey 48:420, 1951.

4. Duffy, B. J., and Howland, J. W.: Radiophosphorus (P^{32}) in diagnosis and treatment, New York J. Med. 52:551, 1952.
5. Erf, L. A.: Radiophosphorus as the treatment of choice in primary polycythemia, Am. J. Med. 1:362, 1946.
6. Hall, B. E., *et al.:* Radioactive phosphorus in the treatment of polycythemia vera, Am. J. M. Sc. 209:712, 1945.
7. Hall, B. E.: *Therapeutic Use of Radiophosphorus in Polycythemia Vera, Leukemia, and Allied Diseases: Use of Isotopes in Biology and Medicine* (Madison: University of Wisconsin Press, 1948). p. 353.
8. Lawrence, J. H.: Therapy with radioactive isotopes, J. Kansas Med. Soc. (Cancer supp.) 52:7A, September, 1951.
9. ———; Berlin, N. I., and Huff, R. L.: Nature and treatment of polycythemia, Medicine 32:323, 1953.
10. Lawrence, J. H.: Treatment of chronic leukemia, M. Clin. North America 38:525, 1954.
11. Low-Beer, B. V.; Blais, R. S., and Scofield, N. E.: Estimation of dosage for intravenously administered P^{32}, Am. J. Roentgenol. 67:28, 1952.
12. Marshak, A.: Effects of x-ray and neutrons on mouse lymphoma chromosomes in different states of the nuclear cycle, Radiology 39:621, 1942.
13. Osgood, E. E.: Titrated, regularly spaced radioactive phosphorus or spray roentgen therapy of leukemias, A.M.A. Arch. Int. Med. 87:329, 1951.
14. ——— and Seaman, A. J.: Treatment of chronic leukemias: Results of therapy by titrated, regularly spaced total body radioactive phosphorus, or roentgen irradiation, J.A.M.A. 150:1372, 1952.
15. Reinhard, E. H., *et al.:* Radioactive phosphorus as a therapeutic agent, J. Lab. & Clin. Med. 31:107, 1946.
16. Wasserman, L. R.; Rashkoff, I. A., and Yoh, T. F.: The use of radioactive and stable isotopes in hematology, J. Mt. Sinai Hosp. 17:1037, 1951.
17. Wasserman, L. R.: Polycythemia vera, Bull. New York Acad. Med. 30:343, 1954.
18. Wiseman, B. K., *et al.:* The treatment of polycythemia vera with radioactive phosphorus, Ann. Int. Med. 34:311, 1951.

CHAPTER 10

Cancer Therapy

A. CANCER OF THE THYROID

IF A CARCINOMA OF THE THYROID has retained sufficient hormonal activity to accumulate iodine, it may pick up enough radioiodine (I^{131}) to destroy itself. Carcinomas of the thyroid may be classified, according to pathology, into the following three groups, which may also be used for purposes of judging I^{131} uptake.

1. *Papillary carcinoma,* constituting about 50 per cent of all cancers (1), is the most benign variety. This type of cancer may be subdivided (2) into (*a*) predominantly papillary cancers, (*b*) mixed papillary and follicular cancers and (*c*) predominantly follicular cancers. Some uptake has been demonstrated (1) in 28 per cent of the papillary cancers, but in the true papillary tumor there is not sufficient uptake to warrant I^{131} therapy.

2. *Follicular carcinoma,* divided into (*a*) invasive and (*b*) encapsulated cancers, comprises about 10 per cent of all cancers. In this form, there is an attempt at the reproduction of normal colloid-containing follicles, and there is some uptake in 74 per cent of the cases, which is frequently adequate for therapeutic consideration.

3. *Undifferentiated* or *solid cancer* constitutes 30 per cent, and *Hürthle cells tumor,* 9 per cent, of the total. Some of the solid tumors contain some functioning follicles and have selective uptake; this uptake, however, is rarely enough to be of help but may be sufficient to justify investigation.

1. Indications for Therapy

Of all the patients with cancer of the thyroid, less than 10 per cent are treatable with I^{131} (1, 3). The basic indication for I^{131} therapy is a tumor which cannot be removed surgically but which can pick up, or can be induced to pick up, I^{131}.

Therapy with I^{131} is of no value as a prophylactic measure. The destruction by internal irradiation is produced primarily by beta rays with a maximum effective range of only 3 mm. The cross-fire effect of each discrete center of radiation deposited within a small tumor diminishes as the tumor diminishes in size, so that more accumulation is necessary in a tumor 1 mm. in diameter than in one 3 mm. in diameter. At cellular size, it would be impossible for a tumor to collect sufficient I^{131} to destroy itself. Even if a large mass of normal thyroid receives a destructive dose, frequently the outer 1 or 2 mm. will survive because of less cross-fire effect. From this consideration alone, the question arises whether it is possible at any time to destroy completely all thyroid tissue, especially if its I^{131} uptake is as low as it is in cancer of the thyroid.

One can rule out, for treatment with I^{131}, all patients in whom the tumor has been removed surgically and who have no clinical evidence of recurrence or metastases and all patients who have histologically proved true papillary carcinomas or undifferentiated carcinoma. There is so much overlap between follicular tumors which may be amenable to treatment and the relatively benign papillary tumors and the more malignant, undifferentiated tumors that one should not rely on the histologic appearance of a single microscopic section. In other words, one may rule out all patients with any type of malignancy in which there is no evidence anywhere of follicle formation. After these categories of patients have been eliminated, there will be left no more than 20 per cent of patients for whom investigation with the use of I^{131} will be warranted. Of these, about half will be found acceptable for treatment with I^{131} (4). King (5), from his personal experience and a review of the literature, finds that most investigators agree that 10–15 per cent of all carcinomas of the thyroid should be treated with I^{131} and that improvement will be obtained in 15–25 per cent of treated cases. Unfortunately, according to these figures, no more than 1 patient in 20 with carcinoma of the thyroid will receive any benefit from internal radiotherapy.

2. DEMONSTRATION OF UPTAKE

To determine the percentage of I^{131} uptake by a thyroid tumor, it is advisable to administer a fairly large tracer dose, which will vary from 100 to 2,000 μc., with 500 μc. as the ordinary top limit. It must be remembered that, if a large tracer dose is given to a patient routinely before a thyroidectomy or before a biopsy of the neck, a great deal of the material will be concentrated in the adjacent normal thyroid tissue, and the surgeon's fingers will receive repeated dangerous doses of radiation. A tracer dose should not be given preceding an operation in a neck that contains normal or active thyroid tissue except for a specific purpose; even then, the dose should be as small as circumstances will permit.

Uptake can be quantitatively estimated by five methods, as follows:

1. The first is directional counting over a metastatic lesion elsewhere than in the neck or over a metastatic lesion in the neck after complete ablation of the thyroid gland. For this purpose, it is best to use a well-shielded scintillation counter with a focusing collimator. The quantity of radiation per gram found in the tumor tissue will have to be estimated rather crudely from the apparent size and depth of the tumor.

2. A scintigram following ablation of the thyroid gland, using millicurie-sized tracer doses.

3. A biopsy, followed by an autoradiograph, will demonstrate uptakes down to 2 μc./gm. This method has the advantage of indicating the degree of distribution. Quantitative measurement, however, is difficult.

4. Retention of I^{131} in the tumorous tissue as calculated from urinary excretion, is the most applicable method in a patient whose thyroid gland has been completely destroyed. It does not, however, consider the total mass of the metastases. A concentration of the retained I^{131} in the malignant tissue could vary enormously with identical percentages of retention. Rawson and

his colleagues (6) have found that a urinary excretion of less than 40 per cent of a tracer dose in a thyroidectomized patient is a good indication for I^{131} therapy.

5. A large tracer dose, a biopsy, digestion of the tissue and calculation of the radioactivity per gram constitute by far the simplest and the best method, when feasible. Following a tracer dose, a generous biopsy specimen is removed and dissolved in 6N NaOH. The solution is placed in a test tube, then in a calibrated well-type scintillation counter, and assayed for radioactivity. Seidlin (7) believes that, for radioiodine to have a cancerocidal effect, a concentration of 0.03 per cent of the administered dose per gram of tissue should be demonstrated. It is certainly unlikely that any uptake below this level would be effective. It is generally conceded that the hyperplastic radiosensitive gland of the exophthalmic goiter requires a concentration of 100 μc./gm. for partial destruction. Since the effective half-life of I^{131} in cancerous tissue is probably less than in the hyperplastic thyroid, one can hardly expect smaller concentrations to be effective. At a concentration of even 0.1 per cent/gm. of tumor, a therapeutic dose of 100 mc. would be needed to deliver 100 μc./gm.

3. Increased Uptake

Total ablation of the thyroid is a prerequisite in internal radiotherapy. It has a twofold indication: to eliminate the more vigorous competitive capacity of the normal thyroid to trap the therapeutive dose, and to stimulate the tumorous tissue to greater hormone activity. A total thyroidectomy will sometimes initiate and frequently increase the uptake of metastatic follicular carcinoma (8). Rall and his co-workers (9) found that a thyroidectomy increased uptake in 60 per cent of cases; thiouracil therapy in 70 per cent; and thyroid-stimulating hormone in 31 per cent. The operative procedure of a total thyroidectomy is not a simple one and carries with it a high incidence of parathyroid tetany, as well as recurrent laryngeal nerve injury. This is particularly true if there has been a previous subtotal thyroidectomy. Ablation with I^{131} is not so quickly and completely accomplished as by surgery, but it does not require a comparably high degree of professional skill. For all practical purposes, it can be accomplished by administering a preliminary dose of 50–75 mc. and waiting an interval of 4–8 weeks.

Antithyroid therapy has been used by Rawson and his colleagues (6). In 42 patients a marked to maximum function was induced in 25 after administration of 1–1.5 gm. of thiouracil daily for 30 days to 3 years. These investigators have found it to be most beneficial in those patients who had at least some uptake in the metastases following total thyroidectomy.

Thyroid-stimulating hormone (TSH), as used by Rall and his colleagues (9), increased the uptake in 5 of 16 patients. From experimental evidence obtained from euthyroid patients, it can be assumed that a 10 unit intramuscular injection of TSH will produce the maximum increase in uptake at the end of 24 hours.

Most investigators have found that, unless the tumor has an original strong avidity for iodine, increases in the uptake obtained from antithyroid therapy and TSH are not large enough to be of clinical usefulness.

4. Dosage Regimen

Two general methods of treatment with I^{131} have been advocated in thyroid cancer. In the method usually accepted, the tumor is stimulated to its greatest functional capacity and a carefully calculated maximum dose is administered in an effort to destroy the tumor without fatality to the patient. In the second method, repeated small doses (30 mc. twice monthly) are administered empirically in the hope of destroying the tumor little by little. Serious objections have been raised against the second method because a small dose of radiation may destroy only the functional capacity of the tumor without interfering with its regenerative tendencies. Furthermore, a large dose of radiation delivered at once is more effective than when delivered fractionally. On the other hand, some follicles in a follicular or alveolar carcinoma, or even in a normal thyroid, may pick up iodine; and other follicles of an identical nature may not (1).

Uptake is known to be of irregular distribution, and the administration of a large dose does not mean total destruction. These facts make multiple doses necessary, whether they are large or small. No matter how logical or how correct is the basic contention in favor of infrequent large single doses, there remains the observation that repeated smaller doses have at times had a profound palliative effect.

Marinelli and Hill (10) found that a dose of 100 mc. of I^{131} produced 108 roentgen-equivalents-physical of general body radiation. Seidlin (4) found that the figure varied from 25 to 228 rep/100 mc. administered. Actually, because of variation in uptake by the metastases and variations in the turnover rate of the accumulated I^{131}, body radiation varies too much to predict safe radiation without a preliminary check of the blood of each patient (7). Individual doses as high as 200 mc. and total doses as high as 2,000 mc. have been given without adverse effect. However, without accurate blood I^{131} studies, a single dose should not exceed 100 mc., and the dose should not be repeated without examination for hemapoietic injury. Care should be painstaking, as the total dosage rises above 500 mc. Trunnell and his associates (11) reported a fatal case of pancytopenia following a total dosage of 638 mc. occurring a month after a single dose of 250 mc. As doses are repeated, it is imperative to watch for persistent leukopenia, which Seidlin (4) found in two patients—one with a total dosage of 1,000 mc. over an 8-month period and the other with 450 mc. in 6 months.

Pochin (12) advises the following regimen:

1. There should be total ablation of the normal thyroid by surgery or by a dose of 80 mc. of I^{131}.

2. If little or no uptake is demonstrable at tumor sites with the onset of myxedema, allow the myxedema to persist and repeat the tests for uptake in 1 or 2 months.

3. Give doses of 150 mc. at intervals initially of 6–8 weeks, but later at 6 months or 1 year, as evidence is obtained of a decrease in the remaining amount of functioning tumor tissue. The patient is given thyroxine or thyroid extract* from 48 hours after each dose until 4 weeks before the next dose.

King (5) recommends a similar routine, as follows:

1. Thyroid ablation with 50 mc. (surgical ablation is preferred).

---

* Tri-iodothyronine would be better, in that its effect begins more quickly and disappears more quickly.

2. Initial dose, 100–200 mc.
3. Subsequent doses of 100 mc. every 3–6 months until—
    a) Metastasis disappears.
    b) Metastasis uptake is zero.
    c) Hematopoiesis is depressed.
4. Total dose varies from 500 to 2,000 mc.

Catz and his associates (13) present another facet in cancer therapy, with these recommendations:

1. Surgical ablation of all accessible thyroid tissue, normal or malignant.
2. Maintenance of the patient in a euthyroid state with exogenous medication.
3. Administration of 10 units of TSH daily for 5–7 days, followed by the administration of 1–2 mc. of I^{131}.* This is followed by scintigrams of the neck and chest.
4. A therapeutic dose of 40–100 mc. if there is any evidence of collection of I^{131} by residual thyroid tissue in the neck or in metastatic sites.
5. Seven days later, repeat scintigram to verify the localization.
6. Repeat scintigrams with TSH without discontinuing thyroid or thyroxine medication.

Possible untoward effects are discussed under therapy of hyperthyroidism in Chapter 8. In general, only a few complications, other than depression of the hemapoietic system, have been encountered. A preliminary dose of 50–76 mc. may produce thyroiditis in an intact normal gland or lobe. Mild radiation sickness and transient parotitis are sometimes encountered. A localized ulcer of the urinary bladder has been reported in one patient. Amenorrhea has occurred after I^{131} therapy in three women under the age of 41. One patient died of a myeloid leukemia after I^{131} treatment of a carcinoma of the thyroid. The last three effects may or may not have been attributable to the I^{131}.

Rall and his co-workers (14) have reviewed the course of cancer of the thyroid with pulmonary metastases treated with I^{131} in 15 cases. Two patients died from what was presumed to be radia-

---

* Experimental evidence indicates that the maximum effect of TSH is obtained by a single injection of 10 units and is not increased by repeated injections.

tion pneumonitis. In 4 other patients, there was x-ray evidence of pulmonary fibrosis. Crile and Wilson (15) reported transformation of low-grade papillary carcinoma of thyroid to anaplastic carcinoma after treatment with I^{131}.

5. TECHNIQUE OF ADMINISTRATION

a) MATERIAL.—Dose, in millicuries, of sodium radioiodide (NaI^{131}) and water.

b) APPARATUS.—A list of the apparatus needed is herewith given (see Fig. 42):

> Lead shield
> Glass beaker

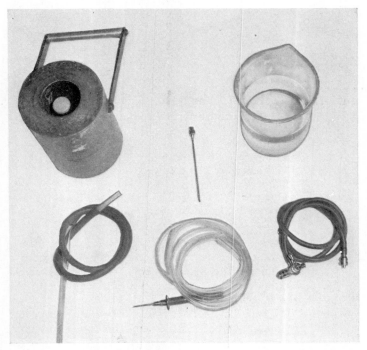

FIG. 42.—Apparatus for administration of therapeutic dose of I^{131}. (See list above and on p. 222.)

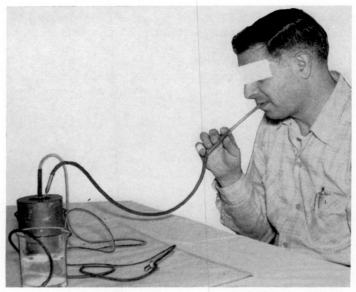

Fig. 43.—Administration of therapeutic dose of I[131].

Plastic straw
Plastic needle adaptor (B–D)
Plastic tubing, 2 ft., ⅛ in. deep
Three-way stopcock
One needle, 15 gauge, with ¾ in. shaft
One needle, 15 gauge, with 3 in. shaft
Rubber tubing, 2 ft.

c) PROCEDURE.—A procedure is described for those laboratories in which the therapeutic dose is delivered from a single container. The dose may be left in the lead shield and shipping container received from the supplier, or the dose may be transferred to the lead shield or pot as illustrated in Figure 42. In either case, the following procedure will give a minimum of radiation exposure to the personnel.

1. Place the rubber tubing in the glass beaker, which has been filled with tap water.

2. Connect the tubing to the three-way stopcock, one end of which is exposed to the air. Connect the other end to a plastic tube, which in turn should be connected to a plastic adapter to which is attached a 15 gauge needle, ¾ in. long, inserted into the therapeutic dose bottle.

3. Using remote-handling tongs, insert the other 15 gauge needle, 3 in. long, into the dose bottle; and connect, through a plastic adapter into rubber tubing, 2 ft. in length, to the patient's side, which has connected to it a plastic straw.

4. Expose the three-way stopcock to the air and have the patient suck up the radioactive material from the bottle. Then connect the three-way stopcock to the tap-water end and flush the therapeutic dose bottle with water.

This procedure holds the exposure to both personnel and patient to a minimum (Fig. 43) and is simply applied when one uses a single container bottle.

Alternative Technique of Administration of Solution NaI[131]

If several therapeutic doses are to be removed from the same vessel, a different technique will be required, as follows:

1. Place the vial in a lead container which will hold the vial rather snugly; place the container, in turn, within a lead enclosure.

2. From behind the lead, remove the stopper from the vial or bottle of NaI[131].

3. Pipette the solution out by a distant pipette, a homemade one or one of commercial variety. In either form of pipette there is a long column of air between the suction apparatus and the liquid in the pipette, which interferes with accuracy. If the tip of the pipette is inserted at a level of, say, 3 cm. below the surface of liquid in the vial and if the solution is aspirated into the pipette to the desired level, then, as the pipette is withdrawn and the pressure of 3 cm. of water is released, the amount of air in the aspirating apparatus permits the liquid in the pipette to drop to a slightly lower level. Practice may compensate for

this error, but it would be better to use a system with less potential of gaseous expansion. Absolute accuracy, fortunately, is not too important except in an investigative problem demanding it. The method is not satisfactory in measuring quantities to be diluted for use as a stock solution for tracer doses. In such a case, it is best to wait until most of the shipment has been used and then extract the remainder through a more closely coupled system.

If the pipette is viewed through a mirror, the radiation hazard to the face is reduced, but at the expense of accuracy.

4. After the therapeutic dose has been withdrawn, empty it into a small container (a ½ oz. waxed paper cup is satisfactory). A small vessel has been specified because it should remain in a portable lead container with walls ½ in. or more in thickness. A large drinking cup necessitates an exceedingly heavy container. The lead container should give protection and permit handling of the therapeutic dose at a distance.

5. Have the patient pick up the cup himself and take the drink while leaning over a sink.

6. Have the patient rinse the cup three times and then throw it into a waste receptacle. If the patient is tremulous, spillage may occur; it is then better to have him drink the dose through a glass tube or straw or place the solution into a larger vessel.

7. After the patient takes the drink, send him promptly on his way. Do not stand directly in front of the patient during any conversation, for he may spray radioactive droplets during speech. Once he has taken the drink, the patient has a tendency to talk the matter over; and the technician, considering the mission accomplished, may disregard the fact that 10 or 25 mc. of I^{131} inside the patient represents a hazard similar to 10–25 mc. in a glass beaker on an open bench.

Capsule Technique

Secondary suppliers now furnish any ordinary dose of I^{131} in capsule form, similar to the capsule form of the tracer dose. If only one patient is to be treated, it is much simpler to order the requisite amount in a capsule, which will be shipped in a small lead container. All that one need do then is to open the container, empty the capsule into a paper cup, which is in the patient's hand, and have him swallow it.

6. RESULTS

Seidlin (7) studied 65 patients with metastatic thyroid carcinoma. Of these, 13 received I^{131} therapy, with the following results: Among 6 patients still living at follow-up, 1 patient was improved somewhat and 5 were greatly improved. Of 7 who had died, 5 had shown initial improvement; 2 no improvement.

Rawson and his associates (6) reported that, of 35 treated, 10 showed sustained improvement; 10 transitory improvement; 8 were unimproved; and 7 had been treated too recently to ascertain the results.

Sheline and Miller (16) reported, in 1957, their results in the treatment of carcinoma of thyroid from 1938 to 1959. There were, in all, 124 patients; of these, 86 were investigated for possible treatment with I^{131} and 23 were selected, of which 18 completed treatment. In general, these investigators gave 100 mc. monthly as long as there was evidence of uptake. Of the 18 treated cases, 11 showed arrest or regression of the tumor.

B. INTRACAVITARY THERAPY

Intracavitary Injection of Radioactive Colloidal Gold

When colloidal radiogold (Au^{198}) is injected into a serous cavity, a large part of it becomes fixed to the serous lining; some of it is engulfed by phagocytes; and some becomes attached to the malignant cells in the fluid (17). Some gold penetrates into the tumor and into the normal tissue, and a small quantity is picked up by the blood stream or lymphatic system and deposited in the spleen and liver (18). Appreciable amounts may pass from one serous cavity into the other (19), but none is excreted in the feces or urine. The effective radiation is due largely to a beta ray of 0.38 Mev with a maximum penetration of 3.8 mm. and a half-range of 0.4 mm. There is some cancerocidal effect on the cancer cells free in the fluid and a little superficial injury to the tumor surface. There is some superficial fibrosis and some capillary injury as well. None of the pathologic changes are serious, and none account satisfactorily for the beta ray's inhibitory influence on malignant effusion.

Intracavitary injection of colloidal Au[198] for a carcinomatous effusion is intended not as a cancerocidal agent but only as a means of reducing the amount of effusion. It is indicated in patients with carcinomatosis of the pleura, peritoneum or pericardium who are in relatively good condition and who have no important symptoms except those related to fluid accumulation which requires repeated aspirations (20).

In terminal patients the injection of Au[198] is more frequently lethal than palliative. It is of little value when the abdomen is filled with large nodular masses of cancer. The effusion must be of a malignant origin, as proved by biopsy or the presence of free cancer cells. Radioactive gold has been used frequently by means of immediate postoperative abdominal instillation in patients with carcinoma of the ovary, especially in a pseudomucinous variety where there has been rupture or satellite growths.

1. DOSAGE REGIMEN

The initial maximum dose for the pleural cavity is 75 mc., and for the abdominal cavity, 150 mc. A good result was obtained (21) in one pericardial effusion with 12.2 mc. and in one with 100 mc.; there was no improvement (22) in one with 90 mc. There seems to be a more profound systemic reaction if the injection is into a relatively normal cavity (17) than into a cavity surrounded by thick fibrotic cancer. If the initial dose is not effective, subsequent doses probably should not exceed 100 mc. for the chest and 250 mc. for the abdomen. A total dose of 500 mc. necessitates considerable caution.

2. UNTOWARD REACTIONS

A systemic reaction characterized by nausea and vomiting may occur in 12–24 hours, followed by weakness and malaise for the next 2 or 3 days. There may be an adynamic ileus or at times the converse, resulting in diarrhea. Marrow depression is slight but does occur, especially with repeated large doses.

3. End Results

Recent reports and surveys (23–26) permit the following generalizations of the end results: About one third of all patients treated will be dead of the disease within 2 months. A third will have definite diminution in fluid collection from one injection. A third will obtain moderate improvement or will require repeated injections. All but a few patients will be dead of the disease within a year. There is no evidence that Au^{198} increases morbidity, nor is there any evidence that it lengthens life expectancy. It is purely a palliative agent.

4. Technique of Administration

a) MATERIAL.—Radioactive gold (Au^{198})* in the amount of 50–150 mc. will be required.

b) EQUIPMENT.—The following list comprises the necessary apparatus:

> An apparatus for intravenous injection
> Lead pot†
> Two No. 19 needles, 5 in. shaft
> Plastic needle adapter (B–D)
> One No. 19 needle, 2-in. shaft
> Polyethylene catheter (sterile), 3 ft. long, to fit
> over No. 19 needle

c) PROCEDURE.—The technique described here may be used whenever a paracentesis or a thoracentesis is performed on the patient before the administration of Au^{198}:

1. Place the patient in a supine position. Insert the polyethylene catheter through the trocar needle and then remove the trocar, leaving the sterile catheter in place, at least 6 in. within the cavity. Cross-tape the catheter in a fixed position on the patient.

2. Insert the other end of the catheter over the No. 19 needle, and connect it through the adapter and needle arrangement, as shown in Figure 44.

---

* Source: Abbott Laboratories, Oak Ridge, Tennessee.
† Source: Tracerlab, Inc., Richmond, California.

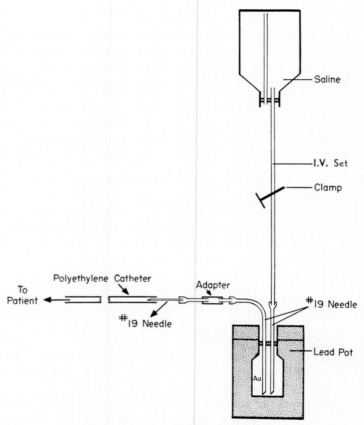

FIG. 44.—Intracavitary infusion method for Au[198].

3. Unclamp the intravenous setup. The saline solution
   will then flush through the bottle of Au[198] and into the
   patient.

   With the materials cited, this procedure will take
   between 2 and 3 minutes. Normally, from 150 to 200 cc.
   of saline solution is ample to flush the bottle containing
   the Au[198] completely.

4. Stop the infusion of the gold as soon as the solution from the container is seen to be clear.

5. Remove the polyethylene catheter from the patient and discard it, with the adapter, into a waxed paper bag. Save the needles for decontamination and future use.

6. Cross-tape the hole through which the catheter was inserted into the patient, to reduce leakage. Apply gauze bandages over this area for the absorption of possible fluid leakage.

7. Rotate the patient from side to side every 15 minutes for 1½ hours after administering the dose.

8. Complete a dosage chart for radiation safety purposes, as shown in Chapter 19 (p. 368).

Intracavitary Use of Radioactive Colloidal Chromic Phosphate

If colloidal radiochromic phosphate ($CrP^{32}O_4$) is substituted for colloidal radiogold, administration can be simplified. Since P^{32} has no gamma emission, it is a convenient isotope to handle. Its half-life of 14.3 days, combined with a beta emission of 1.7 Mev, permits considerable ionizing radiation from a relatively small amount of isotope, small enough so that it may be used on an outpatient basis. Its colloidal physiologic characteristics are similar (27) to those of Au^{198}.

1. TECHNIQUE OF ADMINISTRATION

a) DOSAGE.—The dose is approximately 7 mc., with a maximum of 20 mc. for the chest and from 10–30 mc. for the abdomen. Multiple doses up to six have been given.

b) PROCEDURE.—Administration is as follows:

1. Before the stopper is removed, shake the vial in which the material is shipped.

2. Draw up into a shielded syringe the prescribed amount of colloidal suspension. A lucite covering, ½ in. thick, will suffice.

3. Withdraw the fluid from the abdomen through a large trocar. Then pass a small catheter through the trocar,

which is removed, the catheter being left within the abdomen. The catheter must fit snugly or leakage will be troublesome.

4. Connect a 500 cc. bottle of saline solution to the catheter. After the flow has started, inject the tubing with the colloidal suspension and flush it into the abdomen. To avoid leakage from the trocar wound, the patient should be supine during the injection.

5. If necessary, after the intra-abdominal catheter has been removed, suture the trocar wound snugly.

6. Instruct the patient to move his position frequently, from upright to lying, from side to side and from front to back.

If an intrapleural injection is contemplated, aspirate the chest and inject the suspension through the same needle.

2. UNTOWARD EFFECTS AND RESULTS

Radiation sickness has been observed with doses of 15 mc., but there has been no noteworthy effect on the hemopoietic system. There is some excretion of P^{32} in the urine. It is possible—in animals, at least—to have puddling of colloidal conglomerates, with resultant excessive local reaction. The colloidal suspension is not so uniform or so stable as that of gold.

An evaluation of the clinical intracavitary use of $CrP^{32}O_4$ has been made by Jaffe (28). He injected the material intrapleurally into 30 patients with carcinomatous pleural effusion and obtained good results in about two thirds of them. He also gave intraperitoneal injections to 20 patients with carcinomatous ascites, with improvement in 12 and no improvement in 8 patients. Jacobs (29) gave it in 41 patients with pleural effusion, with good results in 60.9 per cent of the patients; and to 16 patients with carcinomatous ascites, with 31 per cent good results.

C. PROSTATE THERAPY

The incidence of cancer of the prostate has been rising in direct proportion to the prolonged survival rate. A solution to the clinical problems of occurrence, diagnosis and treatment of prostatic cancer, therefore, is more urgently needed than formerly. Inasmuch as early evidence of prostatic cancer represents one of the most frequent examples of cancer in situ, for it is usually in a relatively small area of tissue and increases within the fascial configuration of the prostatic tissues, interstitial irradiation lends itself particularly well to the destruction of this lesion.

Theoretically, if ionizing radiation could be given locally in and about the tumor, the neoplasm could be destroyed in a rather simple manner and with few side effects. At present, cancer of the prostate is being treated by interstitial injection of radiogold (Au^{198}) and radiophosphorus (P^{32}). Recent experimental work indicates that radioyttrium (Y^{91}) might be added to one or both of these substances with the hope of achieving better distribution and a possible pickup by the regional lymphatics.

The clinical results obtained from intraprostatic injection of Au^{198} have been encouraging insofar as disappearance and control of the local lesion is concerned. Gold seems to be somewhat more effective than phosphorus. This is because gold has an additional component of gamma radiation, while phosphorus emits beta radiation solely.

1. TECHNIQUE OF ADMINISTRATION

Improved techniques have almost completely overcome the early high incidence of vesicle and rectal injury accompanying both external and local treatment of the prostatic area.

Although the reports of Flocks (30) and of Burns and his associates (31) stress better results in the treatment of prostatic cancer by transvesicle and retropubic injection, it appears that such a radical procedure is unnecessary in most instances. Perineal injection, properly performed, can accomplish equally satisfactory results without the necessity of a wide suprapubic exposure of the bladder and bladder neck. The perineal method has the advantage of being a relatively minor procedure which can be repeated frequently without discomfiture or danger to the patient.

In prostate therapy, effort is directed toward overcoming the difficulties encountered in other types of radiation therapy. The interstitial injection of radioisotopes offers a possibility of positive cure in early cases and a worthwhile palliative measure even in relatively advanced instances of the disease.

a) MATERIAL.—In interstitial irradiation with radioisotopes, a solution containing the radioactive material is distributed through the tissue mass. The radioisotope must be used in a form that is insoluble in the fluids of the tissue, in order to minimize its removal from the site of injection. Inasmuch as the radiation effect results predominantly from beta particles which have a maximum range of a few millimeters in tissue, it is desirable that the particle size be small so as to provide essentially point sources of irradiation. Small particle size also aids in obtaining distribution through the tissue mass, although it may contribute to a more rapid removal of the material from the injection site. A colloidal solution of Au^{198} with particle sizes in the range of 0.003–0.007 μ has been most widely used for interstitial irradiation of the prostate. The material is inert chemically and is insoluble in tissue fluids. Radiogold decays with a half-life of 65 hours. A beta particle with a maximum energy of 0.98 Mev and gamma radiation with energies of 0.12 and 0.41 Mev are produced in the process. During the complete decay of 1 μc. of Au^{198} per gram of tissue, 76 rep are delivered by the beta particles. The exact radiation delivered by the gamma rays depends on the size of the gland, but it is ordinarily assumed to be about 10 per cent of the beta dose.

Colloidal radiogold* may be obtained commercially with specific activities of 3–15 mc./mg. The concentration of the solutions varies from 20 to 30 mc./ml. The solution is sterile and pyrogenfree.

b) APPARATUS.—Two main pieces of apparatus are required for the procedure: a device with which a measured volume of Au^{198} may be diluted with saline solution without hazardous exposure to the operator, and a shielded syringe by which the solution may be injected into the prostate.

A device† for measuring and diluting the Au^{198} without the

* Abbott Laboratories, Oak Ridge, Tennessee.
† The idea for this apparatus was originally suggested by Theodore Fields and Ervin Kaplan.

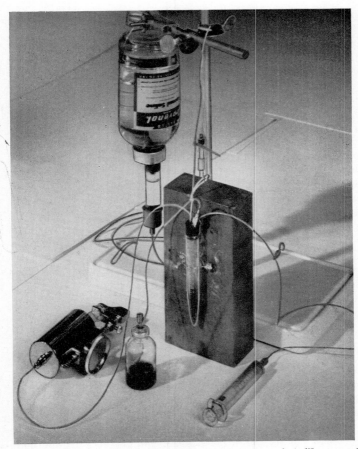

FIG. 45.—Apparatus for measurement and dilution of Au[198] removed from lead shield. (See text for description of parts.)

lead shield for protection of personnel is shown in Figure 45. It consists of a graduated 15 ml. conical centrifuge tube provided with a rubber stopper, through which pass four lengths of 0.86 mm. I.D. polyethylene tubing. One of the tubes is introduced into the bottle of Au^{198} remotely, through a short 13 gauge needle. A ¾ in. needle serves as an airway. The second tube is attached through an adapter to a bottle of normal saline solution to which has been added 150 turbidity units of hyaluronidase and 1 ml. of 1:1,000 epinephrine/100 ml. of solution. The third tube is attached by an adapter to a sterile 20 ml. syringe provided with a three-way stopcock. The side arm of the stopcock is attached to a cotton air filter. The fourth tube, which reaches to the bottom of the centrifuge tube, is used for withdrawing the diluted gold into the shielded syringe. The ampule containing the gold is placed in a lead shield with a slit through which the polyethylene tubing passes. The shield and centrifuge tube are placed in a lead shield built of 2 in. lead bricks, shown in Figure 46 and 47. A light source and concave mirror permit the graduations on the centrifuge tube and liquid level to be viewed without exposure to radiation.

All transferring of liquid is carried out without use of pressure, minimizing the possibility of contamination from failure of connections.

Before assembly, the centrifuge tube is sterilized by heat, and the rubber stopper and polyethylene tubing are sterilized by soaking in Zephiran® (1:1,000), followed by rinsing with sterile saline solution. The tubing for withdrawing the gold into the shielded syringe is wrapped in a sterile towel to maintain sterility of the exterior of the tubing and needle.

The apparatus is simple and may be fabricated in any hospital. Views of the apparatus in place in the lead shield are shown in Figures 46 and 47.

The shielded syringe shown in Figures 48 and 49 was designed by Flocks (30) and is available commercially.* It consists of a 5 ml. Luer-Lok syringe surrounded by 1.3 cm. of lead. A rack and pinion permits the required pressure to be exerted on the syringe for forcing the radioactive solution into the prostate.

---

* Mills Hospital Supply, Chicago, Illinois.

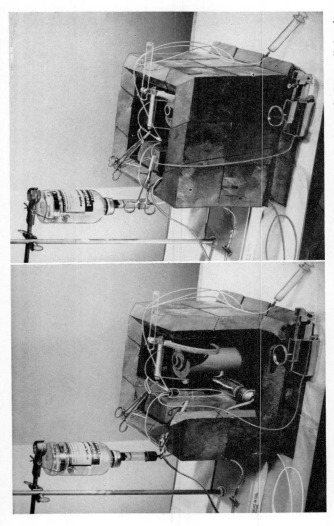

Fig. 46 (*left*).—Apparatus for measurement and dilution of Au¹⁹⁸ in place in lead shield. One wall has been removed to permit relationship of parts within the enclosure to be visualized.

Fig. 47 (*right*).—Completely assembled apparatus.

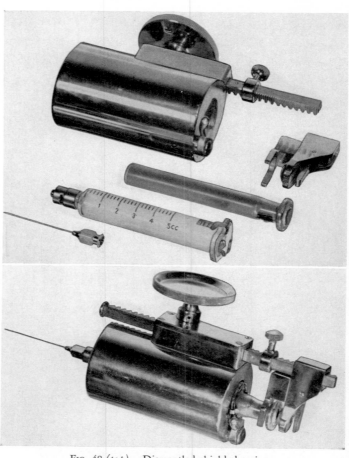

FIG. 48 (*top*).—Dismantled shielded syringe.
FIG. 49 (*bottom*).—Assembled shielded syringe.

c) Procedure for Handling Apparatus.—The technique is as given below:

1. With clamps on the tubing leading to the saline solution and to the shielded syringe, transfer the desired volume of gold into the centrifuge tube by drawing back on the plunger of the transfer syringe and reducing the pressure in the system.

2. Then clamp the tubing leading from the gold and expel the air from the transfer syringe through the side arm of the three-way stopcock.

3. Release the clamp on the tube leading to saline solution and draw into the centrifuge tube the required amount of saline solution to dilute the gold.

4. After the saline tubing has been clamped, again discharge the air from the transfer syringe through the three-way stopcock and release the clamp on the tube to the shielded syringe, which has not been attached to the syringe. Draw the air carefully through the mixture in the centrifuge tube by withdrawing the plunger on the transfer syringe. Since the tubing to the shielded syringe reaches to the bottom of the centrifuge tube, the air bubbles will mix the solution in the tube.

5. Attach the shielded syringe to the tubing and fill the syringe with the radioactive solution.

6. Expel the air from the syringe back into the tubing before removing the shielded syringe.

2. Other Dosage Schedules

In their early work, Flocks and his co-workers (30) used the following dosage schedules: for prostates weighing between 20 and 35 gm., 3 mc./gm.; from 35 to 70 gm. glands, 2 mc./gm.; from 75 to 150 gm. glands, 1 mc./gm. The largest dose was limited to 150 mc. to avoid excessive gamma irradiation of the rectum. Twenty millicuries were injected into the seminal vesicles. Subsequently the dose was reduced to 1–1.6 mc./gm. and the amount injected into the seminal vesicles reduced to 10 mc. Because results with this schedule were not so good as in the original series, these investigators advocated 2 mc./gm. for glands weighing between 20 and 60 gm. and 1 mc./gm. for larger glands, with a maximum of 150 mc.

Burns and his co-workers (31) initially used 1 mc./gm. without mention of an upper dosage limit. Later they advocated using from 0.5 to 0.7 mc./gm.

O'Conor and Bulkley (32) have used 2 mc./gm. for glands weighing up to 50 gm., and 1 mc./gm. for larger glands, with an upper limit of 150 mc.

The radioactive material is injected in a volume of 8–20 ml., depending on the size of the gland.

3. Surgical Approach

a) Suprapubic Approach.—The bladder is opened through the usual suprapubic incision, and the bladder neck and prostate are visualized intravesically. The dose required is estimated on the findings at surgery. The 22 gauge, 3 in. needle is inserted into the center of the tumor tissue and the Au[198] injected as the needle is moved throughout the tumor mass. Attempts are made to distribute the radioactive material uniformly through the tumor tissue and prostate gland. Several needle punctures are made to reach the apex and lateral lobes of the prostate. An injection of 8–10 mc. is made through a separate puncture into the region of the seminal vesicles. Care should be exercised, when injecting in this area, to prevent a spread of the material to the rectal wall. The bladder is closed rapidly by the first assistant, a suprapubic catheter being left in place.

b) Perineal Approach.—O'Conor and Bulkley (32) favor the perineal approach in most cases because it involves only a minor procedure, with little morbidity and short hospitalization. The results are comparable to those following suprapubic injection. The patient is placed in the lithotomy position; and, guided by a finger in the rectum, the operator introduces 22 gauge spinal needles through the perineum into the tumor mass. In order to obtain distribution throughout the entire mass, from two to five needles are used, depending on the size of the tumor. After all the needles are in place, 4 ml. of Au[198] are injected through each needle while it is being moved and withdrawn. A Foley catheter is left indwelling and is clamped off.

Postoperatively, the urine is collected and the bottles are sent to the radioisotope unit for assay and disposal. All dressings and linen are kept in the room, to be surveyed for radioactivity before removal.

4. RESULTS

a) DISTRIBUTION.—Little quantitative data are available on the distribution of Au^{198} after intraprostatic injection in the human being. In the dog (33) 10.5 per cent was found in the prostate a week after infiltration of the gland. Most of the remaining activity was found in the pelvis, where it apparently had been carried by direct extension along fascial planes or by the lymphatics. The regional lymph nodes were found to have appreciable activity. The Au^{198} content of the liver, spleen, marrow and lung was low.

b) RADIATION EFFECTS.—In the dog the time course of radiation effects in the prostate have been followed at intervals up to 3 months. In the early period there was an acute suppurative reaction with exudate in the glands and connective tissue. Only small areas of hemorrhage and necrosis were seen. Healing became apparent at 5 or 6 weeks, with scar formation, decrease in the number of glands and hyalinization. The difficulty of achieving uniform distribution of activity throughout the gland was quite apparent; islands of normal glandular tissue remained surrounded by areas of complete destruction.

c) CLINICAL RESULTS.—Although only fragmentary data are available regarding the course of radiation effect in man, the results would probably not differ greatly from that observed in the dog.

d) PROSTATE.—There is a rapid decrease in the size of the gland in almost all cases, often within a period of a month. There is little or no urethral or vesical irritation. Chronic bleeding and sloughing following transurethral resection for prostatic carcinoma may cease when the patients are subsequently injected with Au^{198}. On postinjection biopsy, from 20 to 30 per cent of the patients are found to have no evidence of neoplasm (32). Of 50 cases followed from 6 to 17 months, in which there was extension of the neoplasm outside the capsule of the prostate but no evidence of distant metastases, Kerr, Flocks, Elkins and

Culp (34) reported that 27 were alive and well with no evidence of disease of the prostate, and 7 were dead but had not shown evidence of prostatic disease. Among those who had shown evidence of the disease, 8 were alive and 8 were dead.

e) GASTROINTESTINAL TRACT.—Irradiation of the prostate with Au^{198} produced some degree of radiation proctitis in about a third of the cases, according to the early work of Flocks and his co-workers (30, 34). In most instances the complication was adequately handled medically, but in some patients the involvement was so severe as to require surgical intervention and a colostomy. The incidence and severity of proctitis were related to the dose injected into the prostate and seminal vesicles, and represented a major consideration in limiting the amount of radioactive material used. The more recent techniques of injection, avoiding deposition of material near the rectal wall, have almost eliminated this complication.

f) HEMOPOIETIC SYSTEM.—Although there has been a report of some degree of leukopenia occurring at various intervals following irradiation, no serious depression of marrow activity for prolonged periods has been reported following the intraprostatic injection of Au^{198}.

REFERENCES

1. Fitzgerald, P. J., and Foote, W. W., Jr.: Function of various types of thyroid carcinoma as revealed by radioautographic demonstration of radioactive iodine (I^{131}), J. Clin. Endocrinol. 9:1153, 1949.
2. Woolner, L. B., *et al.*: Panel discussion on classification and pathologic findings in thyroid carcinoma, Meeting American Goiter Association, Chicago, 1959.
3. Meckstroth, C. V., and Curtis, G. M.: Criteria for therapy of malignant thyroid lesions with I^{131}, A.M.A. Arch. Surg. 67:187, 1953.
4. Seidlin, S. M.: Radioiodine in treatment of metastatic thyroid carcinoma, M. Clin. North America 36:1, 1952.
5. King, E. R.: Present status of radioiodine in thyroid disease, M. Ann. District of Columbia 25:473, 1956.
6. Rawson, R. W.; Rall, J. E., and Robbins, J.: Uses and misuses of radioactive iodine in treatment of cancer of thyroid, A.M.A. Arch. Int. Med. 92:299, 1953.
7. Seidlin, S. M.: Blood radioiodine concentration and blood radiation dosage during I^{131} therapy for metastatic cancer, J. Clin. Endocrinol. 12:1197, 1952.
8. Dobyns, B. M., and Maloof, F.: Study and treatment of 119 cases of

carcinoma of thyroid with radioactive iodine, J. Clin. Endocrinol. 11:1323, 1951.

9. Rall, J. E., *et al.:* Use of thiouracil in treatment of metastatic carcinoma of thyroid with radioiodine, J. Clin. Endocrinol. 11:1273, 1951.

10. Marinelli, L., and Hill, R. F.: Radiation dosimetry in treatment of functional thyroid carcinoma with I^{131}, Radiology 55:494, 1950.

11. Trunnell, J. B., *et al.:* Treatment of metastatic thyroid cancer with radioactive iodine: Credits and debits, J. Clin. Endocrinol. 9:1138, 1949.

12. Pochin, E. E.: Place of radioactive iodine in treatment of thyroid disease, Postgrad. M. J. 33:317, 1957.

13. Catz, B., *et al.:* Treatment of cancer of thyroid postoperative with suppressive thyroid medication, radioactive iodine, and thyroid-stimulating hormone, Cancer 12:371, 1959.

14. Rall, J. E., *et al.:* Radiation pneumonitis and fibrosis; complication of radioiodine treatment of pulmonary metastases from cancer of thyroid, J. Clin. Endocrinol. 17:1263, 1957.

15. Crile, G., Jr., and Wilson, D. H.: Transformation of low grade papillary carcinoma of thyroid to anaplastic carcinoma after treatment with radioiodine, Surg., Gynec. & Obst. 108:557, 1959.

16. Sheline, G. E., and Miller, E. R.: Studies with radioiodine: Evaluation of radioiodine treatment of carcinoma of thyroid, Radiology 69:527, 1957.

17. Andrews, G. A., *et al.:* Intracavity colloidal radiogold in treatment of effusions caused by malignant neoplasms, Ann. Surg. 137:375, 1953.

18. ———, ———, and Kniseley, R. M.: Metabolism and distribution of colloidal Au^{198} injected into serous cavities for treatment of effusions associated with malignant neoplasms, Cancer 6:294, 1953.

19. Cowan, I. J., *et al.:* Transport of radioactive colloidal gold between serous cavities, Surg., Gynec. & Obst. 98:721, 1954.

20. Rose, R. G.; Osborne, M. P., and Stevens, W. B.: Intracavitary administration of radioactive colloidal gold, New England J. Med. 247:663, 1952.

21. Bachman, K. P., *et al.:* Radioactive gold instilled intrapericardially: Report of a case, Ann. Int. Med. 40:811, 1954.

22. Seaman, W. B.; Sherman, A. I., and Bonebrake, M.: Radioactive gold in treatment of malignant effusions, J.A.M.A. 153:630, 1953.

23. Weed, J. C., and Borrazal, D. F.: Management of ovarian carcinoma in 123 patients, with particular emphasis on prophylactic use of radioactive gold, South. M. J. 52:278, 1959.

24. Hahn, F. F.; Meneeley, G. R., and Carother, E. L.: Use of gold and silver-coated radioactive gold colloids in palliation of ascites and pleural effusion, Brit. J. Radiol. 31:242, 1958.

25. Seal, S. H., *et al.:* Treatment of malignant effusions with radioactive

colloidal gold (Au[198]): Review of 66 cases, Am. J. Obst. & Gynec. 75:1027, 1958.

26. Fickhardt, T.; Jacobs, E. L., and Savage, D. J.: Colloidal radiogold in malignant effusions and early ovarian carcinoma, South African M. J. 32:5, 1958.

27. McCormick, J. B., *et al.:* Tissue distribution of injected radioactive colloidal chromic phosphate (CrP[32]O$_4$), A.M.A. Arch. Path. 58:187, 1954.

28. Jaffe, H. L.: Interstitial use of radioactive chromic phosphates in therapy: Symposium: Radioisotopes in medicine (Oak Ridge, Tenn.: Institute of Nuclear Studies, September 1953).

29. Jacobs, M. L.: Radioactive colloidal chromic phosphate to control pleural effusion and ascites, J.A.M.A. 166:597, 1958.

30. Flocks, R. H.: Treatment of carcinoma of the prostate, J. Urol. 70:491, 1953.

31. Burns, E.; Judalgo, J. U., and Nieset, R.: Radioactive gold in the treatment of advanced carcinoma of the prostate and bladder: Preliminary results in 24 cases, J. Louisiana State M. Soc. 105:99, 1953.

32. O'Conor, V. J., and Bulkley, G. J.: Private communication.

33. Cooper, J. A. D.; Bulkley, G. J., and O'Conor, V. J.: Intraprostatic injection of radioactive colloids: I. Distribution and excretion following injection in the dog, J. Urol. 71:624, 1954.

34. Kerr, H. D., *et al.:* The treatment of moderately advanced carcinoma of the prostate with radioactive gold, Am. J. Roentgenol. 69:969, 1953.

CHAPTER 11

Cardiac Therapy

THE RELATIONSHIP BETWEEN hyperthyroidism and myocardial and coronary insufficiency has long been known. Blumgart and his co-workers have elaborated the rationale for treating the euthyroid intractable cardiac patient by thyroidectomy. The cardiac output is geared to metabolic demand. In the euthyroid person the circulatory demand may exceed the ability of an impaired myocardium or an atherosclerotic coronary tree to respond to the peripheral circulatory need. By inducing a hypothyroid state the cardiac output is decreased along with the speed of circulation, the pulse rate and the circulating blood volume. If sufficient cardiac reserve remains, it may meet the lowered requirements in the decreased metabolic state of hypothyroidism.

Surgical extirpation of the thyroid gland was attempted in chronic cardiac patients about 20 years ago but was never generally adopted because such patients were poor surgical risks. With the advent of antithyroid drugs, interest in a medical approach was reawakened, and it has been further stimulated by the availability of radioiodine (I^{131}).

A. MATERIAL

With proper dosage of I^{131}, euthyroid patients may be made effectively hypothyroid with little morbidity and low mortality. See Chapters 10, 14 and 15 for further details on materials and apparatus.

B. SELECTION OF PATIENTS

The cardiac patient most likely to show improvement from I^{131} destruction of thyroid function should satisfy several criteria, as follows: (1) The patient in congestive heart failure must evidence some cardiac reserve by an ability to improve under intensive conservative therapy or while at rest. (2) The clinical state of angina or congestive failure should be well stabilized, preferably over a 6-month period. (3) It is highly desirable for the therapist, or a close associate who is familiar with the therapist's criteria for selection of patients, to have observed the patient for a period of several months. Those patients with rapidly progressing heart disease will prove disappointing because they may not survive the period between therapy and the onset of hypothyroidism.

Knowledge of the level of thyroid function is a prerequisite for calculating I^{131} dosage; I^{131} pickup by the thyroid should exceed 12 per cent in 24 hours. The basal metabolic rate should be above minus 10 per cent. The patient with heart disease who is already hypothyroid cannot be expected to benefit if a small decrease in thyroid function results in myxedema. Pretreatment evaluation should be comprehensive to substantiate both the diagnosis and the status of the patient. Co-operation of the patient is essential, for refusal of follow-up substitution therapy with desiccated thyroid may result in myxedema in addition to the existing cardiac condition.

C. DETERMINATION OF DOSAGE OF RADIOIODINE

The amount of I^{131} necessary to destroy effectively the thyroid gland in euthyroid patients is approximately 40,000 rep/gm. tissue, although the sensitivity to radiation may vary widely and cannot be predicted. The ability of the thyroid to concentrate I^{131} must be determined by thyroid tracer study (see Chapter 1). The effective half-life of I^{131} in the thyroid need not be ascertained, although this is academically desirable. Table 27, which gives the approximate dosage for varying degrees of concentration of I^{131}, uses a thyroid of 25 gm. as normal.

TABLE 27.—Approximate Dosage of I¹³¹ in Millicuries to Deliver 40,000 Rep/Gm. Tissue to the Normal-Sized Thyroid Gland

Percentage Concentration in Thyroid in 24 Hours	Total Single Dosage I¹³¹ in Mc.	or	Dosage I¹³¹ Mc. per Week for 3 Weeks*
15	44		20
20	33		18
25	27		16
30	22		14
35	20		12
40	16.5		10

* Increased total dosage based on decreased pickup of second and third doses.

D. ADMINISTRATION OF RADIOIODINE

The total amount of I^{131} that can be expected to be effective is noted in Table 27. It is not desirable to give the total dosage at one time. A too rapid destruction of the thyroid gland will lead to temporary hypermetabolism and a reasonable incidence of radiation thyroiditis. The incidence will be decreased by using the weekly dosage schedule. Retention of the I^{131} of the second and third dose is depressed by the initial treatment.

E. SIDE EFFECTS

Thyroiditis and transient hypermetabolism are the most frequent side effects resulting from the use of I^{131}. Thyroiditis may be adequately treated in most instances by ice-bag application and minor analgesics. Any observed depression of hematopoiesis is of minor nature.

F. PATIENT'S COURSE AFTER THERAPY

A gradual decrease of the patient's metabolic rate can be expected over a period of 2–6 months if therapy is effective. The early signs of myxedema may become apparent: increase in weight, puffiness about the eyes, dryness of the skin and hair, voice changes, lethargy, paresthesias and arthralgias of the extremities. Before the development of myxedema the symptoms and signs of angina and congestive failure usually become somewhat alleviated. If improvement is immediate or too rapid, a psychogenic factor must be considered.

G. MAINTENANCE ON THYROID

At the early signs of myxedema the patient should receive daily doses of desiccated thyroid, starting with ⅛ grain per day. The dosage of thyroid may be gradually increased if it is necessary to maintain the patient at an optimal level between the myxedema level and the level at which the cardiac symptoms would be troublesome. This optimum level is ordinarily secured when the basal metabolic rate is maintained at about minus 25. Securing this level takes skill on the part of the clinician and may not be possible at all in some instances. If the patient is receiving desiccated thyroid, metabolic status should be evaluated by determining the basal metabolic rate and serum cholesterol levels.

When little clinical improvement is noted or signs of myxedema do not appear, a thyroid function study of I^{131} uptake should be repeated 3 months after the last treatment. The course of I^{131} therapy is repeated if indicated. Dosage is determined on the basis of the current I^{131} uptake.

H. RESULTS

Blumgart and his associates (8) have presented the results of treatment with I^{131} in 720 cases of angina pectoris and 350 cases of congestive heart failure. In angina pectoris patients, 40 per cent of the results were classified as excellent, 35 per cent as good and 25 per cent as not worthwhile. Of the cases of congestive heart failure, 23 per cent of the results were excellent, 38 per cent were good and 39 per cent not worthwhile. An excellent result is defined thus ". . . the patient is markedly improved over pre-treatment status, with either no recurrence of symptoms or a marked decrease in the frequency and severity of angina pectoris or congestive failure, despite markedly increased activity." A good result is defined: ". . . definite improvement with a decrease in frequency and severity of attacks of angina pectoris or congestive failure on the same or increased activity as before treatment" (8).

REFERENCES

1. Ben-Asher, S.: Further observations on the treatment of the anginal syndrome with thiouracil, Am. Heart J. 33:490, 1947.
2. Blumgart, H. L.: The velocity of blood flow in health and disease: The velocity of blood flow in man and its relation to other measurements of the circulation, Medicine 10:1, 1951.
3. ————, and Freedberg, A. S.: Lewis A. Conner Memorial Lecture: The heart and the thyroid, with particular reference to I¹³¹ treatment of heart disease, Circulation 6:222, 1952.
4. ————; ————, and Buka, R. B.: Treatment of euthyroid cardiac patients by producing myxedema with radioactive iodine, Proc. Soc. Exper. Biol. & Med. 67:190, 1948.
5. ————, and Kurland, G. S.: Hypothyroidism produced by radioactive iodine (I¹³¹) in the treatment of euthyroid patients with angina pectoris and congestive failure: Early results in various types of cardiovascular disease and associated pathologic states, Circulation 1:1105, 1950.
6. ————; Freedberg, A. S., and Kurland, G. S.: Treatment of incapacitated euthyroid cardiac patients by producing hypothyroidism with radioactive iodine, New England J. Med. 245:83, 1951.
7. ————; ————, and ————: Hypercholesterolemia, myxedema and atherosclerosis, Am. J. Med. 14:665, 1953.
8. ————; ———— and ————: The treatment of incapacitated euthyroid cardiac patients with radioactive iodine, Proc. 103d Annual Meeting A.M.A., San Francisco, June, 1954.
9. ————; Gargill, S. L., and Gilligan, D. R.: Studies on the velocity of blood flow: XIII. The circulatory response to thyrotoxicosis, J. Clin. Invest. 9:69, 1930.
10. ————, ———— and ————: Studies on the velocity of blood flow: XIV. The circulation in myxedema with a comparison of the velocity of blood flow in myxedema and thyrotoxicosis, J. Clin. Invest. 9:91, 1930.
11. ————; Levine, S. A., and Berlin, D. D.: Congestive heart failure and angina pectoris: The therapeutic effect of thyroidectomy on patients without clinical or pathologic evidence of thyroid toxicity, Arch. Int. Med. 51:866, 1933.
12. ————, et al.: Therapeutic effect of total ablation of normal thyroid on congestive heart failure and angina pectoris: III. Early results in various types of cardiovascular disease and coincident pathologic states without clinical or pathologic evidence of thyroid toxicity, Arch. Int. Med. 52:165, 1933.

13. Freedberg, A. S., *et al.:* The treatment of euthyroid cardiac patients with intractable angina pectoris and congestive failure with radioactive iodine, J. Clin. Endocrinol. 10:1270, 1950.
14. Hollander, G., and Mandelbaum, H.: The treatment of angina pectoris with propylthiouracil, Ann. Int. Med. 28:1150, 1948.
15. Jaffe, H. L., *et al.:* Radioiodine in treatment of advanced heart disease: End results in one hundred patients, J.A.M.A. 151:716, 1953.
16. Kurland, G. S.; Schneckloth, R. E., and Freedberg, A. S.: The heart in I[131] induced myxedema: Comparison of the roentgenographic and electrocardiographic findings before and after the induction of myxedema, New England J. Med. 249:215, 1953.
17. Parsons, W. H., and Purks, W. K.: Total thyroidectomy for heart disease, Ann. Surg. 105:722, 1937.
18. Raab, W.: Thiouracil treatment of angina pectoris: Rationale and results, J.A.M.A. 128:249, 1945.
19. Schoenwald, G.: Treatment of angina pectoris by reduction of basal metabolism, Brit. M. J. 1:251, 1948.
20. Wolferth, C. C.; Chamberlain, R. H., and Mead, J. J.: Radioactive iodine in the treatment of angina pectoris, Pennsylvania M. J. 54:352, 1951.

CHAPTER 12

External Beta Radiation with a Strontium-90 Applicator

SOURCES OF BETA RAYS, such as radium, radon and radium D and E, have been used in external radiation therapy for almost half a century. With the development of nuclear reactors during recent years, large numbers of artificial radioactive substances have become available. Many difficulties in obtaining and handling such sources have been overcome, and a wider use of external beta radiation is to be expected. Beta rays penetrate only a few millimeters of tissue, and therefore their effectiveness in external radiation therapy is confined to superficial lesions, particularly to those of the skin and cornea (1).

A strontium-90 beta-ray applicator was first designed and described by Friedell, Thomas and Krohmer (2), of Western Reserve University in Cleveland, Ohio, in 1950. Strontium-90 was selected because of its long half-life of 25 years, the sufficient energy of the beta particle, the absence of any accompanying gamma radiation and the ease of manipulation of this source.

Friedell and his co-workers (3) emphasized that, in order to use the applicator effectively, certain principles established in radiation therapy should serve as guidance. This applied to physical, as well as to radiobiologic, considerations. Dosages should be expressed in roentgen equivalents (rep) and not in millicuries per second. Other physical factors, such as strength of source, treatment time, field size and areas, number of treatments, and surface and depth dose, should be known to the operator and recorded. The dose should be recorded according to area treated. Recording as "total dose" the addition of doses received by several areas is meaningless.

In considering the radiobiologic factors, it should be kept in mind that the erythema threshold of the Sr[90] applicator is approximately 325 rep. Skin erythema studies with the Phillips contact tube, radioruthenium (Ru[106]), Ra D and E, and Sr[90] resulted in comparable reactions despite the different quality of radiation (3). Studies of the skin erythema as a base for biologic calibration seem more logical than studies of the minimal inflammatory reaction of the animal eye, which, according to Wilson (4), is observed after approximately 35,000 rep. Friedell (3) pointed out that "the skin studies help in relating the beta radiation dosage used for eye conditions to radiation dosage used in general therapeutics."

The depth dose for the Sr[90] applicator is shown in Table 28.

TABLE 28.—DEPTH DOSE FOR SR[90] APPLICATOR

Depth	Per Cent	Depth	Per Cent
0 mm.	100	3 mm.	9
1 mm.	41	4 mm.	4
2 mm.	19	5 mm.	1

In determining therapeutic doses in roentgen equivalents and planning a treatment program for a given case, one should be aware of the underlying radiobiologic factors, primarily the age of the process and its location. It is well known that young and growing tissue cells are more radiosensitive than mature and well-differentiated cells and that a deep-seated lesion will require larger doses to the surface because of the rapid attenuation of the beta radiation.

A. MATERIAL

Strontium is an alkaline earth metal. Four stable isotopes are known: Sr[84, 86, 87, 88]. The atomic weight of thirteen known radioactive isotopes of Sr ranges from 81 to 97. These isotopes are fission products and are also produced in the cyclotron by the bombardment of Sr metal or oxide.

Strontium-89, with a half-life of 55 days, is widely used in biologic research; it is a pure beta emitter with a maximum energy of 1.52 Mev. Strontium-90 has a half-life of 25 years; it emits a beta particle with a maximum energy of 0.65 Mev. It decays to yttrium-90, which emits a beta particle with a maximum energy of 2.16 Mev. Although yttrium-90 has a half-life of 60 hours and decays to the stable zirconium, in the applicator both radioactive elements are in equilibrium, so that the penetrating radiation is that of yttrium-90 beta particles.

B. APPARATUS

A 40 mc. applicator,* delivering 38 rep/sec., was used. The applicator, a beta-emitting plaque, contains the nuclides Sr^{90} in equilibrium with Yt^{90}. The protective cover of 100 mg./cm.^{2} absorbs 97 per cent of the beta particles of Sr^{90} and 40 per cent of the beta particle of Yt^{90}. Because of this filtration, the Yt spectrum is actually almost pure, with a maximum energy of 2.16 Mev.

The applicator (Fig. 50) has a shaft 6¾ in. long with a circular Plexiglas protective shield that is 4 in. in diameter and ¼ in. thick. The plaque has an outside diameter of 12.7 mm. and an active diameter of 7.8 mm. It is covered by 2 mils of stainless steel and 10 mils of aluminum and is hermetically sealed.

The Sr^{90} applicator may be used only by applicants approved by the United States Atomic Energy Commission: "The physician must be a qualified therapeutic radiologist or a qualified specialist in ophthalmology or dermatology (diploma of the appropriate board will be accepted as evidence of such qualification), with a minimum of three years' experience as a therapeutic radiologist or a specialist in ophthalmology or dermatology. Such experience must include the use of beta rays or soft x-rays in the treatment of superficial lesions, and the applicant must furnish evidence of training and experience in beta-ray dosimetry."

Manufacturers supply the user with an instruction manual containing a certificate of the output of the applicator in roentgen equivalents at the time of purchase, a radioautography of the

* Manufactured by Tracerlab, Inc., Richmond, California, and by Technical Operations, Inc., Arlington, Massachusetts.

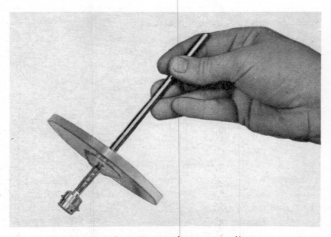

FIG. 50.—Strontium-90 beta-ray applicator.

plaque and a statement that there is no detectable leak of activity to the exterior. Every 12 months the applicator has to be sent to the manufacturer for remeasurement of the surface dosage rate, for inspection for leakage and for a renewal of the certificate.

C. PROCEDURE

The procedure is simple. However, certain rules should be strictly followed in order to assure protection to the operator, the patient and the personnel and to guarantee the delivery of a given dose to the selected area. The following preparations are recommended:

a) APPLICATOR:

    1. Remove the applicator from the shield housing. Hold it with one hand at the stem and direct the source away from the person at all times.

    2. Clean the applicator. Prepare a tray with three sterile gauze pads: one saturated with 70 per cent alcohol; the second with normal saline solution; the third dry. The

surface of the plaque should be thoroughly brought in contact with these pads, in the order described.

3. Place the applicator into the upright auxiliary shield housing (Fig. 51).

4. Have a chart prepared, giving the time required for

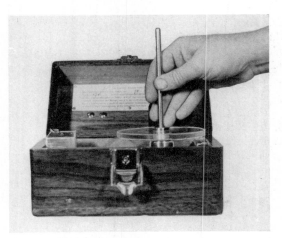

FIG. 51.—Strontium-90 beta-ray applicator placed in upright auxiliary shield housing.

from 100 to 1,000 rep surface dose, and from 1,000 to 10,000 rep.

b) OTHER INSTRUMENTS:

1. Have a sterilized eye speculum ready for use.

2. Have an assistant help with a stop watch to assure proper timing.

3. If an eye speculum cannot be used, employ a long tongue depressor to elevate the upper eyelid or to lower the lower eyelid. The tongue depressor may be lengthened by using two wooden tongue depressors overlapping 1 in. at the ends and fastened together by adhesive tape.

4. Have a good light source available—either a flashlight

or a lamp—in order to assure proper positioning of the plaque.

c) PATIENT.—The patients should be instructed to keep both eyes open during the time of treatment. The nontreated eye should be held fixed at a selected object to assure proper radiation of a selected field. The patients should be examined with the slit lamp and ophthalmoscope. If more than one field has to be treated, it is advisable to divide the globe of the eye into four quarters and treat at 3, 6, 9 and 12 o'clock with the limbus as center.

1. Have the patient lie on a treatment table.
2. Anesthetize the eye with 0.5 per cent pontocaine solution and wait until it has taken effect.
3. Insert the eye speculum.
4. Remove the applicator from the auxiliary shield housing and bring the surface of the plaque in direct, but gentle, contact with the area to be treated, holding the applicator with one hand at the stem and supporting the elbow with the other hand, in order to secure a steady positioning.
5. After treatment has been terminated, clean the source again, as described, and place it into the housing.
6. Remove the eye speculum.

Good records, including progress notes, are essential. Patients with eye disturbances should be treated in consultation with the ophthalmologist.

d) OTHER CONDITIONS.—In cases of treatment of other than eye lesions, such as small superficial tumors of the skin and mucous membranes, the plaque should be brought into direct contact with the lesion. No special shielding is required.

D. RESULTS

At the Cook County Hospital, Chicago, Radiation Center, in co-operation with the Eye Department, a total of 80 lesions on 77 patients, were treated during a 3-year period. In general, the suggestions of Friedell and his co-workers (1, 2, 3) were followed with regard to indications, treatment technique and dosages. The treatments were fractionated either once or twice a week. The single dose varied from a minimum of 600 rep to a maximum of 2,000 rep.

It is beyond the scope of this manual to detail the different

TABLE 29.—EVALUATION OF RESULTS

DIAGNOSIS	NO. OF CASES	AVG. TO-TAL DOSE IN REP	DOUBT-FUL	NO CHANGE	RESULTS		
					Fair	Good	Excel.
Postoperative pterygium ..	33	5,200	2	..	2	2	27
Corneal vascularizations ..	20	6,200	3	..	1	11	5
Episcleritis	5	4,200	..	1	1	..	3
Postoperative granuloma ..	4	8,400	..	..	..	..	4
Keratitis	4	7,200	2	..	..	1	1
Postoperative corneal transplants	2	6,000	..	..	..	2	..
Port-wine marks	2	2,750	..	2	..	..	..
Keloid scars	2	7,000	..	..	..	..	2
Epithelial downgrowth	2	6,500	..	2	..	..	..
Phlyctenulosis	2	1,500	1	..	..	1	..
Tuberculous keratitis	1	8,000	..	..	..	..	1
Vernal catarrh	1	6,000	..	..	..	..	1
Pterygium	1	6,000	..	..	..	..	1
Pseudopterygium	1	6,000	..	..	..	..	1
Total	80	....	8	5	4	17	46

conditions suitable for beta radiation. For further information on the subject, reference may be made to the bibliographical references at the end of the chapter.

E. DISCUSSION OF EXPERIENCE

a) POSTOPERATIVE PTERYGIUM.—Surgery followed by beta irradiation has been called the treatment of choice in this condition. The first treatment should be given from 4 to 6 days after surgery. Excellent healing of wounds has followed this form of treatment, with no recurrences. Lenticular changes which could have been due to irradiation have not been observed.

b) CORNEAL VASCULARIZATIONS.—The results of beta irradiation depend greatly on the age of the blood vessels and their location; the best results are seen in the young and growing vessels. It is difficult to obliterate long-standing vascularizations even with high dosages.

c) EPISCLERITIS.—Patients with episcleritis may profit from radiation therapy.

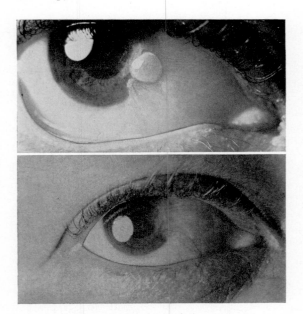

FIG. 52 (*top*).—Postoperative granuloma before treatment.

FIG. 53 (*bottom*).—Postoperative granuloma after beta radiation (five months after last treatment). Total dose to surface, 10,000 rep (five treatments, one each week, 2,000 rep each). Total dose to base of tumor, 4,000 rep.

d) POSTOPERATIVE GRANULOMA.—Granulomas following surgery respond well, and no recurrences have been observed after beta irradiation. About 4,000 rep should be delivered to the base of the granuloma. Flattening of the lesions will usually begin from 2 to 3 weeks after the last treatment (Figs. 52 and 53).

e) POSTOPERATIVE CORNEAL TRANSPLANTS.—Postoperative

corneal transplants heal better, and vascularization of the transplant can be prevented, if external beta irradiation is given in time—if possible, not later than 2 weeks after surgery.

f) PORT-WINE MARKS.—Port-wine marks do not respond sufficiently to justify beta irradiation.

g) KELOID SCARS.—If keloid scars are small and can be treated soon after surgery, they are suitable for treatment, particularly in the region of the sclera, conjunctiva and eyelids.

h) EPITHELIAL DOWNGROWTH.—Beta irradiation is not recommended for epithelial downgrowth after cataract operations, because of the rapid fall-off of the dose. In these cases, contact irradiation offers promising results.

i) PHLYCTENULOSIS, TUBERCULOUS KERATITIS, VERNAL CATARRH AND PTERYGIUM.—Cases of phlyctenulosis, tuberculous keratitis, vernal catarrh and pterygium have been treated with some success by others. The authors have had only one case of each type and in each the results were excellent.

j) SUPERFICIAL MALIGNANCIES.—Because of the low depth dose of the Sr^{90} applicator, the Philips contact tube is preferred for superficial malignancies of the cornea or sclera.

REFERENCES

1. Friedell, H. L.; Thomas, C. I., and Krohmer, J. S.: Beta-ray application to the eye, Am. J. Ophth. 33:525, 1950.
2. ———, ——— and ———: Description of an Sr^{90} beta-ray applicator and its use on the eye, Am. J. Roentgenol. 65, 2:232, 1951.
3. ———, ——— and ———: An evaluation of the clinical use of a strontium^{90} beta-ray applicator with a review of the underlying principles, Am. J. Roentgenol. 71, 1:25, 1954.
4. Wilson, F. M.: Applicators for beta irradiation of eye: Review and comparison, Am. J. Ophth. 35:645, 1952.
5. Candlin, F. T., and Levine, M. H.: The use of beta radiation on corneal lesions in the dog, N. Am. Veterinarian 33:632, 1952.
6. Catcott, E. J.; Tharp, V. L., and Johnson, L. E.: Beta ray therapy in ocular diseases of animals, J. Am. Vet. M. A. 122, 912:172, 1953.
7. Hughes, W. F., Jr.: Beta radiation therapy in ophthalmology, Tr. Am. Ophth. Soc. 50:469, 1953.
8. Krohmer, J. S.: Physical measurements on various beta-ray applicators, Am. J. Roentgenol. 66, 5:791, 1951.
9. Wilson, F. M., and Wilson, J. W.: Radioactive strontium therapy of the eye, A.M.A. Arch. Ophth. 48:686, 1952.
10. Wilson, F. M.: Sr^{90} beta irradiation of the eye, Quart. Bull. Indiana Univ. M. Center 13:91, 1952.

PART III

PLANNING AND OPERATING
THE RADIOISOTOPE LABORATORY

CHAPTER 13

Chronologic and Physics Review

A MODEST AMOUNT of chronologic and physics background material is presented here for a better understanding and appreciation of the described techniques. The reader is directed to the references for a thorough and exhaustive coverage of the subjects.

A. CHRONOLOGIC REVIEW

In the period from 1896 to 1939 the following noteworthy advances became known and served as the basis for the future use of radioactive materials.

1. The atom was described as consisting of a nucleus surrounded by electrons. The latter determined the chemical properties of the nucleus, and the nucleus seemed immune to any external forces.

2. Some atoms, particularly those above lead in the periodic table, were found to have nuclei which spontaneously and randomly emitted energy in particular ways. Some emitted electrons (called "beta particles"), and others emitted heavier particles ("alpha particles"). The latter were identified in charge and mass with the helium nuclei. With both, very penetrating radiations, called "gamma rays," were emitted. These were found to be uncharged and similar to radio waves but of much shorter wavelength.

3. The phenomenon of nuclear disintegration became firmly established. It was found possible to change the nature of stable nuclei by firing alpha particles or accelerated hydrogen nuclei (protons) into target materials.

4. Some of these nuclear reactions resulted in the formation of artificial radioactivities. It was found that bombardment of high-energy particles from accelerators could make many targets and materials radioactive.

5. Some nuclear reactions caused the formation of an uncharged particle called a "neutron" (mass approximately equal to a proton). This particle did not exist long because it, in turn, traveled until it hit some nucleus and caused another nuclear reaction.

6. It was soon discovered that most elements absorbed neutrons and became radioactive.

7. Fission (disintegration) of uranium by neutrons was discovered, the product of which is a lot of energy, about 2½ neutrons/fission and radioactive isotopes of many lighter elements. These extra neutrons enable a chain reaction to be maintained and form the basis of a nuclear reactor. Targets and materials can be placed into this reactor to make artificial radioactive elements (radioisotopes), as described above (paragraph 4). The obvious diagnostic and therapeutic techniques followed, in which chemicals were utilized, tagged with elements emitting radiation.

It is interesting to reflect that approximately fifty years elapsed between the first studies with radioactivity by Becquerel to the first clinical applications of radioisotopes other than radium. The enormous impetus given studies in nuclear physics in the 1940's by arms development caused a similar increase in medical applications of nuclear physics. Radioisotopes produced by the bombardment of accelerated protons or deuterons from the cyclotron were the first radiochemicals employed.

Some of the earlier and more important studies of radioiodine (I^{131}) were made by Hamilton and Soley in 1939 on the use of I^{131} for iodine metabolism; by Hertz and Roberts in 1942 on the application of I^{131} in the therapy of Graves' disease; by Blumgart in 1948 in the treatment of cardiac patients by producing myxedema with I^{131}; and by Seidlin and Marinelli in 1945 in the treatment of adenocarcinoma of the thyroid with I^{131}.

The medical applications of radiophosphorus (P^{32}) were pioneered by J. H. Lawrence in 1940 in his report on the use of P^{32} in the treatment of leukemia and polycythemia; by Kenny in 1942 on the use of radioactive chromic phosphate colloid for intracavitary application; and by B. Selverstone in 1948 on the use of P^{32} for the localization of intracranial tumors at surgery.

Paul Hahn pioneered (1945) in the therapeutic use of radioactive colloidal gold, and in 1948 W. G. Myers reported on the use of radiocobalt (Co^{60}) in various forms for therapeutic purposes. Other diagnostic and therapeutic applications were also begun: brain tumor localization studies by G. Moore in 1948, metabolism of radioiron by Paul Hahn and his co-workers in 1938, and the rates of absorption of radiosodium in normal human subjects by J. Hamilton in 1937.

B. ATOMIC STRUCTURE

The atom, as depicted by Bohr and others, consists of a nucleus around which a number of negatively charged particles revolve. These particles, called "electrons," move in certain orbits around the nucleus. Any change in the normal location of these electrons will cause either absorption or emission of electromagnetic energy (e.g., light, x-rays). The orbits are divided into subgroups, called "shells," which are labeled K, L, M, . . . , in the order of increasing distance from the nucleus. They contain a maximum number of electrons in each shell. The K level contains a maximum of 2 electrons; the L level, 8 electrons; and succeeding levels hold as many as 32 electrons. The electrons in the outermost shell are called the *valence electrons;* these determine the chemical behavior of the atom. Atoms having as many as 101 electrons have been discovered or artificially produced.

The nucleus contains positively charged protons equal in number and charge to the number of negative electrons, resulting in an atom with no net charge. The proton has a mass 1,840 times that of the electron, or 1.68×10^{-24} gm., so that practically all of the mass of an atom is concentrated in the nucleus. In addition, all nuclei (except hydrogen) contain uncharged particles ("neutrons") of mass slightly larger than that of the proton. The attraction of these particles for each other is important in making ordinary nuclei stable against the highly repulsive electrical forces of the protons.

Atoms Grouped According to Number of Outer (Valence) Electrons

	I	II	III	IV	V	VI	VII	VIII		
1	1 H 1.0080							2 He 4.003		
2	3 Li 6.940	4 Be 9.013	5 B 10.82	6 C 12.011	7 N 14.008	8 O 16.0000	9 F 19.00	10 Ne 20.183		
3	11 Na 22.991	12 Mg 24.32	13 Al 26.98	14 Si 28.09	15 P 30.975	16 S 32.066	17 Cl 35.457	18 A 39.944		
4	19 K 39.100	20 Ca 40.08	21 Sc 44.96	22 Ti 47.90	23 V 50.95	24 Cr 52.01	25 Mn 54.94	26 Fe 55.85	27 Co 58.94	28 Ni 58.71
	29 Cu 63.54	30 Zn 65.38	31 Ga 69.72	32 Ge 72.60	33 As 74.91	34 Se 78.96	35 Br 79.916	36 Kr 83.80		
5	37 Rb 85.48	38 Sr 87.63	39 Y 88.92	40 Zr 91.22	41 Nb 92.91	42 Mo 95.95	43 Tc 99.	44 Ru 101.1	45 Rh 102.91	46 Pd 106.4
	47 Ag 107.880	48 Cd 112.41	49 In 114.82	50 Sn 118.70	51 Sb 121.76	52 Te 127.61	53 I 126.91	54 Xe 131.30		
6	55 Cs 132.91	56 Ba 137.36	57 La 138.92	72 Hf 178.50	73 Ta 180.95	74 W 183.86	75 Re 186.22	76 Os 190.2	77 Ir 192.2	78 Pt 195.09
	79 Au 197.0	80 Hg 200.61	81 Tl 204.39	82 Pb 207.21	83 Bi 209.00	84 Po 209	85 At 210	86 Rn 222.		
7	87 Fr 223	88 Ra 226.05	89 Ac 227.							

The Rare Earths

6	58 Ce 140.13	59 Pr 140.92	60 Nd 144.27	61 Pm 145.	62 Sm 150.35	63 Eu 152.0	64 Gd 157.26	65 Tb 158.93	66 Dy 162.51	67 Ho 164.94	68 Er 167.27	69 Tm 168.94	70 Yb 173.04	71 Lu 174.99
7	90 Th 232.05	91 Pa 231.	92 U 238.07	93 Np 237	94 Pu 244	95 Am 243.	96 Cm 248	97 Bk 247	98 Cf 251	99 E 254	100 Fm 253	101 Mv 256	102	103

FIG. 54.—Periodic Table of the Atoms (1956).

264

C. PERIODIC TABLE

In 1870 Mendelyeev introduced a table in which the known elements were arranged in a series of groups. The elements in each vertical group were chemically related in that they generally behaved similarly in chemical reactions. Subsequently it was noted that each group of elements had a similar number of valence electrons (electrons in the outer shell) (Fig. 54). The elements are consecutively listed in the order of ascending atomic numbers, the atomic number being the total number of protons in the nucleus. The mass number is the total number of neutrons and protons in the nucleus; but it will be noticed that the atomic weights of many of the chemical elements are not integers (as they should be), since atomic weights are expressed on a scale in which protons and neutrons deviate slightly from unit mass. These elements are made up of isotopes, which are the same element with the same atomic number but with varying atomic mass, i.e., a different number of neutrons. For example, the element nitrogen has atomic weight 14.008 because it is made up of 99.635 per cent of isotope N^{14} and 0.365 per cent of isotope N^{15}. There are isotopes that differ in mass number but have the same atomic weight. Such isotopes are called *isobars,* of which neon, with atomic number 10 and weight 21, and sodium, with atomic number 11 and weight 21, are typical examples.

D. SYMBOLS

It is necessary to have a technical shorthand for designating the commonly used terms in medical nuclear physics. The abbreviations for each element, as given in the periodic table, are well known. The subscript before the abbreviation gives the atomic number *(Z),* and the superscript after the abbreviation designates the mass number *(A).* For example, $_6C^{14}$ is carbon with 6 protons and 6 electrons, a mass number of 14 and 8 neutrons $(14 - 6)$.

The electron is sometimes written as $_{-1}e^0$, depicting a charge of -1 and a mass number of zero. The neutron is written as $_0n^1$, designating a zero charge and mass of 1. The proton is written as $_1H^1$, showing it to be the nucleus of the hydrogen atom with a mass number of 1 and an atomic number or charge of 1.

E. RADIOACTIVITY

Soon after the discovery of x-rays by Röntgen, Becquerel (in 1896) found that some compounds of uranium emit rays similar to the x-rays. These compounds and other naturally occurring substances (generally with high Z) emit such rays spontaneously, independent of external environment (heat, light, electric or magnetic fields). These rays have certain basic characteristics, depending on their mass, velocity, charge and energy.

The nucleus of an atom is held together by a balance of forces, some acting as cohesive forces and some as repulsive forces. These include, among others, coulombic forces (repulsion of like electrical charges) and attraction of neutrons and protons for each other by a specific nuclear force the nature of which is not yet completely understood. When a nucleus exists in which the forces are not well balanced, there is spontaneous emission of radiation in an effort of the nucleus to return to a balanced position or stable configuration. All naturally existing elements of atomic number greater than 83 and mass number greater than 209 (bismuth) are unstable or radioactive.

One of the heaviest particles emitted from the nucleus is the alpha (α) particle. It consists of the nucleus of a helium atom with a positive charge of 2 and a mass of 4 (2 neutrons and 2 protons). The range in air of these particles commonly varies from 3 to 8 cm., depending on their emission energy. Their velocities vary as the square root of their energies. An atom giving off such a particle will have its atomic number reduced by 2 and its mass by 4. For example, when uranium isotope U^{238} of $Z = 92$ and $A = 238$ gives off an alpha particle, it decays into Th^{234} of $Z = 90$ and $A = 234$. The alpha particles are easily stopped by a few sheets of paper and have a range of a few microns in tissue (skin).

Another particle emitted from the nucleus is the beta particle (β^- or $_{-1}e^0$). It does not exist free in the nucleus but results from the transformation of a neutron into a proton within the nucleus. Simultaneously with the emission of the beta particle there occurs the emission of a neutrino ($_0v^0$), which has negligible mass and no charge and is theoretically necessary in accounting for the various energies that beta particles possess when leaving the nucleus. The beta particle is an electron of negative charge and a mass 1/1,840 that of the proton or hydrogen nucleus—in fact, is simply an electron of nuclear origin. Following the emission of a beta particle, the nucleus is left with the same mass number and an atomic number one greater than before. The velocities of beta particles can approach 95 per cent the velocity of light, and these particles may have a maximum range of several meters in air and up to 10 mm. in tissue. It is known that the energies of the beta particles emitted by a single isotope range in a continuum from zero to a finite maximum. The maximum energy is a characteristic of the emitting substance. It has been found that there will be a peak energy distribution of these electrons at a value of $E = E_{max}/3$.

Often, a gamma (γ) ray will be emitted along with a beta particle. The emission of the beta particle may still leave the nucleus in an excited state, and additional energy must be released to have a stable nucleus. This energy may be released in a form of electromagnetic radiation such as gamma rays, which are identical with x-rays except as to origin, the gamma rays being emitted from the nucleus. Gamma rays are emitted in definite energy values and with a velocity equal to that of light. They are absorbed in an exponential manner, to be described later.

There are other types of radiations and decay processes, such as isomeric transition, internal conversion, positron emission and electron capture. None of these processes is common in the isotopes described in this manual, and the reader is directed to the bibliography at the end of the chapter for a complete description of all types.

F. ARTIFICIAL RADIOACTIVITY

It is seen from the foregoing that when the nucleus of a heavy element is in an unstable state there can be emitted an assortment of radiations. An unstable nucleus can be created by injecting into a stable nucleus one or more protons or neutrons. The nucleus will then become radioactive, and by radiation emission will return to a stable configuration. In practice, the addition of particles to nuclei can be made either through the neutrons provided by a nuclear reactor or by the protons provided by an accelerator, such as the cyclotron. It has sometimes been found more feasible to use some of the by-products of the uranium fission normally occurring in nuclear fission than to use particle-injecting devices.

To understand how these by-products are obtained, it is necessary to have a general view of the fission process. In fission the uranium (U^{235}) nucleus absorbs a neutron and fissions into two approximately equal parts (fission products). The resulting atoms have atomic numbers (Z) much lower than the original U^{235}. Since fission can occur in many different ways, many different kinds of fission products can be formed. The atomic numbers of the fission products produced in sizable yields range from $Z = 140$ (cerium) to $Z = 95$ (molybdenum). The fission products are unstable because of a surplus of neutrons.

As discussed above, a nucleus with a surplus of neutrons will generally emit negative beta particles until it reverts to an isotope which has a stable balance of protons and neutrons. In this fissioning process there will be given up, for each 1,000 gm. of U^{235}, about 989 gm. of fission products, 10 gm. of neutrons, 100 mg. of radiation from the decay products and 700 mg. of kinetic energy. Iodine-131 is one of the fission products of relatively high yield, approximately 2.8 per cent of the total. By chemical separation it is possible under elaborate radiation safety precautions, to isolate the I^{131} fraction of the fission products and to process this element for medical application.

It is thus possible to obtain a radioactive isotope of almost any element and to use it clinically. Considerations in the selection of radioisotopes include such items as their half-lives or decay rates, the energy of their radiations, their absorption coefficients in matter, and other factors, which will be briefly described.

G. CHARACTERISTICS AND EFFECTS OF RADIOACTIVITY

The medical user is primarily concerned with the phenomenon of ionization as an effect due to radioactivity. It is this effect which enables him to detect the presence of a radioisotope and to use it as a therapeutic agent. Ionization is the process or result of any process by which a neutral atom or molecule acquires either a positive or a negative charge. The charged atom or molecule is called an "ion." Ionization by radiation (alpha particle, beta particle, gamma ray, etc.) depends on the velocity, charge and mass of the radiation and the density of the media through which it is passing.

Charged particles, such as alpha and beta particles, can cause ionization in the atoms through which they pass by the physical dislocation of an electron from its natural orbit. There will be a specific number of these ionization events taking place per unit path length in the medium traversed until the maximum range is reached. The number of such events is also determined by the medium's characteristic energy requirement for making an ion pair; for example, the average energy loss per ion pair in air is about 32.5 ev, and an incident beta particle of 1 Mev will produce in air $1.0 \times 10^6/32.5$, or 3.08×10^4, ion pairs. (See Appendix A, Glossary, for definitions of terms.)

Electromagnetic radiation, such as x- or gamma radiation, reacts with matter in one of the following manners, depending on the energy of the radiation:

1. PHOTOELECTRIC EFFECT

The photoelectric effect is predominant in tissue at energies less than 0.5 Mev. Herein the gamma ray is incident upon an atomic electron and delivers all its energy to it while simultaneously removing it completely from the atom. If the energy of the incident particle is greater than the energy required for removal, the additional energy is imparted to the electron in the form of kinetic energy. This fact is expressed in the equation

$$E_\gamma = E_\beta + \text{K.E.}$$

where E_β (binding energy) is the energy needed to remove the electron from its orbit, K.E. is the kinetic energy of the ejected electron and E_γ is the total energy of the incident photon or gamma ray.

2. COMPTON EFFECT

The Compton effect is predominant between 0.5 and 5.0 Mev in tissue. Here, as a result of a collision between a photon and an electron, the two are scattered at an angle $(\emptyset)$ to the trajectory of the primary photon. Compton treated the photon as if it were a particle having mass. He concluded that there should be a change in wavelength of the incident photon given by

$$\Delta\lambda = 0.024 \ (1 - \cos \emptyset)$$

In the Compton process the products are an energetic electron and a scattered gamma ray whose energy is less than that of the incident gamma ray. The scattered gamma ray may in turn be Compton scattered, so that in effect the energy of the scattered photon is continually reduced until it falls into the range of the photoelectric effect, after which the latter process occurs.

3. PAIR PRODUCTION

Pair product effect is important in tissue at photon energies greater than 10 Mev. Therein, a high-energy gamma ray in the vicinity of a nucleus will suddenly give up all its energy and form a positive and a negative electron pair. Because the rest mass of a single electron corresponds to an energy of 0.51 Mev, the combined kinetic energies of the positive and negative electrons is given by the equation

$$\text{K.E.} = E - 1.02 \ \text{Mev}$$

The effect of the gamma and the x-radiation on tissue is the result of ionization by the electrons released when the photon interacts (i.e., the photoelectron, the Compton electron or the electron pair).

H. ABSORPTION

The foregoing processes determine the absorption of radiation in matter. Radioactive charged particles have a maximum range in matter; i.e., they do not penetrate beyond a certain distance characteristic of the medium, the particle and its energy. This is in sharp contrast with photon radiation (x, γ), which has no maximum range but is attenuated in an exponential manner. The range of beta particles can be approximated by

$$R = 0.546 \text{ Em} - 0.16$$

where R is the maximum range in grams per square centimeter and Em is the maximum energy of beta particles in million electron volts.

Gamma rays are absorbed by any or all the processes described. This intensity loss can be described by the equation

$$I = I_0 e^{-\mu X}$$

where I = intensity of the gamma rays after passage through absorber

I_0 = intensity of gamma rays before entering absorbing medium

μ = absorption coefficient, and

X = thickness of absorbing medium.

The magnitude of the absorption coefficient μ depends on the photon energy and on the medium.

It is more convenient to describe absorption in terms of a half-value layer. This is the thickness X of any absorbing material required to reduce the incident gamma-ray intensity to one half of the incident intensity; i.e., $I_{1/2} = \frac{1}{2}I_0$. It can be shown that this value is equal to $0.693/\mu$. For example, the linear absorption coefficient μ for I^{131} in tissue is 0.033 cm.$^{-1}$, or a half-value layer of 0.693/0.033 cm.$^{-1}$, or 21 cm. If a flux of gamma rays were incident on the surface of a body, at a depth of 21 cm. there would be one half of this quantity; and at a depth of 42 cm. there would be one fourth of this initial intensity, owing to absorption. These are important considerations in radioisotope therapy.

I. DECAY

As mentioned above, the radioactive atoms decay into another nucleus. This process takes place at a definite rate, and it tends to be longer for isotopes having low energy and low atomic number. If N_0 is the number of radioactive nuclei present at zero time, then

$$N = N_0 e^{-\lambda t}$$

where N is the number of nuclei present after a time t, and λ is the decay constant which is a measure of the rapidity with which the nuclei decay. A large value of λ corresponds to rapid decay;

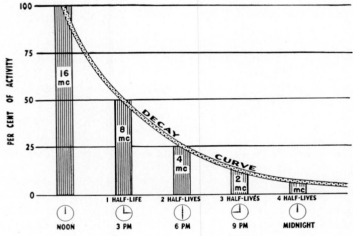

FIG. 55.—The meaning of half-life.

a small λ to a slow decay. The equation is an exponential one (Fig. 55); but when plotted on semilogarithmic paper (logarithmic ordinate and linear abscissa), it yields a straight line.

As in the case of the exponential absorption of gamma rays, it is more convenient to ascribe to an isotope a half-life than a decay constant. The half-life $(T_{1/2})$ is the period of time required for the decay of a radioisotope to one half of its original quantity. It is derived from the decay constant by the following equation:

$$T_{1/2} = 0.693/\lambda$$

For example, I^{131} has a half-life of 8.1 days. In this period of time, one half of the initial activity will have decayed away. In

16.2 days there will only be a fourth of the initial activity present, and so forth.

J. INVERSE SQUARE LAW

Reception of radiation from an emitting source is decreased by absorption in the intervening medium or by the position (geometry) of the source with respect to its receiver. Light rays and gamma rays obey the same laws of electromagnetic radiation; that is, with no absorption, the received intensity varies inversely as the square of the distance. This law is strictly valid only for point sources but is approximately correct provided the distance of the receiver (tissue or detector) from the source is at least three times the source dimensions.

The intensity of radiation per unit area received at a distance r from a point source is given by

$$I = N/4\pi r^2$$

where N is the disintegration rate of the source in photons per unit time and I is the intensity received at the distance r in photons per time per unit area.

With a detector of prescribed area, it is thus possible to estimate the proportion of emitted photons which are incident upon the area. Because of scattering effects, this relationship is, in general an oversimplification; but it can be used as an approximation for many practical applications.

Herein

$$G = A/4\pi r^2$$

where G = proportion of emitted photons entering detector,

A = detection area, and

r = distance from point source.

REFERENCES

1. Glasser, O., et al.: *Physical Foundations of Radiology* (New York: Paul B. Hoeber, Inc., 1952).
2. Lapp, R. E., and Andrews, H. L.: *Nuclear Radiation Physics* (New York: Prentice-Hall, Inc., 1954).
3. Pollard, E., and Davidson, W. L.: *Applied Nuclear Physics* (New York: John Wiley & Sons, Inc., 1951).
4. Siri, W. E.: *Isotopic Tracers and Nuclear Radiations* (New York: McGraw-Hill Book Company, Inc., 1949).

CHAPTER 14

Establishing the Laboratory

A. ESTIMATING DEMAND

THE ADVISABILITY OF INSTALLING a radioisotope laboratory in a general hospital depends primarily on (1) the desire and feasibility of carrying on clinical or nonclinical research, (2) the number of patients with thyroid disease in the community and (3) the size and character of the institution. There are only two reasons for the use of radioisotopes in a general hospital: one is for the purpose of research; the other is solely for clinical application.

1. RESEARCH APPLICATION

A radioisotope laboratory is a necessity in any institution—of whatever size—in which research, whether animal research or human clinical, constitutes even a small part of the institution's activity. It is a mistake, however, to set up a radioisotope laboratory in the hope that it will inspire the staff to enter investigative fields. On the other hand, a single enthusiastic staff member who has the time and who has a record of proved sustained interest in research is sufficient to warrant the establishment of a laboratory as a functioning tool to further his scientific curiosity.

The co-operation of the clinical pathologist is a second requirement. Without his help and without access to his department, research would be difficult in the average community hospital. In most hospitals there are no funds to finance research, and in many hospitals the pathologist finds it highly unprofitable to lend his facilities for unremunerative investigations. The same difficulty may arise without the co-operative effort of the roentgenologist.

2. Clinical Application

The radioisotope laboratory is useful primarily in the diagnosis and treatment of hyperthyroidism, which constitute its sustaining activity. The use of a tracer dose of iodine-131 is a helpful diagnostic procedure but is not a mandatory test. Except in a few instances, the basal metabolic rate is an equally reliable test. The clinical need for a laboratory in a hospital is in direct proportion to the number of patients with hyperthyroidism who are available for therapy. This can be readily calculated by adding up the number of patients with toxic diffuse or exophthalmic goiter in the community who are operated on during a single year and assuming that approximately the number arrived at will be treated in the future with I^{131}. At the outset, even one exophthalmic goiter patient a week who is available for treatment will justify setting up a laboratory.

To be sure, I^{131} is useful in the treatment of carcinoma of the thyroid, but this is not a common disease and the need of a laboratory for its treatment will not be valid unless the institution has a large goitrous population from which to draw its patients.

An occasional patient with angina pectoris is benefited greatly by the production of hypothyroidism with I^{131}. The number of patients who will be treated with I^{131} will depend on the enthusiasm of the internist, but normally the number will not be large.

The treatment of choice in polycythemia probably is phosphorus-32. Again, this is not a common disease, so that only in the event of a large potential population or in a specialized practice will the cases mount sufficiently to justify a laboratory for this reason. Although P^{32} is helpful in chronic leukemia, its advantages over roentgen therapy are not great enough to replace it entirely, even when P^{32} is available.

Blood-volume studies with isotopes have many clinical applications but will be used by only a few clinicians.

The intracavitary injection of radioactive colloids will be indicated frequently throughout the year in almost any community. The use of radioactive needles and seeds containing gold-198 and cobalt-60 is applicable when there is a consistently large flow of cancer patients through the institution. However, teletherapy and therapy by the use of fixed radioisotopes in the form of needles, seeds and external applicators are functions of the radiology department and are not to be included in the field of a general radioisotope laboratory.

3. CONCLUSION

It is unlikely that a radioisotope laboratory will prove to be a useful clinical venture in a general hospital of under 200-bed capacity unless the hospital draws an uncommonly high percentage of hyperthyroid patients. In a hospital of at least 400-bed capacity, a radioisotope laboratory will usually prove to be a helpful ancillary facility. If the hospital is inclined to research or is a part of a large medical center, the radioisotope laboratory is a necessity.

B. FACILITIES

For clinical, as well as research, purposes the radioisotope laboratory in an ordinary general hospital will not be a large installation; it will be one that may be housed in two or three rooms. It is most advantageously placed near the other laboratories, with access from a common waiting room and with one receptionist for all laboratories. In most small hospitals the roentgenologist will be the most competent person to head the radioisotope laboratory, which may become an integral part of the radiology department. If the radioisotope laboratory is not engaged primarily in external radiation therapy, it will be professionally more closely associated with the clinical pathology laboratory and would then best be placed in juxtaposition to it. In practice, inasmuch as the radioisotope laboratory will be installed in an already established institution, it will have to be situated wherever a place can be found.

The requirements of the parent institution will vary. Therefore, in order to be specific, let us assume that a laboratory for relatively low-level radioactivity is to be installed and equipped

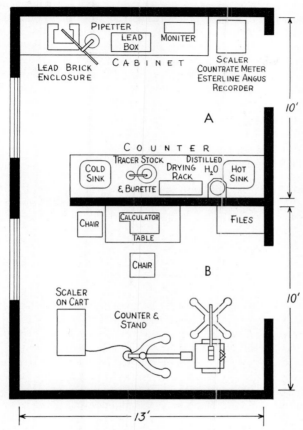

FIG. 56.—Plan for a hospital radioisotope laboratory.

as cheaply as possible in an ordinary general hospital of 350-bed capacity for the purpose of providing routine clinical and research facilities.

The minimum space necessary is two rooms, of about 10 × 12 ft. each. As shown in Figure 56, the rooms may be side by side with a connecting doorway, or they may be on opposite sides of a hallway. Ordinary hospital rooms will suffice. In at least one room, there must be access to the water and sewerage systems. Alterations will consist chiefly in rearranging the plumbing and in adding electrical outlets, which should be installed in such numbers that any portion of either room has ready access to a double-outlet.

One room, Room A (Fig. 56), should be a *"hot"* laboratory. It will be used for the receiving, handling and storage of all radioisotopes and for their preparation and administration, whether in tracer or therapeutic quantities. Biologic samples may be prepared and counted in this room, provided the background is kept low and the counters are adequately shielded. Theoretically, it is not considered advisable to measure biologic radiation in the same room in which radioisotopes are prepared and stored; nevertheless, in the ordinary hospital the method has some merit in that it compels the technician to shield all radiation sources properly. If they are not shielded, the radiation sources will be promptly brought to his attention by the excessively high background of his counting equipment. If there is a great deal of low-level counting, it may be advisable to install a small counting room at a distance. In most circumstances, however, two adjacent rooms will suffice.

Room A should contain two sinks, with 20 sq. ft. of counter space and 20 cu. ft. of storage space in the underlying drawers and cabinets. One sink, to be used for *hot* material, should be deep enough to control splashing. The other sink should be kept *clean*—that is, no contaminated material should be permitted in it. How this basic equipment is arranged makes little difference. The sinks, with part of the working-table surface, may be separated; but usually, because of the plumbing, it is cheaper and more convenient to place them at opposite ends of a long counter. The use of radioisotopes does not require that the counter and sinks be of stainless steel; but from the point of view of general utility, stainless steel is advisable. Manufacturers of kitchen cabinets furnish so many designs and sizes that almost any type of sink or counter can readily be assembled at a relatively low cost, compared with the cost of specifically designed laboratory equipment.

Enamel paint is preferred for the walls. A fume hood is not a necessity unless the heating or evaporating of radioactive mix-

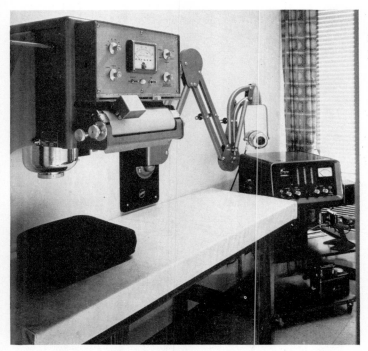

FIG. 57.—Small office laboratory for thyroid diagnosis and therapy. This side of the office is equipped with a scanner, a scintillation counter hanging from the wall on a movable arm, a scaler and a monitor. (See also Fig. 58.)

tures at frequent intervals, or the handling of boiling liquids or dusty material, is intended. If the floor is of wood or concrete, it should be covered with asphalt or battleship linoleum.

Room B (Fig. 56), is used for all clinical work directly involving patients, as well as to house the files, working desk and mechanical calculator. It contains a directional scintillation counter and scaler for uptake studies. If necessary, the secretary's desk and typewriter may also be placed in this room. The mechanical calculator is not a necessity, especially if one uses a decade scaler instead of the binary scaler.

The cost of equipping Room A, including sinks, a scaler, a count-rate meter, a recorder, a monitor and also a well-type scintillation counter, will be approximately $3,000. Room B, including a scaler, directional scintillation counter with stand, type-

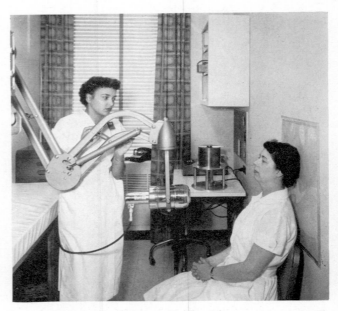

Fig. 58.—Other side of the small office laboratory shown in Figure 57. The patient sits with head against the wall. The counter is swung out in front of the patient's neck. In the background, there is a well-type scintillation counter, and behind it, the calculator.

writer, desks, cabinets and chairs, will cost about $2,000. A scanner will cost from $3,300 to $5,000 extra.

In a private office, where both space and money are used more economically than in hospitals or governmental institutions, a laboratory designed principally for thyroid diagnosis and treatment can be set up in smaller quarters and for less money. Figures 57 and 58 depict a more compact arrangement in a room 11 × 6 ft. On one side of the room (Fig. 57), is the scanner,

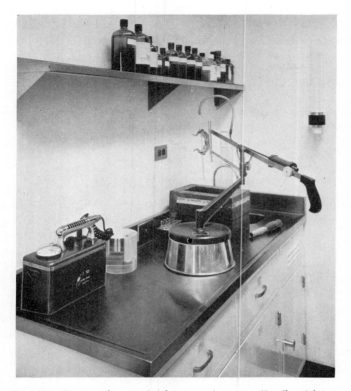

FIG. 59.—Corner of general laboratory (near small office laboratory shown in Figures 57 and 58), in which is placed a kitchen type of counter containing a small sink at one end. Placed on the counter are a lead brick enclosure, a remote pipetter, a phantom and a survey meter.

a scintillation counter hanging from the wall on a movable arm, a scaler and a monitor. On the other side of the room (Fig. 58), against the opposite wall, the patient for thyroid uptake study sits on a chair with his head resting against the wall. The counter is swung out across the room in front of his neck. On the desk in the background is a well-type scintillation counter, and behind it is located the calculator. The total cost for this equipment and furniture is $6,500. The essential instruments—monitor, scaler, counter, and moveable arm—come to approximately $2,000. The remaining equipment needed is the scanner, calculator, desk and table. In an adjoining room, used for a general laboratory, there is, in one corner (Fig. 59), a small sink and stainless steel counter holding a lead brick enclosure and a distant pipetter, leaving a few square feet of table surface to hold accessories and to be used for working space. Cabinets beneath the sink give adequate storage space. This latter room, including sink, counter, pipetter and all accessories, will cost approximately $1,000.

C. STORING AND SHIELDING EQUIPMENT

Radioactive isotopes are delivered to the laboratory in quantities of tens of millicuries rather than hundreds of millicuries. Most shipments can be stored in a lead container having small volume and 1 in. thick walls. The container is placed in a far corner of the room; or, if it holds a large amount of radioactivity (above 10 mc.), it is placed behind a barrier of 2 in. lead bricks. The quantity of radioactivity on hand will largely depend on the speed with which the isotopes are used or dispensed. The simplest way to reduce excess radiation is to order the exact amount of radioisotope that is required and then use it immediately on arrival. If radioactive material is not kept on hand, there is no need for elaborate storage facilities.

Lead bricks, either interlocking or rectangular, are a necessity. The bricks are very useful for forming a small four-walled enclosure within which millicurie quantities may be stored (Fig. 59). In it are placed all material which may be active enough to create a health hazard or which might unduly raise the background of the counters—indeed, into this enclosure goes everything that is *hot,* whether the material is to be used or is waiting out its period of decay.

A lead box with ½ in. thick walls is a handy place to store tracer doses or beta emitters. A small lead carrying case with 1 in. walls is also useful; larger storage containers may be necessary.*

---

* All of these items may be obtained from Atomic Accessories, Inc., 244–02 Jamaica Ave., Bellerose, New York.

The 24-hour collection and transportation of urine from a hospital patient following a therapeutic dose presents the most difficult problem in health protection and is advisable only for research purposes. If the patient is ambulatory, he might collect it himself and carry it, under supervision, to the laboratory unshielded. If hospital personnel are continually handling such

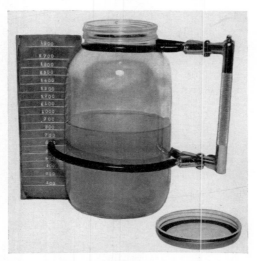

Fig. 60.—A urine bottle with bottle holder used in operating rooms to handle flasks of boiling water. Beside it is a movable gauge to measure the quantity.

urine, it will have to be collected and transported behind 1 or 2 in. of lead. After surrounding the collecting vessel with an adequate layer of lead, a heavy-machinery mover may be needed to transport it. With this exception, storage containers of small capacity and relatively light weight will suffice.

HOLDING TOOLS.—In a laboratory handling low-level isotopes, it is not necessary to invest in elaborate and expensive holding equipment. It is not wise, however, to pick up any receptacle containing radioisotopes directly with the hands. There is little danger of injurious radiation from a few microcuries of I^{131} so long as the contamination is recognized and immediately washed away; but it is best to maintain the habit of a "sterile" technique, regardless of the quantity involved. If the operator must pick up vessels containing radioisotopes with the hands, he should wear gloves. A heavy type of rubber glove is cheaper and safer than the thin latex surgical gloves.

The simplest holding tool,* such as is used in factories to pick up and hold small bolts, rivets and the like, is serviceable in the radioisotope laboratory. It comes in various lengths up to 20 in., with rigid or with pliable tubing. By pushing the plunger, a forked spring can be placed around the neck of small flasks, test tubes, bottles and vials. When the plunger is released, the object is held firmly in place. Larger, more elaborate and sturdier holding tools can be obtained from Atomic Accessories, Inc.† Figure 60 shows a bottle holder used in hospital central supply departments for picking up bottles of boiling water. It can also be used to handle large bottles containing radioactive liquid.

PIPETTERS.—Atomic Accessories, Inc., and Tracerlab, Inc.,‡ supply an excellent remote pipetting device. Micropipettes, microsyringe pipette controls and the "Propipette" can be obtained from Atomic Accessories, Inc.

D. PROCUREMENT OF RADIOISOTOPES

All radioisotopes are obtained through permission of the Isotope Extension, Division of Civilian Application, U. S. Atomic Energy Commission, Washington, D.C. The hospital proposing to establish a laboratory takes the following steps: (1) forms a Medical Isotopes Committee, (2) establishes a laboratory,§ (3) requests an isotope allocation on Forms AEC-313 and AEC-313a and (4) receives an allocation from the Isotopes Extension.

Each allocation is for a specific radioisotope, to be used for a specific purpose, setting a definite maximum quantity of the

---

* Bonney Tool & Forge Co., Allentown, Pennsylvania.

† Atomic Accessories, Inc., 244–02 Jamaica Ave., Bellerose, New York.

‡ Tracerlab, Inc., 1601 Trapelo Road, Waltham, Massachusetts.

§ It is possible to establish the laboratory after the allocation has been obtained, by submitting with Form AEC-313 sufficient evidence of intention to establish the laboratory, which will include diagrams of the intended area and a list of the equipment to be procured.

radioisotope which may be kept on hand. A few of the larger institutions may secure a general allocation which permits storing of any amount of most isotopes.

A *secondary supplier* is any person or persons to whom an allocation has been issued, specifically entitling him to receive radioisotopes for processing and synthesis for distribution to the holder of specific use allocations. A *distributor* is defined by the Atomic Energy Commission as a person or group operating AEC-owned laboratories under a contract with the Commission and engaged in the distribution of radioisotopes for the Commission. At present, almost all radioactive chemicals are produced by secondary suppliers. Only a few larger clinical laboratories are in a position to process the material, as it is received from the Union Carbide and Carbon Corporation,* according to acceptable *U. S. Pharmacopoeia* standards.

The Union Carbide and Carbon Corporation, acting as contractor for the Oak Ridge National Laboratory of the Atomic Energy Commission, is the principal distributor of the basic radioisotopes. Service irradiation of units is also made by Brookhaven National Laboratory, Argonne National Laboratory and the Materials Testing Reactor.

Most hospital laboratories transmit their allocation Form AEC-374 to a secondary supplier.

While radioisotopes may be obtained directly from the Union Carbide and Carbon Corporation at Oak Ridge, as indicated in the *Catalogue & Price List of Radioisotopes* issued by the Corporation, the materials supplied by the Corporation must be checked for identity and carefully assayed by the user before administration. Shipments of I^{131} and P^{32} from Oak Ridge now carry a notice stating that the material is pharmaceutically unrefined and that the radiochemical purity should be established and individual doses precisely calibrated. In short, the material does not conform to the requirements recently adopted by the *U. S. Pharmacopoeia* (USP, XV, 1955) and by the *New and Nonofficial Remedies* (NNR) of the Council on Pharmacy and Chemistry of the American Medical Association. In the near future, radioisotopes

---

* Oak Ridge National Laboratory, Union Carbide Nuclear Company, P. O. Box P, Oak Ridge, Tennessee.

will be distributed under the auspices of the Federal Food and Drug Administration. It is expected that FDA regulations will require processing beyond the capabilities of an ordinary general hospital.

The principal sources of radioisotopes in the United States are herewith listed:

Original Source of Almost All Radioisotopes:

Oak Ridge National Laboratory
Union Carbide Nuclear Company
P. O. Box P
Oak Ridge, Tennessee

Partial List of Secondary Suppliers for Hospitals:

Abbott Laboratories	E. R. Squibb & Sons
Oak Ridge, Tennessee	Georges Road
	New Brunswick, New Jersey
Nuclear Consultants	Volk Radiochemical Company
9842 Manchester Road	5412 N. Clark Street
St. Louis, Missouri	Chicago 40, Illinois

E. PERSONNEL

The Isotope Extension of the U.S. Atomic Energy Commission, in a circular entitled *Radioisotope Procurement Procedures; The Medical Use of Radioisotopes: Recommendations and Requirements by the AEC . . . ,* has stated in detail the requirements preliminary to the establishment of an isotope laboratory. The basic organization is diagrammatically represented in Figure 61.

F. FINANCING

The cost of a radioisotope installation varies from a few thousand to several hundred thousand dollars. The simplest arrangement, designed to do only tracer studies for thyroid disease, can be established in any ordinary hospital room at a cost of no more than $2,000. A laboratory designed for tracer studies, internal therapy, blood volume studies, animal analysis and all clinically useful types of radioactive measurement (except "scinti-scanning") can be put in operation for $7,000. This amount includes costs for: alterations; installing sinks, counters, tables and filing cabinets; glassware, lead bricks and containers; and a calculating machine, as well as the electronic equipment, including an end-window scintillation counter with supporting arm and

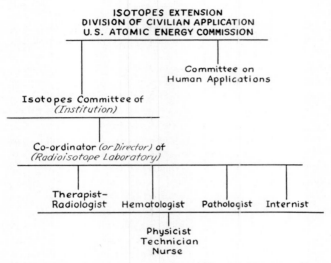

FIG. 61.—Table of organization of medical procurement and use of radioisotopes.

stand, a well-type scintillation counter, a directional counter, monitor and scaler. With such a laboratory, which would accommodate only one full-time technician, any necessary type of radiation measurement could be made. Additional equipment would permit enlarged service but, with few exceptions, would not improve the quality.

If the laboratory is to make its own way financially, it must do so almost entirely on the fees obtained through diagnostic thyroid tracer doses and through therapeutic doses of I^{131}. The basic unit described, with a full-time technician devoting half his time to practical clinical duties and half to investigation, will cost about $1,000 a month to maintain. This sum will be divided about as follows:

1. Rent for space, including light and heat; telephone; billing; accounting; cleaning; etc. .... $ 300
2. Technical and stenographic help 400
3. Supplies, repairs and new equipment 300

$1,000

To cover these expenses adequately, it will be necessary to perform approximately 50 tracer tests a month, at $10 a test, and to treat 10 exophthalmic goiter patients, at from $50 to $75 each. Without such a flow of patients the laboratory will not be self-sustaining, let alone have any surplus to satisfy the director of the laboratory. Fees vary enormously, those cited probably represent less than what the laboratory services are worth, and they are less than the average charge in most institutions.

Therapy for cancer of the thyroid will be administered, in most instances, for only a little more than the cost of the material. A return of $2.00 for each millicurie administered would be a reasonable charge; but even this will often be more than the patient can pay. Intracavitary injections for carcinoma of the pleura or peritoneum are in the same category. The fees cited are solely laboratory fees, and do not include medical care. Unfortunately, only rarely are any of these costs covered by health insurance. Radioisotope therapy is too new to be included in insurance policies, and the insurance companies are not eager to append riders for this coverage.

In a general hospital, the facilities of the laboratory are presumably available to all the physicians in the institution. Normally, the director of the laboratory will check the patients who are to be treated and will determine the dosage to be given; the patient will then return to the referring physician for further care.

CHAPTER 15

Radioactive Materials for Medical Use

A. PROPERTIES AND PREPARATION OF PHARMACEUTICALS

WHEN RADIOISOTOPES WERE FIRST INTRODUCED into experimental medicine, the problems presented by production, handling and radioassay overshadowed the pharmaceutical aspects. The Atomic Energy Commission early emphasized that the materials supplied by them were to be regarded as "bulk chemicals" requiring characterization, identification, assay and, if necessary, further purification before use. Commercial groups soon moved to provide such services, supplying properly processed radiopharmaceuticals, ready for use by those holding appropriate AEC licenses. Most isotope users now elect, in making their license applications, to specify that they will procure their supplies from such secondary suppliers.

A number of radioactive preparations must now be marketed under effective new drug applications. Some of these have been included in the *U. S. Pharmacopoeia* (USP), Fifteenth Revision, and additional ones will be added to the forthcoming revision. These USP monographs set up rigorous standards of purity and composition which must be met by all products marketed thereunder. Details of radioassay procedures are given there in detail.

The participation of private industry has also resulted in the development and production of a considerable variety of tagged compounds designed to make possible new isotopic diagnostic and therapeutic procedures. The more important of these will be described in subsequent sections.

Improved packaging—and, in particular, the invention of techniques for supplying individual doses in capsule form—has done much to make possible the safe use of isotopes in the average hospital.

Because of the broad experience and excellent instrumentation devoted to problems of purity and radioassay, these commercial preparations have achieved an excellent record of reliability. Several groups, as well as the U. S. Bureau of Standards, do supply carefully reassayed analytical samples which provide a relatively simple and effective way of calibrating equipment. With the number of counts to be expected from a given activity accurately known, one can quickly check any gross error in shipments received or in samples prepared in the laboratory.

Some of the preparations now available are listed below:

1. SODIUM RADIOIODIDE SOLUTIONS (I^{131}) USP

Sodium radioiodide is supplied as a clear solution having a pH of between 7.0 and 8.5. It is essentially carrier free, and it is kept reduced by bisulfite or ascorbic acid. A bacteriostatic agent such as benzyl alcohol and a color for identification may be added.

Such solutions are required to contain not less than 95 per cent, nor more than 105 per cent, of the labeled activity at the stated time of assay. Absence of other chemical forms of I^{131} is established by paper chromatography, using 75 per cent methanol as the eluting agent.

Assay is officially carried out by beta counting versus known standards, although gamma counting provides a more practical way of checking the activity of solutions being employed.

Pharmaceutical Forms

A. Multiple-dose vials for diagnostic use, containing 250 μc. in 10 ml. of water. These are sterile, since in certain procedures the solution is given parenterally.

B. Individual-dose or multiple-dose vials for therapy or for the preparation of solutions for diagnosis or synthetic purposes. Amounts up to 50 μc. are usually supplied in less than 10 ml.

volume. Solutions for oral use are in screw-capped bottles; other solutions, in rubber-capped vials.

2. Encapsulated Sodium Radioiodine (I^{131})

These capsules are prepared by the evaporation of an alcoholic solution of carrier-free iodide on the interior wall of a gelatin capsule. The activity remains firmly attached; and, especially if the unit is sealed, the capsules provide an extremely convenient and safe way of handling and administering both diagnostic and therapeutic doses. The capsules are assayed individually during manufacture and are normally within ±3 per cent of the stated value on the specified assay date. They are color coded to facilitate identification of a given lot and are shipped in advance of the official calibration date.

Pharmaceutical Forms

A. Diagnostic capsules calibrated at 10, 15, 25 and 50 μc. (Several activities may be secured in a given shipment and used as the assay approximates that preferred by the user.)

B. Therapeutic capsules. These customarily are provided in units of 1, 2, 3 and 5 mc. A proper combination of such capsules is employed to approximate the desired therapeutic dosage.

3. Sodium Radiophosphate (P^{32}) USP

Sodium radiophosphate is a clear solution of Na_2HPO_4, which may darken on standing, owing to radiation effects. It is usually adjusted to a pH of 5–8 with sodium acetate and contains up to 0.2 mg. of carrier phosphate to facilitate handling. Assay is by beta counting of evaporated samples and intercomparison with standard samples. Capsules are also currently available.

Pharmaceutical Forms

A. The sterile solution is isotonic and the activity is about 2 mc./ml. The oral solution is packaged in screw-capped bottles, containing either a single dose or sufficient activity for several doses. For repeat therapy, a group of bottles may be secured so adjusted as to provide the same dosage on successive specified days.

B. Capsules prepared in activities of 1–2 and 3 mc., or as specified by the user.

4. SODIUM RADIOCHROMATE (CR⁵¹)

Radiochromate is primarily used for the tagging of red cells, which are then employed for estimating red cell mass and/or the determining of the total circulating blood volume.

For such purposes, it is essential that the specific activity should be high—at least 5–15 mc./mg. Such a solution, prepared by the peroxide oxidation of $CrCl_3$, is essentially colorless. It is sterile, contains a preservative and has a pH of between 5 and 7.

For greatest tagging efficiency, sterile vials are available containing a special formula ACD solution. The blood and chromate are added directly to these, where tagging takes place.

Where chromic chloride is required, it may be easily secured by the addition of ascorbic acid to the above chromate solution.

Pharmaceutical Form

Multiple-dose vials of a sterile solution containing about 0.5 mc./ml., with an activity of 10–15 mc./mg.

5. IODINATED HUMAN SERUM ALBUMIN (IHSA) (I¹³¹)

This is a biologic preparation secured by the careful iodination of purified USP albumin. The past history of the albumin, the mode and extent of iodination and the radiation exposure during and after iodination are all important in determining the stability and clinical usefulness of the ultimate product.

Iodination is usually carried out at 10°, in a slightly alkaline medium, by the dropwise addition of very dilute hypochlorite to a mixture of iodide and the protein. Unbound iodide is removed by an ion exchange column, and the product is sterilized by a Seitz filtration. Benzyl alcohol is added as a preservative. Each lot is tested in animals to insure the absence of pyrogens.

The amount of combined iodine does not exceed 1 atom per 60,000 molecular weight and, on the average, because of the

excess of albumin used, is actually much less than this. The biologic half-life of good material will be of the order of 15–20
days. For such studies of metabolic rates, a form protected against
internal radiation by the addition of a fivefold excess of protein
should be employed. Supplies should be kept at 2°–10° C.; and
under these conditions, they may be used over a period of 3–4
weeks.

The amount of free iodide is determined by filter-paper chromatography, using 75 per cent alcohol, and should not exceed
1–1.5 per cent.

Iodinated globulins, prepared in the same way, are available.

Pharmaceutical Form

Sterile pyrogen-free solution having an activity of 250–750
μc./cc., in a rubber-capped multiple-dose vial. Albumin content,
10 mg./cc. or more.

6. Iodinated Triolein (I^{131}); Iodinated Oleic Acid (I^{131})

Iodinated triolein is prepared by the action of iodine monochloride on a highly purified monounsaturated fat, triolein in a
CCl_4 solution. After removal of the solvent and any free iodide,
the resultant is diluted with peanut oil to an activity of about
1 mc./ml. The iodine bond is relatively stable in the digestive
tract but is liberated as the molecule is metabolized in the blood
stream and tissues.

Iodinated oleic acid is prepared in a similar manner and has
similar properties.

A. Multiple-dose vials containing a solution of the reagents
in peanut oil to give an activity of about 1 mc./ml.

B. Capsules containing 25–100 μc. accompanied by a suitable
I^{131} reference standard.

7. L-Thyronine (T4) and L-Tri-iodothyronine (T3) I^{131}

Preparation is carried out by the exchange of the respective
crystalline synthetic hormones with I^{131} under carefully controlled

conditions. Since such reactions always result in a mixture of products, purification must be effected by column and/or paper-strip chromatography.

Owing to the high specific activity required, radiation damage can easily take place. This is in part prevented by the use of 50 per cent propylene glycol as a solvent. Packages should be refrigerated or even frozen during storage, and they should not be used longer than 2 weeks.

Pharmaceutical Form

Multiple-dose vials containing 0.5–0.6 mc./ml. of 50 per cent propylene glycol. Dilutions may be made into saline solution. Specific activity, 10–50 mc./mg.

8. RADIOCYANOCOBALAMINE (Co^{60} OR Co^{58})

Radiocyanocobalamine is prepared by the growth of the organism Streptomyces griseus in the presence of cobalt salts, and it is purified by a complex system of extractions. Since absorption from the gastrointestinal tract is markedly dependent on the specific activity, this should be kept as constant as possible, preferably in the range of 600–1,000 $\mu c./mg.$ of vitamin B_{12}. This is much easier in the case of the Co^{60} product because of the longer half-life of the isotope.

The dose required for the Schilling test is usually 0.5 $\mu c.$ and may be less if special counting equipment is available. Units containing the inactive vitamin B_{12} and the intrinsic factor required in the test are available.

Pharmaceutical Forms

A. Multiple-dose vials of a sterile isotonic solution of radiocyanocobalamine containing 1 $\mu c./ml.$ Specific activity, about 1,000 $\mu c./mg.$ of vitamin B_{12}.

B. Capsules containing 0.5 $\mu c.$ and a specific activity of about 750 $\mu c./mg.$

9. MISCELLANEOUS I^{131}-LABELED DIAGNOSTIC AGENTS

There are now available, either as stock items or as special preparations, a number of I^{131} reagents which have specific distribution or excretion patterns in the body. Through their use, together with the use of suitable external counting systems, it becomes possible to study liver and kidney functions, circulation times and mechanisms, et cetera, very simply and often quite effectively. Among the products are:

Diodrast® (iodopyracet)	Kidney function
Rose bengal	Liver function
Urokon® (acetrizoate)	Kidney function
Miokon® (diprotrizoate)	Kidney function
Hypaque® (diatrizoate)	Kidney function
Teridax®	Gallbladder studies
Cholografin®	Gallbladder studies
4-Iodo-antipyrene	Total body water

Pharmaceutical Forms

All are available as sterile solutions; 100–1,000 μc./ml. and specific activity around 100 μc./mg.

10. RADIOGOLD (Au^{198}) COLLOID

Colloidal radiogold is a cherry-red solution stable toward aging, and reasonably stable to heat, but unstable to metallic salts. The particle size is about 0.005 μ. It may be diluted with water, pectin or local anesthetics.

Pharmaceutical Forms

Single-dose or multiple-dose vials having an activity of 20–50 mc./cc. at time of preparation and a specific activity of 4–5 mc./mg. of Au^{198}. The solution is sterile and contains pyrogen-free gelatin as the stabilizing agent.

11. STERILE CHROMIC RADIOPHOSPHATE (P^{32}) SUSPENSION

This is a rather coarse colloid, the particle size ranging from 0.2 to 4.0 μ. The suspending agent is usually 25–50 per cent glucose. It is produced by the precipitation of a hydrated form, ignition to confer insolubility and grinding to an appropriate state. When dialyzed against phosphate solution, the exchangeable P^{32} should not exceed 2 per cent. Before withdrawal of supplies, the container should be thoroughly shaken.

Pharmaceutical Form

Sterile suspension containing about 2 mc./cc. of P^{32} and 3–6 mc./mg. of $CoPO_4$.

B. PREPARATION OF LABELED COMPOUNDS

Practical considerations and some procedural details are presented here for the physician who is contemplating preparing his own radioisotopic compounds or having a chemist prepare them. The information here should also be of value to the physician who wishes to devise a new clinical use for radioisotopes and wishes to estimate the feasibility of obtaining the desired labeled compound.

There are three general methods for preparing labeled compounds: biosynthesis, chemical synthesis and synthesis by nuclear activation of atoms.

1. Biosynthesis

Biosynthesis involves three steps: (1) administration of an isotopic compound to a living organism, (2) conversion by the organism to the desired compound and (3) isolation of the compound in pure state.

a) Usefulness of the Method.—Biosynthesis is preferred when the desired substance is difficult or impossible to prepare by chemical means. Such substances include: proteins; complex carbohydrates (starch, glycogen, inulin); complex lipids (lecithin, cerebrosides); nucleic acids; antibiotics; alkaloids; and many other substances. Even relatively simple compounds, such as the amino acids, sugars and purines, may often be prepared more easily by biosynthesis. One advantage of this method, when plants are used as the synthesizing organism, is that simple, cheap isotopic compounds can be used as the starting material. Plants ordinarily grow on carbon dioxide (C^{14}), water (tritium), sulfate (S^{35}), phosphate (P^{32}) and a variety of trace elements. Although animals usually require more complex starting materials, they, too, can incorporate the simple isotopic compounds into many substances. For example, animals fix carbon dioxide into several amino acids, glucose, purines and pyrimidines.

b) LIMITATIONS OF THE METHOD.—For the most part, the method is restricted to the preparation of substances that occur normally in living organisms. However, organisms are not entirely strict about this and will usually make unnatural modifications if furnished with an unnatural precursor. Thus, unnatural isotopic penicillins can be prepared by including in the penicillium medium the desired radioactive acid residue.

Another limitation is in the specific activity that can be attained. As may be expected, there is a limit to the irradiation that an organism can withstand. A specific activity of 0.7 mc./gm. of carbon has been reported for plants grown in a greenhouse atmosphere of $C^{14}O_2$ (1, 2), and the Schwarz Laboratories has been furnishing C^{14} and S^{35} yeast cells with a specific activity of 100 mc./gm. The specific activity from a biosynthesis is also limited by the presence of preformed living matter in the organism. If a seed or spore is the starting organism and an isotopic medium is used, this dilution is minor. However, if a later stage in the plant or a growing animal is used, there will be somewhat more dilution. In the case of an animal, there will be a tendency toward greater dilution because of the need to continually furnish an external diet.

The dilution effect of using an organism can sometimes be overcome by using a specially oriented organism for just a short time. For example, C^{14}-labeled starch and glucose have been prepared by incubating a previously starved Turkish tobacco leaf in an atmosphere of labeled carbon dioxide (3). Not only is the waste of side reactions minimized this way, but the short exposure time reduces the importance of radiation effects and much higher specific activities can be obtained.

An additional restrictive factor in biosynthesis is that there is usually a great deal of diversion of the isotope into side products, and a large investment in isotopic starting material may be necessary. However, this point is unimportant with the trace elements. It is necessary, of course, to examine various organisms to learn which will give the best yield of the desired compound. It may be possible to locate some persons or organizations who are interested in the other labeled compounds and who will share the expense and effort of isolation.

c) ENZYMES FOR CERTAIN CHEMICAL STEPS.—A special type of biosynthesis which has many points in its favor is the use of enzymes for certain chemical steps. A surprising variety of enzymes is now available commercially* and there are many that can be simply prepared in crude but useful form.

The physician would do well to re-examine the biochemistry textbooks before consulting an organic chemist. Enzymes are frequently not so particular about their substrates as are living things, and therefore many unnatural compounds can be prepared.

2. CHEMICAL SYNTHESIS

The method generally used for preparing labeled compounds is chemical synthesis. In weighing the practicability of a proposed synthetic route, several factors must be considered.

a) YIELD.—The yield is an important question, the importance depending on the cost of the isotope used. Most radioisotopes are rather expensive, especially when the keeping qualities are considered. Unfortunately, most chemical processes have been developed with the wrong yield in mind, the details being biased in favor of the normally more expensive starting material. Carbon dioxide, for example, until recently has not been an expensive item.

When several steps are involved, losses must inevitably occur at each step. It is therefore desirable to pick a route that will incorporate the radioisotopic element toward the end. The same conclusion is reached when the decay characteristics of the radioisotope are taken into account. A stock of a fast-decaying radioisotopic compound cannot be kept long; but a stock of the penultimate compound in the series of steps can be stored if the radioisotope is incorporated in the last step.

A device peculiar to isotope work which is useful in improving the yield is called *dilution scavenging*. In crystallizing, for example, some loss of material is always encountered, part of the

---

* Three prominent suppliers are: Sigma Chemical Company, St. Louis 18, Missouri; Worthington Biochemical Corporation, Freehold, New Jersey; and Mann Research Laboratories, New York 6, New York.

material staying in solution in the mother liquor. A great deal of this isotopic material can be recovered by adding the same compound—nonisotopic—to the mother liquor and crystallizing again. The second crop, to be sure, has a lower specific activity.

b) SPECIFIC ACTIVITY.—Generally, the specific activity should be as high as possible so that the dosage will be minimal, in the physiologic range. Especially important are therapeutic doses, in which it is desired to deliver a maximum amount of activity to a given volume. In the case of I^{131}, for instance, syntheses have been restricted to iodination of phenols, aromatic amines and double bonds, because these go efficiently and readily on a microscale. Other methods of introducing iodine into organic compounds, such as the Sandmeyer reaction, require excessive dilution of the iodine or investment in a large amount of radio-iodine. In the case of many elements, the unused isotope can be recovered and used again; with C^{14}, it is often difficult to recover because dilution with C^{12} may take place.

c) MICROMETHODS; AVOIDANCE OF TRANSFERS.—In order to minimize losses and the need to dilute the isotope, micromethods and avoidance of transfers are necessary. Whenever possible, successive steps should be carried out in the same vessel. When it is necessary to transfer material, it may be possible to use rinses and, if necessary, subsequent evaporation to bring the volume down again (4).

d) PURITY.—Chemical purity of the isotopic compound is not always synonymous with isotopic purity, particularly if a deliberate dilution has been made at the last step, as in dilution scavenging. It may be that an appreciable fraction of the radioactivity is due to the presence of another compound, even though its weight may be a small fraction of the total. When ordinary methods of chemical analysis are not sensitive enough, such as when the nature of the impurity is unknown, chromatographic analysis represents a general method of testing for isotopic impurities. Chromatography is also a valuable method for the isolations involved in biosynthesis.

Chromatography is a method of separating substances, such as a desired compound and its contaminants, by dissolving the mixture in a suitable solvent and pouring the solution into a glass tube filled with a suitable powder, such as activated charcoal, alumina, silica gel or an ion-exchange resin. The liquid is allowed to percolate through the powder and is then followed by more solvent. The liquid effluent from the chromatographic column is collected in serial portions, and with some luck the needed compound will be found in those portions that are free from the contaminants. Such a procedure often gives 100 per cent recovery of pure material. One simply analyzes all the serial fractions from the column for radioactivity. All the activity should be found in those fractions that contain the desired compound, and in amounts that are strictly proportional to the concentrations.

Even easier and faster is paper chromatography, an extraordinary method of chromatography which eliminates the powder and the glass tube and instead uses a rectangular sheet of filter paper. The solution of material to be analyzed is applied as a small drop near one end of the sheet, and the solvent is evaporated off. The paper is then lowered into a glass cylinder containing at the bottom a suitable solvent; a support system keeps the paper vertical so that only the bottom part of the paper is immersed. As the solvent rises by capillary action through the paper, it carries with it the various substances present in the dried spot, each at a different speed. If the solvent was properly chosen, each substance present will form a single, round spot, separate from the other substances, and the radioactive spots can be located by a scanning Geiger counter. A radioisotopically pure substance will reveal only one spot.

Several books describing the various types of chromatography are now available (5, 6, 7).

Storage of the final product is a problem, the seriousness of which has only recently been realized. There are the usual chemical factors peculiar to each compound. Iodine compounds, for example, should be kept cold and away from light, acids and oxidizing agents. However, the radiations from any decomposing atoms inevitably cause a certain amount of destruction of the remaining material. The amount of destruction will depend not only on the isotope but on the nature of the compound. In the case of C^{14} compounds, the self-destruction seems to involve a chain reaction which results in more breakdown than would be expected from the number and energy of the disintegrations suffered (8, 9). Within a few months an appreciable fraction of the labeled compound may be lost. Workers in the field have been slow to realize this, and commercial sources still furnish their labeled materials without noting the shelf storage time or taking precautions to reduce the damage.

Only dilution can reduce the damage to stored compounds, and the easiest way to accomplish dilution is by reducing the specific activity. Alternatively, the compound may be diluted by storing it in solution, but there is the possibility that free radicals formed from the solvent will have a deleterious effect. The safest method is dilution with an inert, finely powdered solid, such as analytic grade celite. The isotopic compound can be dissolved in a volatile solvent, mixed with an appropriate amount of celite, which gives an apparently dry powder, and then dried in a desiccator or oven. Care must be taken to dry the mixture slowly, using a thinly spread sample, since sudden evolution of solvent vapor may widely disperse the radioactive material. Celite is recommended because of its inertness, its large capacity for liquids, its low adsorptive power, which permits ready dissolving-out of the compound, and its low solubility.

e) RADIATION EXPOSURE.—Radiation exposure to the operator must be considered in working with some radioisotopes. In trial runs only small amounts of activity need be handled, but practical work may require dangerous amounts. This means choosing reactions and apparatus which can be controlled from a distance or for short periods of time. Some of the suitable protective techniques are described elsewhere, particularly in Chapter 4 of this book. Mention may be made here of long flexible fingers,* long tongs or solenoids. Solenoids, readily available electromagnets which operate on ordinary house current, are ideal for allowing transfer of solutions; they permit the use of rubber tubing instead of glass stopcocks (10, 11).

For finer control of small movements, a Selsyn motor can be used. In general, stirring motors are used instead of hand-operated stirring rods, electric heaters instead of Bunsen burners, and so on. A window for direct observation can be made readily

---

* Available from Aircraft Specialties, Inc., 415 Howard Street, Lapeer, Michigan.

from a hollow glass brick by drilling a hole in the side, placing the hole side up, and filling the brick with saturated zinc bromide solution.

f) PYROGENS.—The presence of pyrogens in solutions to be injected into animals must be considered. Pyrogens are little-known water-soluble substances, probably lipopolysaccharides, which produce fever and chills on injection. They are produced by many bacteria and molds and may be found even in distilled water which has been allowed to stand. Pharmaceutical companies take great pains to ensure the absence of pyrogens, and any person who prepares isotopic compounds for injection, particularly for human injection, is equally responsible. Sterilization and filtration do not remove all pyrogens.

Many of the purification steps involved in a synthesis will eliminate pyrogens. For example, pyrogens will not develop in dry powders or in solutions that do not allow microbial growth. When possible, the final compound should be dissolved in commercially available pyrogen-free water or saline solution. Pyrogen-free water can be prepared by freshly distilling water from a freshly cleaned still.

Murray and Williams (11) have collected and condensed the procedures for synthesizing a very large number of isotopic compounds. Their first volume describes the synthesis of carbon-labeled compounds, and the second describes the synthesis of organic compounds labeled with isotopic halogens, hydrogen, nitrogen, phosphorus and sulfur.

3. SYNTHESIS BY NUCLEAR ACTIVATION

When a nuclear reaction takes place, either in an atomic pile or in an atom undergoing radioactive decay, the individual atom involved in the reaction has a great deal of energy, which results in the breaking and forming of chemical bonds. In this way, new chemicals are formed; and, under the correct conditions, one might get the desired compound without any need for chemical manipulation except for isolation. Thus, one can expose a mixture of lithium carbonate and an organic compound to neutron bombardment in an atomic pile and end up with the same organic compound, now containing tritium atoms in place of some of the hydrogen atoms (12, 13). The tritium atoms arise from the conversion of lithium atoms. In this way, reserpine, a complex alkaloid of high activity in the central nervous system, has been produced with an activity of 225,000 disintegrations per minute per milligram (dpm/mg.) by 3 days' irradiation. Benzoic acid is a much more suitable starting material, since it yields specific activity of 10,000,000 dpm/mg.

A more convenient approach was recently devised by Wilzbach (14), who showed that a high density of tritium results in exchange of tritium with many hydrogen atoms on adjacent molecules. In this procedure, the compound to be labeled is simply left for a period of several days in a glass vessel filled with tritium gas. The specific activities that have been obtained range between 1 and 100 mc./gm., depending on the compound. The exposure step is now carried out commercially,* and so it is not necessary for the investigator to purchase and handle the large amount of tritium needed. Not all organic compounds can be labeled in this way; but the method is, indeed, very generally useful (15), especially since simple methods of counting tritium have been developed (16, 17).

Nuclear activation has also been described for C^{14}-labeling (18) and should be useful with other isotopes also.

In all such drastic procedures, there is some breakdown of the compound introduced, owing to radiation effects, and there is also some production of new radioactive compounds. It is necessary to carry out a rigorous removal of the impurities, particularly the radioactive ones.

Details regarding the labeling with tritium, phosphorus and iodine are described below.

a) TRITIUM.—Hydrogen labeling has its peculiarities. The hydrogen atoms attached to certain atoms—oxygen, nitrogen, sulfur and certain "activated" carbon atoms—exchange with the hydrogen atoms in water at extremely high speed. Thus, it is pointless to prepare acetic acid in which the carboxyl hydrogen is radioactive, since this atom will simply equilibrate itself with the other exchangeable hydrogens in the medium. Besides this type

---

* New England Nuclear Corporation, Boston, Massachusetts, and Tracerlab, Inc., Waltham, Massachusetts.

of exchange, there is enzymatically activated exchange, which occurs in living organisms acting on certain hydrogen atoms ordinarily considered stably bound. For example, the alpha hydrogen atoms in amino acids are soon "washed out," owing to activation by pyridoxal phosphate enzymes. In general, any position adjacent to a carboxyl or ketone group is suspect.

When exchangeable tritium atoms are inadvertently introduced during a synthesis (by biosynthesis in T_2O or Wilzbach labeling), it is necessary to remove these, preferably by equilibrating the compound briefly in water or alcohol and distilling off the solvent. Several repetitions of the equilibration should bring the "loose" radioactivity down to a negligible level.

Biosynthesis and Wilzbach labeling result in substances which are labeled in many or all stable positions. This automatically raises the specific activity per molecule, a factor to remember when comparing the merits of C^{14}, tritium and other types of labeling.

Labeling by exchange is not limited to nuclear activation. Organically bound hydrogen can sometimes be made to exchange with the labeled hydrogen in T_2O, T_2, or T_2SO_4 by heating in the presence of a catalyst, such as a strong acid or platinum. Not all bound atoms exchange to an equal extent. Other methods of incorporating tritium involve addition of T_2 to a double or triple bond in the presence of a metal catalyst, or addition of TBr or T_2O to a double bond. Halogen atoms can be replaced with labeled hydrogen by catalytic reduction with T_2 or by forming the Grignard reagent (R-Mg-Br) and adding T_2O. Tritium-labeled lithium aluminum hydride is excellent for reducing esters or ketones to labeled alcohols. Glascock has prepared a useful book describing tritium synthesis, handling and counting (19).

A factor important in planning tritium synthesis and subsequent application of the labeled compound is the *isotope effect*. Reactions involving isotopic atoms do not go at the same speed that is observed with ordinary atoms. This difference is quite small for most elements but is appreciable with the lighter ones and quite sizable with tritium. Because of this factor, discriminatory effects appear and the specific chemical activity of the labeled group that is formed in a synthesis (or biologic reaction) may not be the same as the specific chemical activity of the corresponding compound with normal hydrogen. Of course, if the reaction uses up *all* of the compound involved, there can be no discrimination between light and heavy hydrogen atoms.

b) PHOSPHORUS.—Phosphorus-32 is medically useful in the form of chromic phosphate, a highly insoluble salt that is used in colloidal suspension. A simple method of preparation for clinical application is given by Morton (20).

A solution of 0.1 M phosphoric acid containing 1.95×10^{-4} moles and radioactive phosphate, as supplied by Oak Ridge, is added to an ordinary glass-stoppered 60 ml. Pyrex bottle, and the chromic phosphate is precipitated by adding 2.00×10^{-4} moles of 0.1 M chromic nitrate. The chromic nitrate is previously standardized by persulfate iodimetry, and the phosphoric acid by titration against alkali.

The suspension, which is now too coarse, is dried by means of an infrared lamp and left overnight at 500° C. After it has cooled, ¼ in. steel balls are added, the bottle is stoppered, and the whole rotated several days. This improvised ball mill produces particles smaller than 1 μ in a day; after 2–4 days, the diameters range around 0.01 μ, which means that the suspension is stable. The suspension is then sterilized by autoclaving and is diluted with sterile saline solution. If the concentrations of the reagents were incorrect, there may be free phosphate; this can be checked by dialysis, since no activity should leave the dialysis sack.

Dialysis is a frequently required device which is easy to use. Visking dialysis tubing* is ordinarily used. This is supplied as a flat tube of cellophane, containing a small amount of glycerol as plasticizer. A length of tubing is cut, one end is moistened, and a good double knot tied near the end. The entire tube is then wetted, the other end opened, and the solution to be dialyzed pipetted in. Now the open end may simply be supported and the tube dipped in a beaker of water; or the open end may be tied well and the whole sack suspended in the water; or again, in the case of high radiation levels, the open end may be attached to a rubber stopper and the solution added by means of a syringe

---

* Available from the Visking Corp., 6733 W. 65th Street, Chicago 38, Illinois.

and needle through the stopper. The stopper should have a groove around the outer middle to help make a tight connection with the tubing by the use of rubber bands. A hole should be drilled from the top of the stopper nearly to the bottom, to make insertion of the needle easier. The needle is removed before dialyzing.

It is usually convenient to add a weight to the bottom of the sack to keep it vertical in the water. A marble may be inserted inside or a weight may be tied on by means of a string. The process of dialysis involves diffusion of small molecules and ions through the cellophane membrane while large molecules (protein, polysaccharides) and colloidal particles remain inside.

Diffusion is a slow process, and directions often call for long periods, totaling 24 hours; however, agitation, inside and outside the sack, will speed up the diffusion. A rocking dialyzer may be used;* the entire unit is slowly rocked back and forth and the marble inside the sack allowed to roll from one end to the other. A simple method, though less efficient, is to stir the outer liquid from above or with a magnetic stirrer.

It is always necessary to dialyze against several changes of water, since *the reduction in concentration of the diffusible material is approximately proportional to the ratio of inner and outer liquid volumes.*

A point that may be important is the purity of the original labeled phosphate. *Carrier-free* isotopic compounds tend to contain traces of radioactive compounds which are due either to the presence of another radioactive element or to the presence of an unknown form of the radioisotope. Measurable amounts of such impurity have been reported as detected in phosphate preparations by means of electrochromatography (21); the same paper also reports the presence in Ca^{45} of a gamma-emitting isotopic material which can also be separated by the same means. Trace impurities of this sort might in some cases introduce a serious problem, particularly where a large dose of isotope is used in a patient and an appreciable amount of long-lived activity (due to the impurity) is retained for a dangerously long period. Simi-

---

* The Omni-Shaker, available from the Laboratory Glass and Instruments Corp., New York 31, New York.

larly, where the excretion of an isotopic material is followed over a long period, the latter part of the period studied may represent the metabolism of the impurity rather than that of the main material. Such impurities probably vary in percentage, and it seems wise to process all carrier-free isotopes to check the purity or to convert the impurity to the proper form (see the next section for more on this neglected point).

c) IODINE.—Iodine-131, presently the most popular of clinically useful radioisotopes, can be incorporated into many compounds in a relatively simple way. Most procedures involve oxidation of the NaI^{131} obtained from Oak Ridge to form free iodine, which then reacts spontaneously with phenols and aromatic amines to yield carbon-bound iodo compounds and, as by-product, hydrogen iodide. As oxidizing agents, sodium nitrite (22), nitric acid (23) and ammonium persulfate (24) have been used. The problem of oxidation has not been examined thoroughly until recently, probably because oxidation of iodide is such a familiar phenomenon in ordinary chemistry. When carrier iodide is added before oxidation, there is little problem; but when the attempt is made to oxidize carrier-free iodide, the question of complete oxidation arises: *There is an equilibrium between the reduced and oxidized forms in which the iodine concentration is proportional to the square of the iodide concentration; consequently, a dilute solution will tend to exist as iodide.* Carrier-free Oak Ridge iodide has been estimated to have a concentration of about 10^{-7} M (25).

Isotopic purity in the starting material is an allied problem. One worker has found that some lots of NaI^{131} contain some butanol-soluble radioactive impurity (26); others have found benzene-soluble impurities and have studied the nature of these materials in further detail (25). It appears likely that carrier-free iodine contains sodium iodate and organic iodine compounds originating from contaminants in trace amounts. These findings may explain, in part, the low isotopic yields which have been reported.

A method has recently been described for preparing pure iodide, carrier-free, from Oak Ridge material (27). The original solution is refluxed for 30 minutes with 200 ml. of 0.01 M ceric bisulfate in 8 M sulfuric acid; this appears to break down the various iodine derivatives to free iodine. Solid ferrous sulfate in 10 per cent excess is added to reduce the ceric bisulfate, and the solution is distilled, the first 15 ml. being collected. This amount contains about 95 per cent of the original radioactivity, probably in the form of iodine and hydrogen iodide. It should be noted that Oak Ridge I^{131} contains sodium sulfite and sodium hydroxide.

A simpler procedure has been used for preparing pure radioiodine (28). Here, the sulfite is removed by acidifying the Oak Ridge radioiodide and refluxing for a while, then KI and KIO_3 are added and the resultant iodine (equilibrated with the I^{131}) is distilled out of the system. This method automatically dilutes the isotope, but for most purposes this is not harmful.

A detailed review of the preparation of I^{131}-labeled compounds has been prepared recently by Taurog and Chaikoff (29).

(1) *Phenols*—The phenols of special interest are proteins, which are phenols by virtue of their tyrosine content. If iodine is added in amounts equivalent to or less than the amount of tyrosine present, all the iodine will substitute onto the aromatic ring; if more iodine than this is added, the imidazole ring of the histidine residues will also be attacked. It is customary to iodinate proteins with a minimum amount of iodine, often 1 or 2 atoms per protein molecule; however, as many as 18 atoms per molecule have been reported to give antibodies still possessing their specific precipitability (30). The number of iodine atoms in a few millicuries of carrier-free iodide is so small that this stipulation can be met even with appreciable addition of inactive iodine.

When the iodination can take place in the presence of the oxidizing agent, the hydrogen iodide formed is oxidized to iodine; thus complete utilization of the investment in radioiodine is permitted. When proteins are iodinated, it is advisable to add a buffer to protect the sensitive molecules against denaturation due to pH changes. Some proteins denature readily at the interface between two phases; therefore, violent agitation, bubbling or shaking with immiscible solvents should generally be avoided.

(2) *Serum Albumin.*—A simple method for efficient iodination of serum albumin has been described (24). Bovine albumin powder, fraction V or dried USP salt-poor human serum albumin may be used. In a typical run with 10–20 mc. iodide,

150 mg. albumin is dissolved in 2 ml. saline phosphate buffer (8.46 gm. NaCl, 7.24 gm. $Na_2HPO_4 \cdot 12H_2O$, and 0.53 gm. $NaH_2PO_4 \cdot H_2O$ diluted to 1,000 ml. with distilled water).

To this solution, in a 35 ml. test tube, is added 2 ml. of 2.5 per cent guanidine hydrochloride and 1 ml. of 0.217 per cent potassium iodide. The radioiodide in 0.5–2 ml. is added next and finally 2 ml. of the oxidizing solution, 10 per cent ammonium persulfate, made up in the saline phosphate. The reacting mixture is left in a hood for 4 hours and then transferred to a sack made from 1 in. dialysis tubing, which is then dialyzed against running tap water for 2 hours. The dialysis removes most or all of the nonprotein material. The sack is then cut open while in a beaker containing 300 ml. saline phosphate. After standing half an hour, the iodinated serum albumin is ready.

Pyrogenic reactions have not been observed. The guanidine, potassium iodide, and persulfate solutions should be prepared fresh. The radioisotopic yield runs from 90 to 95 per cent.

The guanidine hydrochloride probably serves to make the tyrosine groups of the protein a little more accessible, since guanidine salts act to break the hydrogen bonds and salt linkages which hold the polypeptide chains in tight arrangements. A suitable milder agent of this type might be urea. However, there is a certain tendency for such reagents to produce some irreversible denaturation, and it might be better to avoid them where it is necessary to retain maximal identity. Francis, Mulligan and Wormall use the above method but without the guanidine (31).

Where a labeled protein can be precipitated out readily with concentrated ammonium sulfate, one might save time by carrying out several such precipitations to remove the excess radioactive reagent and then dialyze briefly to remove the ammonium sulfate that adheres to the precipitated protein.

The problem of labeling proteins with iodine in such a way that the "true identity" of the protein is preserved is sometimes of considerable importance. When the labeled protein is followed for just a short time, the requirements are not so stringent. However, where immunologic reactions or long periods of time are considered, differences in behavior may appear. McFarlane has studied this by comparing iodinated proteins, iodinated in different ways, with biosynthetically labeled proteins (32). The latter were made by feeding animals radioactive amino acids. McFarlane concludes that the least modification is accomplished by a "jet iodination" technique, a rapid method of mixing which is too complex to describe here. Another suggestion for mild iodination is the use of pure radioiodine mixed with carrier (28). Since no other reagents (particularly oxidants) are added, it is claimed that the protein is less likely to change its structure appreciably.

(3) *Whole Blood Serum.*—Iodination of whole blood serum can be performed (30, 33) by mixing carrier-free iodide with a solution of iodine in potassium iodide, allowing 30 minutes to complete the exchange reaction, then adding the serum in borate buffer and leaving the preparation in an ice bath for 30 minutes. The excess iodine is reduced with sodium thiosulfate and nonprotein material removed by dialysis. The dialysis is made against several portions of cold saline solution. Samples are checked to make sure that the amount of radioactivity in the outer liquid reaches a low level. Cold solutions prevent denaturation. Note also that the dialysis here is made against saline rather than water. With some proteins, it is necessary to maintain a rather specific pH or salt concentration in order to maintain the protein in solution or keep it from denaturing. Sometimes it is safer to dialyze against distilled water rather than tap water, since the small ions in the tap water diffuse into the sack.

(4) *Double Bonds.*—Radioiodine can be incorporated into some organic compounds by addition to double bonds, as in the familiar iodine-number determination for the measurement of fat unsaturation. Some fats have been labeled in this way, by leaving iodine or iodine monochloride with the fat in ether or chloroform overnight (23, 34). The solution is then washed successively with sodium thiosulfate, nonisotopic iodide and water to remove the excess, unreacted I^{131}. The nonisotopic iodide wash is used to dilute and exchange with any radioiodide that may be adsorbed on the apparatus or otherwise held back in the organic layer.

Iodine, like hydrogen, can exchange with the carbon-bound element; for example, thyroxine can be made in the ordinary way with ordinary iodine and then many of the iodine atoms can be replaced (26, 35) by I^{131}. The remaining inorganic iodine is then removed by appropriate washings. Iodide is used, with a trace of iodine as catalytic intermediate, and the pH is controlled at 4.6 and the temperature at 65° C. Exchange, incidentally, is sometimes inadvertently found in the course of experimental handling of labeled iodine compounds and may be avoided by keeping the material away from acid, light, heat and oxidizing agents, all of which might produce a trace of iodine.

(5) *Other Methods of Labeling Proteins.*—Proteins have many functional groups which, like the tyrosine phenol ring, can readily be derivatized with a radioactive reagent. One can use diazotized sulfanilic acid, made from S^{35}-labeled sulfanilic acid, or I^{131}-labeled paraiodobenzoyl chloride (36). Isothiocyanates, now so valuable for introducing a fluorescent group into proteins for visual labeling, could be made with radioactive isotopes. A mild acetylating agent is C^{14}- or H^3-labeled acetic anhydride.

REFERENCES

1. Larson, P. S., and Harlow, E. S.: Some current applications of C^{14} to animal and human physiological research: Studies with tobacco and its constituents, in Extermann, R. C. (ed): *Radioisotopes in Scientific Research,* vol. 3 (New York: Pergamon Press, 1958), p. 62.
2. Scully, N. J., *et al.:* Biosynthesis in C^{14}-labeled plants: Their use in agricultural and biological research, *Proceedings of the International Conference on the Peaceful Uses of Atomic Energy, Geneva, Switzerland,* vol. 15 (New York: United Nations, 1956).
3. Putman, E. W., *et al.:* Preparation of radioactive carbon-labeled sugars by Photosynthesis, J. Biol. Chem. 173:785, 1948.
4. Radin, N. S.: Solvent removal by vacuum evaporation, Anal. Chem. 28:542, 1956.
5. Lederer, E., and Lederer, M.: *Chromatography* (New York: Elsevier Publishing Co., 1957).
6. Block, R. J.; Durrum, E. L., and Zweig, G.: *A Manual of Paper Chromatography and Paper Electrophoresis* (New York: Academic Press, Inc., 1958).
7. Cassidy, H. G.: *Fundamentals of Chromatography* (New York: Interscience Publishers, Inc., 1957).
8. Lemmon, R. M.: Radiation decomposition of carbon-14-labeled compounds, Nucleonics 11:44, 1953.
9. Tolbert, B. M., and Lemmon, R. M.: Radiation decomposition of pure organic compounds, Radiation Res. 3:52, 1955.
10. Radin, N. S.: Dispenser for radioactive solutions, Nucleonics 13:6 and 92, 1955.
11. Murray, A., III, and Williams, D. L.: *Organic Synthesis with Isotopes* (2 vols.; New York: Interscience Publishers, Inc., 1958).

312 THE RADIOISOTOPE LABORATORY

12. Rowland, F. S., and Wolfgang, R.: Tritium-recoil labeling of organic compounds, Nucleonics 14:8 and 58, 1956.
13. ——— and Numerof, P.: Radioactive labeling of reserpine by tritium recoil, Internat. J. Appl. Radiation 1:246, 1957.
14. Wilzbach, J.: Tritium-labeling by exposure of organic compounds to tritium gas, J. Am. Chem. Soc. 79:1013, 1957.
15. *Symposium on Tritium in Tracer Applications* (available from New England Nuclear Corp., Boston).
16. Bell, C. G., Jr., and Hayes, F. N.: *Liquid Scintillation Counting* (New York: Pergamon Press, 1958).
17. Tolbert, B. M.: *Ionization Chamber Assay of Radioactive Gases,* UCRL-3499 (available from Office of Technical Services, U.S. Department of Commerce, Washington, D. C.).
18. Wolf, A. P.: Use of recoiling carbon-14 as a new technique in labeling organic compounds, in Extermann, R. C.: *Radioisotopes in Scientific Research* (New York: Pergamon Press), vol. II (1958), p. 114.
19. Glascock, R. F.: *Isotopic Gas Analysis for Biochemists* (New York: Academic Press, Inc., 1954).
20. Morton, M. E.: Colloidal chromic radiophosphate in high yields for radiotherapy, Nucleonics 10:11 and 92, 1952.
21. Sato, T. R., *et al.:* Electrochromatographic separations of calcium and phosphate ions: Factors influencing separations, Anal. Chem. 25:438, 1953.
22. Pressman, D., and Eisen, H. N.: The zone of localization of antibodies, J. Immunol. 64:273, 1950.
23. Hoffman, M. C.: Radioactive iodine-labeled fat, J. Lab. & Clin. Med. 41:521, 1953.
24. Gilmore, R. C., Jr.; Robbins, Margaret C., and Reid, Allen F.: Labeling bovine and human albumin with I[131], Nucleonics 12:2 and 65, 1954.
25. Kahn, M., and Wahl, A. C.: Some observations on the chemical behavior of iodine at low concentrations, J. Chem. Physics 21:1185, 1953.
26. Larson, F. C.; Coulson, D. M., and Albright, E. C.: Radiochemical method for the determination of microquantities of thyroxine, J. Biol. Chem. 196:45, 1952.
27. Kahn, M.; Freedman, A. J., and Shultz, C. G.: Distillation of carrier-free I[131] activity, Nucleonics 12:7 and 72, 1954.
28. Staub, A.; Springs, V., and Elrick, H.: An improved technique for labelling protein with I[131], Internat. J. Appl. Radiation 2:59, 1957.
29. Taurog, A., and Chaikoff, I. L.: Synthetic and analytic procedures involving I[131]-labeled compounds, in Colowick, S. P., and Kaplan, N. O. (eds.): *Methods in Enzymology,* vol. IV (New York: Academic Press, Inc., 1957), p. 856.
30. Pressman, D., and Sternberger, L. A.: Relative rates of iodination of serum components and the effect of iodination on antibody activity, J. Am. Chem. Soc. 72:2226, 1950.

31. Francis, G. E.; Mulligan, W., and Wormall, A.: Labelling antibodies with I^{131} and S^{35}, Biochem. J. 60:364, 1955.

32. McFarlane, A. S.: Labelling of plasma protein with radioactive iodine, Biochem. J. 62:135, 1956.

33. Cohen, S.: Determination of antibody through the use of I^{131} label: Experiments with equine diphtheria antitoxin, J. Immunol. 67:339, 1951.

34. Rutenberg, A. M; Seligman, A. M., and Fine, J.: Studies with radio-active iodized fat, J. Clin. Invest. 28:1105, 1949.

35. Frieden, E.; Lipsett, M. B., and Winzler, R. J.: Methods for label-ing thyroxine with radioactive iodine, Science 107:353, 1948.

36. Blau, M.; Johnson, A. C., and Pressman, D.: p-Iodobenzoyl groups as a paired label for in vivo protein distribution studies: Specific localization of anti-tissue antibodies, Internat. J. Appl. Radiation 3:217, 1958.

CHAPTER 16

Instructions for Operating Radiation Detection Devices

INSTRUCTIONS FOR OPERATING the necessary radiation sensing elements are presented here for those who are medically trained but who have a minimum of mathematical and electronic background. The tests described should enable appropriate personnel to operate and maintain the radioisotope laboratory; they are not intended to supplant more rigorous nucleonic descriptions in other texts (1, 2, 3). It is presupposed that the reader has an elementary knowledge of radioactivity (4, 5).

The quantity of radioactive material is determined by observing the effects of the emitted radiation as it passes through matter. These effects are ionization and emission of light by excited molecules. The ionization can be detected by ionization chambers, Geiger counters, proportional counters and emulsions (film). The emitted radiation can be detected if it traverses special types of matter called "scintillators." When the ions and light do not emerge from the absorber, all the energy goes into heat, which can be measured with a very sensitive calorimeter.

A. LAURITSEN ELECTROSCOPE*

The Lauritsen electroscope (Figs. 62 and 63) is a basic instrument for the radioisotope laboratory. With it, assays can easily be made of entire shipments of isotopes, of doses given to pa-

---

* Manufactured by Fred C. Henson Co., Pasadena, California.

tients and, in many instances, of samples taken from patients.

The Lauritsen electroscope is essentially a combination of the ionization chamber and the gold-leaf (fiber) electroscope. The ionization chamber is an enclosure consisting of two electrodes: the outer wall, or cathode; and the central collecting electrode, or anode. Between these electrodes gas (usually air) is enclosed, and a collecting voltage is impressed upon the anode. The anode is the mount of the indicating leaf. Before using the electroscope, the fiber is deflected from its rest position through being charged by the application of approximately 100 volts. The rate of dis-

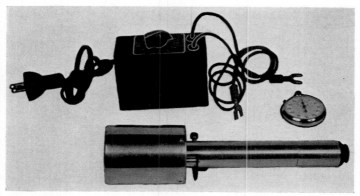

FIG. 62.—Lauritsen electroscope: external view. (Courtesy: Fred C. Henson Co., Pasadena, California.)

charge, or of return to rest position, of the fiber is proportional to the rate of formation of ions in the chamber in which it is mounted. The radiation intensity is measured by determining the time necessary to cause the fiber to discharge a fixed amount. The longer the time, the weaker the radiation source. The fiber is viewed through an eyepiece and a calibrated scale, and a stop watch is used to time the rate of deflection.

a) OPERATING INSTRUCTIONS.—The instrument should preferably be mounted at a considerable distance from scattering (i.e., solid) media in order to prevent secondary radiation from being scattered into the ion chamber. The distance from the room wall to the chamber should be approximately three times the distance from the radiation source to the chamber. It will be most convenient if the electroscope is mounted at eye level above a wood table in the center of a room.

To operate the timer and to provide the light source needed for viewing the quartz fiber, 120 volt, 60 cycle, A.C. current is necessary. In some instances, battery power can be substituted for A.C. power, but for long and continuous use it is preferable to use A.C. power.

The Lauritsen electroscope is easily calibrated by using the radioactive standards supplied periodically by the National Bu-

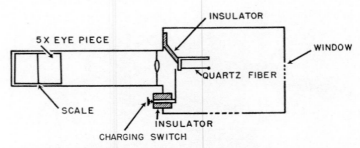

FIG. 63.—Lauritsen electroscope: schematic view. (Courtesy: Fred C. Henson Co., Pasadena, California.)

reau of Standards.* One can simply follow the operating sequence noted below and note the deflection time for a constant degree of deflection of the electroscope fiber. It has been found most convenient to use, as a measurement point, one half (50 divisions) of the full scale and a source-chamber distance of 50 cm. Typical examples for the time of deflection are:

> Iodine-131 = 14.7 minutes/mc./50 divisions/50 cm.
> Iron-59   = 5.9 minutes/mc./50 divisions/50 cm.

It is recommended that each counting procedure be performed a minimum of three times. In this way, spurious effects noticed from faulty insulation, or the momentary passing of radioactive samples (e.g., radium) in the vicinity of the electroscope, can be

---

* Radioactivity Section, National Bureau of Standards, Washington 25, D. C.

eliminated. Because the Lauritsen electroscope is used to calibrate therapeutic doses, the measurements must be accurate to within ± 5 per cent. It will be found that the readings are generally reproducible to better than 1 per cent over the range indicated. Through the use of the same range for all samples, errors due to nonlinearity of the instrument will be eliminated.

b) OPERATION AND SEQUENCES:

1. Before turning on the instrument, set the knob on the power supply at midscale.
2. Turn on the power.
3. Depress the red charging button until it makes contact with the fiber electrode.
4. Observe the position of the fiber and adjust it, by means of the knob on the power supply, to a position just to the left of zero.
5. Release the charging button. The instrument is then ready for operation. It is recommended by the manufacturers that the Lauritsen electroscope be "warmed up" for at least 1 hour before radioactive sources are to be measured; this will eliminate the charge effect on the insulators in this type of device. There is always a slow movement of the quartz fiber across the scale of the viewer even when no radioactive sources are in view; this is due to the background rate produced by cosmic radiation and contamination in the area. The background rate, in most instances, will be less than 1 per cent of the value of the deflection rate resulting from radioactive sources and may be ignored.
6. In those instances in which the deflection rate is rapid, owing to a large amount of contamination, it will be necessary to take a background reading before radioactive sources are counted. The background is subtracted as follows:

$$\frac{1}{T_{sample}} = \frac{1}{T_{total}} - \frac{1}{T_{background}}$$

7. The operative sequence consists of the following:
   (*a*) The quartz fiber should be charged up to a position below zero.

(b) The timing clock should be turned on after the fiber drifts to the zero position. The operator should view the quartz-fiber deflection until it reaches midscale or 50 divisions (full scale 100 divisions).

(c) At this time, the timing clock should be turned off and a record made of the time of deflection. The conversion factor (e.g., for iodine-131 this may be 14.7) is divided by the time lapse, and the quotient is the number of millicuries in the particular sample being tested. This conversion factor may differ for various instruments but remains remarkably constant for any given instrument under conditions of constant geometry and sample preparation.

It is convenient to use a 1 mg. radium source, with an eyelet for insertion of a fine thread, for routine calibration of the Lauritsen electroscope in order to check its accuracy. This electroscope can also be used for the measurement of beta sources under the aluminum window of the instrument, but more accurate results can be secured with an end-window Geiger counter.

B. PORTABLE SURVEY METERS

1. PORTABLE GEIGER COUNTER

The portable Geiger counter* (Fig. 64) is one of the most useful devices for checking radiation safety in the medical radioisotope laboratory. It is helpful in the detection of contamination of equipment, instruments and facilities. Its advantages are its sensitivity and rapid reading time. The instrument contains a Geiger tube,† which delivers an electrical impulse after it has been sensitized by ionizing radiation. This radiation may be either a beta or a gamma ray which has entered the glass window of the Geiger tube (thickness equal to approximately 30 mg./cm.²). The Geiger tube is generally filled with a gas at low pressure

---

* The Geiger-Müller counter, also commonly known as the "G–M counter."

† The Geiger-Müller counter tube, also commonly known as the "G–M tube."

(often an argon and alcohol mixture). This impulse is fed to a simple electronic circuit which integrates these pulses over a short period and indicates the rate at which these pulses are received on an indicating milliammeter. The entire device is battery operated and is small and light in weight. Detailed analysis of the instrument's operation is not presented here, but reference (6) at the end of the chapter may be consulted.

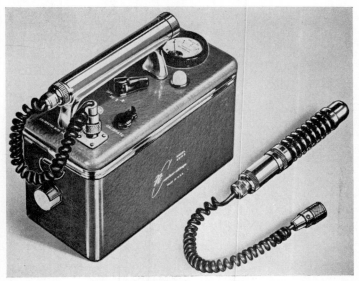

Fig. 64.—Portable Geiger counter: external view. (Courtesy: Nuclear-Chicago.)

The portable Geiger counter is used not for quantitative measurements but only as a qualitative device. The limitations of these sets are: difficulty of reproducing geometry because of lack of rigid mount, and lack of adequate circuit stability. It is not recommended that such an instrument be used for accurate calibration of doses. It should be used solely as a qualitative or indicative type of instrument when contamination or other evidences of radiation (7) is being sought.

The Geiger tube is mounted within a metal probe for ruggedness and protection. The sensitive portion of the counter is exposed behind a screened window in the probe and is ordinarily exposed by moving a closed shield away from this window. To permit distinguishing between beta particles and gamma rays, this shield can be shoved in or out of place. Beta rays will not be detected by the Geiger counter with the shield in place. The probe is attached to the instrument proper by means of a 4 or 5 ft. cable, which allows the operator to scan the less accessible locations, such as corners, ceilings and other areas difficult to reach.

a) OPERATING INSTRUCTIONS.—The portable Geiger counter should be located near the area in which contamination is most frequently found in the clinical radioisotope laboratory—the area near the sinks or radioisotope-dispensing locales of the laboratory. Batteries supply the power for this counter. Generally the battery drain is such that the battery will have a ½ year life if it is used daily for approximately 3 or 4 hours a day. It is important that the device be turned off when not in use.

Although the portable Geiger counter can be calibrated electronically by the use of a pulse generator, electronic pulse generators are not found in the routine clinical radioisotope laboratory, and the subject will not be covered further here. The portable Geiger counter should be calibrated with the use of radioactive sources. A 1 mg. radium source is again recommended. The calibration is done by applying the following formula:

$$\text{Roentgens/hour} = 8.4 \times \text{mc./distance}^2$$

where the source-counter distance is in centimeters. The formula applies only to radium sources in which platinum ½ mm. thick covers the needle. The instrument is usually equipped with a potentiometer adjustment which enables the operator to change the calibration to give an accurate reading, as calculated by use of the formula. This is a simple adjustment and should be done periodically by the operator using the device.

The accuracy of the portable Geiger counter is not any greater than ± 10 per cent of the meter reading. Contributing factors are: variations in response to different energy photons, statistical inaccuracy inherent in the low counting rate and inaccuracy due to the contribution of scattered radiation.

b) OPERATING SEQUENCE.—The switch usually has four positions: 0.2, 2.0 and 20 milliroentgens per hour full scale and an "Off" position. The present maximum radiation tolerance levels are 6.25 mr./hr., and this will be indicated on the least sensitive scale: 20 mr./hr. The cosmic ray background will usually indicate a reading of about 0.05 mr./hr.; this will be noted most obviously on the 0.2 mr./hr. scale. On most of the available portable counters it is possible to use earphones, which are operated by inserting the plug into the jack provided for this purpose. With the phones, it is relatively easy to use the device for surveying an area where the indicating meter cannot be observed continuously.

In operating the portable Geiger counter, the switch should first be turned to the least sensitive scale (20 mr./hr.) to prevent meter damage if a strong radiation field is present. It is not necessary to allow warm-up time, since the device is ready to operate almost instantly after being switched on. If a reading does not appear on the least sensitive scale, the meter should be switched to the other scales until such indication does appear.

The portable Geiger counter is not a rugged device; it should not be dropped, and, in general, should be handled carefully. Tube and battery replacement are required periodically, but the more modern instruments of this type present no problem. In most instruments a Geiger tube is used which has an ordinary life of about 10^{10} counts. It may be possible to purchase a device containing a halogen type of counter tube, a type which has virtually infinite life. This tube has certain limitations, however, which make it a less practical counter than the ordinary argon-alcohol filled Geiger tube.

In a field of very intense radiation, it is a common characteristic of most portable Geiger survey meters that the indicator, instead of reading full scale, will drop to a zero reading. This occurs when the pulses arrive with too short an interval between pulses; the instrument is then unable to distinguish any radiation. The operator should be aware of this serious limitation, which can be noticed when, after the device has been turned on, the indicator swings violently over to full scale and promptly drops down to the zero reading. He should not operate the device for any length of time in this intense field.

2. PORTABLE IONIZATION CHAMBER DEVICES

The ionization chamber device is not as popular as the portable Geiger counter in the clinical radioisotope laboratory, although it has a definite function to perform. As has been noted, the Geiger counter does not function in the presence of very intense radiations—it will give a negative instead of a positive answer. The ionization chamber (Fig. 65), on the other hand, does not

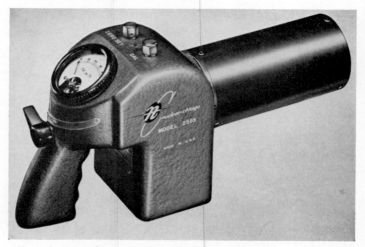

FIG. 65.—Portable ionization chamber: external view. (Courtesy: Nuclear-Chicago.)

exhibit this characteristic and is therefore useful where high radiation levels are encountered, such as after the administration of therapeutic doses of radioisotopes to patients. The sensitivity ranges of the ionization chamber overlap, and it is generally found that this instrument can perform the same radiation measurements as the Geiger counter, although the latter is more sensitive for contamination detection.

The portable ionization chamber consists essentially of a two-electrode system, each system well insulated from the other by means of plastic insulators. The wall of the chamber serves as one electrode, and a center collecting electrode serves as the high-voltage electrode. When ionizing radiation passes through the gas between the electrodes, it produces ion pairs in this gas. Because of the electric field that has been applied across this chamber, these ion pairs are collected, according to their polarity, by one or the other electrodes. If the voltage field is not great enough, some of the ions will recombine before they are collected. A voltage is applied to the chamber which causes a saturation

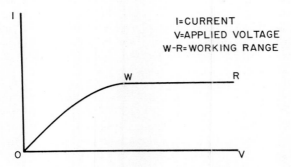

I=CURRENT
V=APPLIED VOLTAGE
W-R=WORKING RANGE

FIG. 66.—Saturation curve, ionization chamber.

collection of ions, or, in other words (Fig. 66), a field which is strong enough to collect all of the ion pairs before they are capable of recombining with one another. The ionization in the chamber is due to photoelectrons, Compton electrons and electron pairs formed in the chamber walls by the incoming photons. One of the factors affecting the number of ion pairs created here is the initial energy of the ionizing radiation; therefore, this type of device gives a quantitative measurement of roentgen dosage.

One of the most common instruments used in this field is a device called a "cutie pie,"* (so-named by the workers of the Atomic Energy Commission). This instrument serves excellently for general area surveying. It is operated by means of a single switch having five positions and is fitted with a pistol-type grip for ease in handling. There is an adjusting position for setting the zero reading of the meter.

---

* Manufactured by Nuclear-Chicago, Chicago, Illinois; Tracerlab, Inc., Richmond, California; and other companies.

The "cutie pie" is primarily intended for the measurement of gamma radiation, but it usually is made with a thin window (approximately 1 mg./cm.²) at the end of its barrel-type ionization chamber. This chamber has a rotary shield permitting the measurement of high-energy beta particles. For the calibration of this device there is an external calibration adjuster. The ranges seen on this type of meter are usually 50, 500 and 5,000 mr./hr. —all full scale.

a) OPERATING INSTRUCTIONS.—The ionization chamber device should be located near the areas of highest possible contamination. It should be taken along whenever techniques are performed which employ large therapeutic doses of radioisotopes. The power supply of the portable ionization chamber is a battery, consisting of one or two 1½ volt cells, often of a mercury type. In addition, there is a B and C supply provided by four 22½ volt batteries of the hearing-aid type. The battery life is approximately 250 hours at an operating rate of 2 hours a day. The meter can be calibrated with the use of the 1 mg. radium source previously described. Here, again, the equation mentioned above (p. 320) is used to calculate the calibration, and the calibration control knob of the "cutie pie" is adjusted to give an accurate reading.

b) OPERATING SEQUENCE:

1. The instrument should be turned to its filament or warm-up position for a period of at least 1 minute.
2. The switch should then be placed on the zero set position, at which time the meter should be adjusted for a zero reading with the potentiometer control.
3. It is recommended that the meter be warmed up for at least 5–10 minutes before actual use.
4. The instrument should be operated on its most sensitive position, which will generally be at 50 mr./hr. full-scale range.

C. THE GEIGER COUNTER

Until the advent of the scintillation counter, the Geiger counter tube (Figs. 67 and 68) was the radiation detection device most frequently used in the medical radioisotope laboratory. Since most of the studies and tests described in this manual employ scintillation counters, some of the uses of the Geiger counter are presented at this point only for the sake of completeness. It is recommended, however, that scintillation counters be used, whenever possible, in preference to Geiger counters. A notable exception is the preferred use of the Geiger counter for internal brain-tumor localization.

The Geiger counter is essentially a two-electrode device. Its operation depends on the creation of electron avalanches within

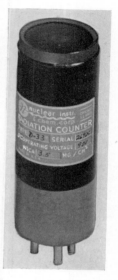

FIG. 67.—End-window Geiger tube: external view. (Courtesy: Nuclear-Chicago.)

the gas of the counter tube. The outer electrode, or cathode, is usually at a ground potential; and the center electrode, or anode, is at a higher potential of approximately 900–1,500 volts, the value depending on the nature of the Geiger tube. Because of the instrument's great sensitivity, even a single ionizing particle is capable of initiating the electron avalanche within the counter tube.

The primary ion pairs (positive ions and free electrons) which are created by this single ionizing radiation begin to move under the influence of the electric field, with the positive ions going to the cathode (negatively charged) and the free electrons going to the anode (positively charged). The counter tube is designed so that the electric field is very intense in the center of the tube (around a central wire). As the electrons move into this region of greatly increasing electric field, they accelerate very rapidly, and they soon acquire sufficient energy to produce additional ion pairs (positive ions and electrons) by colliding with the neutral atoms within the gas. In turn, the secondary electrons produce additional ion pairs. As the electrons travel toward the anode, the positive ions which are formed move toward the

cathode. The total electric charge collected in such an avalanche
is very large, and the result is a tremendous amplification of the
primary ionization. The amplification factor may be as large
as 10^9; i.e., the number of charges collected may be 10^9 times
as large as the number of primary ions.

A common type of Geiger counter is constructed within a
glass envelope. The cathode is made of a copper or higher-
atomic-mass metallic material plated onto the inner wall of the

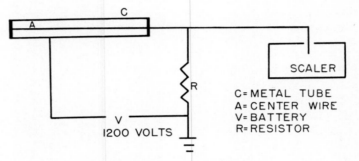

FIG. 68.—Geiger tube: schematic view.

cylindrical glass envelope. Electrical connection is made to the
cathode via a wire sealed into the glass envelope. The center
anode is generally of tungsten wire (about 0.01 in. diameter),
which extends from one end of the glass envelope to the other,
with an external electric lead sealed through the glass. The sensitivity of these counters for gamma rays of a particular energy
is, in the main, determined by the density and atomic number of
the material in the cathode. It will be found that the efficiency
of Geiger counters lies between 0.1 and 1 per cent for the gamma-
ray energies encountered in clinical radioisotope studies.

In using Geiger counters for the measurement of beta radiation, it is essential to modify the thickness of the Geiger counter
wall to allow for the transmission of the beta rays. These particles have a lower penetrating power than gamma rays of the
same energy; therefore, some counters have a window of a thin
material, such as mica or celluloid. The thickness of this window
is commonly described in units of weight per unit area (mg./

cm²). Because beta particles are capable of great ionization, the efficiency of the Geiger counter for detection of such ionizing radiation is approximately 100 per cent; in other words, any beta particle capable of entering the counting chamber of the Geiger counter will ionize the gas and produce a pulse.

There are a number of types of specially designed Geiger counters which may be of use at some time in the clinical radio-isotope laboratory. One special form is the needle-type probe, which is usually a more sensitive and a more useful device than a scintillation counter for the purposes of internal brain-tumor localization. This counter consists of a small probe, 3 mm. outside diameter, with a radioactive sensitive detecting area of approximately 1 cm. in length at the end of the probe. A large-sized barrel, approximately 5 in. from the end of the probe, serves as a reservoir for the gas used in the probe. The counter operates at about 600 volts potential, and some of the more advanced designs are filled with halogen-type mixtures. It is important that the operating instructions for the use of probe Geiger counters be carefully observed, because any overvoltage will cause permanent damage to the counter.

All Geiger counters—or, indeed, any other type of radiation detection device to be used for accurate assay—should not be located near any varying sources of radioactivity. There should also be a relatively constant ambient temperature within the room in which the counter is located. This does not necessitate the use of an air-conditioning system, but large fluctuations in the temperature are undesirable. Some counters may be photosensitive and should therefore be located within a darkened shield, or they may be covered with an opaque surface coating.

As will be noted in the following section on calibration, Geiger counters should be supplied from a stable high-voltage source. This high-voltage supply is usually incorporated within the scaler or rate meter to which the output of the Geiger counter is connected. Because of the variation in sensitivity of the counters for different applied voltages, it is important that the power supply be regulated to ± 1 per cent. In other words, for an operating voltage of approximately 1,000 volts, a ± 1 per cent variation would result in a total fluctuation of the order of ± 10 volts. In general, the counter sensitivity would vary accordingly. It is also desirable that the power supply be of a type that "fails safe"; i.e., when a component fails, the voltage tends to decrease, thus preventing overvoltage in a Geiger tube. In some hospitals, it may be necessary to employ a voltage regulating transformer to the high-voltage supply in order to maintain operation over those periods in which the hospital's service of 110

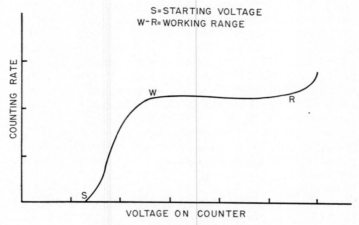

S=STARTING VOLTAGE
W-R= WORKING RANGE

FIG. 69.—Geiger tube: plateau curve.

volts drops below this voltage. This is especially true of old hospital buildings, where sudden line loads drop the voltage.

There is a certain minimum potential required before the counter operates as a Geiger tube. This is the voltage at which the large avalanches begin to form. Above this voltage the size of the individual pulses will increase with an increase in potential, but the number of pulses per unit time for a constant source of radiation should remain virtually the same. As the voltage is increased, this situation will prevail until the voltage reaches a point where there is a continuous discharge across the counter. This type of operation is depicted in Figure 69, in which the counting rate is plotted on the ordinate and the potential is plotted on the abscissa. The value of the potential at which counting begins is called the *starting voltage,* the exact value of which is determined by the input sensitivity of the scaler employed. The horizontal portion of the curve is called the *Geiger plateau* and represents the range over which the counter is used. The slope of this plateau is from 5 to 10 per cent in the commercially available tubes. It extends between 200 and 500 volts, from the beginning of the plateau, depending on the type of counter employed. When the counter is operated at higher voltages, toward the upper end of the plateau, larger pulses result because a greater number of secondary ion pairs are formed. With these pulses, however, there also occurs a more rapid deterioration of the Geiger tube gas, so that the life of the tube is shortened. Whenever a Geiger tube is to be used, the plateau curve should be taken after the input sensitivity of the scaler has been adjusted at its recommended voltage.

Geiger counters should also be tested for such other operating characteristics as resolution time and background rates. For formulas relating to these determinations, the reader is directed to Appendix B. The counting efficiency of Geiger counters for a particular radioactive source depends on a number of factors, including: *(a)* energy distribution of the beta particles, *(b)* absorption of the particles in the sample material and in the walls (or window) of the tube, *(c)* scattering of particles from the sample mount and other solid objects close to the counter and *(d)* the geometric relationship between source and tube window. In order to calibrate the counter, sources of known disintegration rates are necessary. These should have the same energy spectra as the radioactive source to be counted; known amounts of the same source are often used, but "stand-ins" are also available. It is recommended that calibration sources be obtained periodically from the National Bureau of Standards.

Whenever tests are conducted with the use of any radiation detection device, certain inherent errors are introduced by the random nature of radioactive disintegrations. This randomness implies that, if a source is counted several times for the same length of time, each counting interval will yield a different number of counts. In order to utilize the results of a single counting interval, it is necessary to determine the spread of results that would occur if the counting process were repeated again and again for fixed time intervals. By calculating this spread from the results of a single measurement, it is possible to estimate the reliability of the result.

To make such calculations, the standard deviation is used. If N counts are measured in the chosen time interval, then the standard deviation, σ, is equal to $\sqrt{N}$. It is known that statistical fluctuations may be expected, so that a repeated count would yield a number greater than or less than N, but it may also be expected that the new count be within the region of $N \pm t\sigma$. The value of t depends upon the degree of certainty desired. If $t = 1.0$, there is a 68 per cent probability that the new count will be between $N - \sigma$ and $N + \sigma$. If $t = 2.0$, there is a 95 per cent probability that the new count lies in the range $N \pm 2\sigma$; i.e., in many repeated counts, 19 out of 20 results will lie within this range. If $t = 0.67$, there is a 50 per cent probability that the new count lies in the range $N \pm 0.67\sigma$. All of the above methods of expressing the uncertainty are used. When $t = 1$, σ is commonly called the "standard error"; when $t = 2$, 2σ is called the "95 per cent confidence limit"; and when $t = 0.67$, 0.67σ is called the "probable error." The relative error is $t\sigma/N$, or $t/\sqrt{N}$; and the percentage error is $100t/N^{1/2}$. It is obvious that these errors decrease with an increase in N. Thus it can be seen that it is possible to increase the percentage accuracy by either increasing the concentration of the radioactive source with which one is observing a particular procedure or by increasing the total counting time. (See Appendix B.)

a) OPERATING SEQUENCE.—A long warm-up period is not usually required for the operation of a Geiger counter. In some instances it has been noticed that after the high voltage has been turned on, end mica window counters will give an increased counting rate for the first few minutes of operation. It is recommended that with such tubes the counting results taken for the first few minutes be discarded.

It is also recommended that the high-voltage control for Geiger counters be in the minimum position when the high voltage is turned on. This will prevent the possibility of the high voltage overshooting during the warm-up period, which might seriously overvoltage and hence damage the Geiger tube.

In operating the Geiger counter, the clock switch should be set before the "Count-On" switch is operated on the scaler.

In many instances the clock switch is not shunted with a high-capacitance filter, in which case spurious counts will result from the use of the clock switch rather than the scaler switch. More specific information will be given in the operating instructions accompanying the particular device to be used. References at the end of this chapter provide further details.

D. SCINTILLATION COUNTER

The scintillation counter (see Figs. 70, 71 and 72) is the most practical and useful device presently used in the clinical radio-

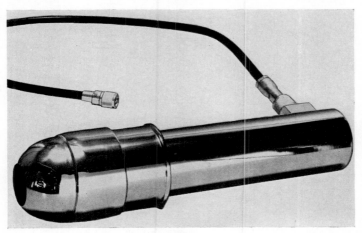

Fig. 70.—Scintillation counter, scanning type. (Courtesy: N. Wood Counter Laboratory, Chicago, Illinois.)

isotope laboratory. It has excellent efficiency, as compared with the Geiger counter, for detection of electromagnetic radiation; moreover, with it the clinician and investigator are enabled to reduce tracer doses for diagnostic studies to a minimum level of radiation hazard.

In brief, the scintillation-counter process consists of the following (8, 9): An ionizing radiation passes through the scintillating crystal and excites electrons within an atom or molecule into higher energy states. In useful scintillations, much of this excited energy is given off in the form of light, which may be detected by a sensitive photomultiplier.

The photomultiplier is a very sensitive type of photocell. Light pulses from the crystal cause the emission of photoelectrons from the sensitive surface called the "photocathode." These electrons are accelerated in an electric field and hit a succession of other

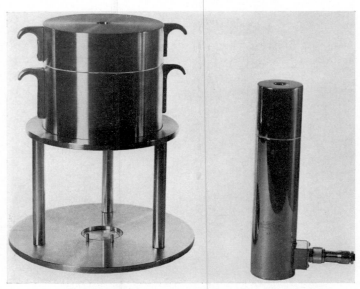

FIG. 71.—Scintillation counter, well type. (Courtesy: N. Wood Counter Laboratory, Chicago, Illinois.)

surfaces, called "dynodes," with secondary emission occurring at each surface. In this secondary emission, for each incident electron hitting one of the surfaces there will be approximately four secondary electrons emitted. If there are eleven stages, there will be an amplification of the order of magnitude of 10^{10}. The output pulse from the photomultiplier is fed into an amplifier or directly into a scaler, depending on the circuits employed.

For clinical purposes it is recommended that the circuit used with the photomultiplier be such as to make its amplification relatively insensitive to variations in high voltage. With such a

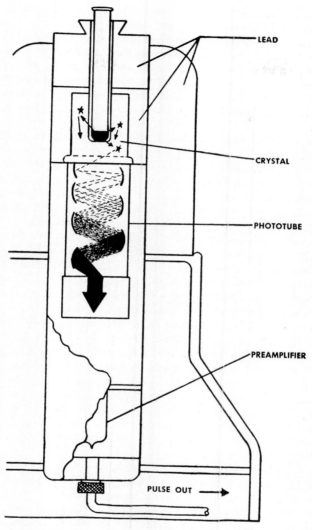

FIG. 72.—Scintillation counter: schematic view. (Courtesy: Nuclear-Chicago.)

circuit, the counting rate does not vary as the high voltage is varied, so that the counter has an "artificial plateau." One of the most useful of such systems is the Morton defocusing circuit, in which one of the dynodes midway in the cascade is permanently biased by a set of batteries or a cold cathode regulator. With this type of defocusing circuit, the photomultiplier can be driven at a high-enough voltage to actuate the ordinary type of Geiger counter scaler; the output pulse is usually greater than 0.25 volts.

To minimize background difficulties the scintillation counter should also be located at great distances from sources of radiation. Because of this counter's great efficiency for the detection of penetrating gamma rays, shielding and separation from sources is even more important than is the case for Geiger counters. Scintillation counters ordinarily require temperature-controlled areas; therefore an air conditioner is recommended.

A well-regulated power supply is essential when the defocusing type of supply for the photomultiplier is not used.

The scintillation counter, inherently a less stable detector than the Geiger counter, requires more frequent calibration. For clinical purposes, comparative measurements are preferable to absolute tests. Aliquots of tracer and therapeutic doses given to the patients should be saved for comparison with samples taken from the patients after they have received these doses. A simple comparison is then possible by dilution and routine counting. It has been found useful to employ cesium-137 (Cs^{137}) standards for the routine calibration of scintillation counters for thyroid-uptake studies. The long half-life of Cs^{137} (37 years) makes this isotope an essentially nondecaying calibration standard, and its energy spectrum is somewhat comparable to that of I^{131}. Similarly, other long-lived radioactive standards can be found for calibrating other isotopes.

The statistics of counting are found in Appendix B.

a) OPERATING SEQUENCE.—A warm-up period is needed. The scintillation-counter circuit should be kept operating continuously during the work week, although it may be shut off over the week end. Under these conditions, the sensitivity is more stable and the counting results more reproducible.

When a defocusing circuit is used, a voltage plateau should

be determined similar to that measured when a Geiger counter is used. The counter should be used at 100 volts above the knee of the plateau for best life characteristics.

The scintillation counter is a rugged device and, with ordinary care, should have a long life. The scintillation phosphor used in most clinical equipment is (thallium activated) sodium iodide, which has a higher sensitivity for gamma measurements than any other commonly employed phosphors.

E. GAS-FLOW COUNTER

In order to detect beta particles of low energy (e.g., those emanating from carbon-14 and sulfur-35), it is necessary to use a gas-flow type of Geiger counter. In this design the sample being counted is actually located within the counting chamber of the Geiger counter. The gaseous mixture, helium and alcohol, flows through the Geiger counter at a pressure slightly in excess of atmospheric pressure. The same principles of operation hold for this type of counter as those described for other Geiger counters. It is recommended that the technician employing a gas-flow counter use a preflush type of counter. In this design there are three positions in which the unknown sample is placed. The sample is inserted in the first position. Then it is rotated to the second position, which consists of a chamber that is being flushed by the helium-alcohol mixture. Next the sample is rotated into the third position, the counting chamber, and the sample may then be counted without delay. This type of gas-flow counter (Fig. 73) is manufactured by several concerns, and the instructions given below apply to most types.

a) OPERATING INSTRUCTIONS.—The gas-flow counter should be located at a considerable distance from the sources of radiation. While it may sometimes be difficult to shield the counter, shielding can often be accomplished simply by placing lead bricks directly above (and, if possible, around) the counting chamber. A well-regulated power supply is not important because a long plateau is associated with this type of counter.

The gas-flow counter presents more problems in preparation of radioisotope samples than do the other types of counters described. The self-absorption of the low-energy beta particles

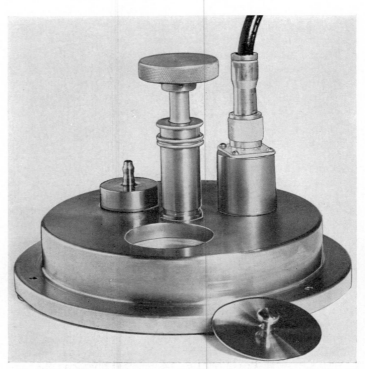

FIG. 73.—Gas-flow counter: external view. (Courtesy: N. Wood Counter Laboratory, Chicago, Illinois.)

within the sample material must be allowed for. It is also essential to reproduce the exact geometric arrangement of the various samples and planchetts on which the samples are mounted within the Geiger chamber. It is recommended that the samples to be plated on the planchetts occupy a small area. This will decrease errors from location of a nonconducting field within a gas-flow counter. The counting planchetts should not have any sharp points on the disks, since these may give rise to spurious counts. Special problems in calibration will not be described here because they differ in each case. There are adequate discussions of this subject in the literature (3, 6).

The same type of statistics that are applicable to the use of Geiger counters applies to the use of gas-flow counters. Discrepancies should be evaluated individually for each counter.

b) OPERATING SEQUENCE.—A gas mixer should accompany the gas-flow counter. Within the mixer there should be absolute ethyl alcohol, to a depth of 1–2 in. A connection between the mixer and the helium tank may be made with plastic tubing. A small bubbler or a flow regulator or indicator may be used to determine the rate of flow of the helium gas through the alcohol mixture. The counter should be flushed thoroughly before use. It should also be tested for leakage, in the following manner: *(a)* clamp the output hose; *(b)* close the tank valve; and *(c)* note whether the pressure indicator at the tank output drops with time. A tight fit should be maintained at all times by using either a silicone or vaseline grease. In some models of this type of counter it is possible to substitute a proportional counter anode for the Geiger counter anode usually supplied. This will enable the technician to have essentially two counters instead of one. The proportional counter can be used for both alpha-particle assay and beta counting.

REFERENCES

1. Yagoda, H.: *Radioactive Measurements with Nuclear Emulsions* (New York: John Wiley & Sons, Inc., 1949).
2. Crowther, J. A.: *Ions, Electrons, and Ionizing Radiations* (London: Edward Arnold & Co., 1938).
3. Rossi, B. B., and Staub, H. H.: *Ionization Chambers and Counters* (New York: McGraw-Hill Book Company, Inc., 1949).
4. Lapp, R. E., and Andrews, H. L.: *Nuclear Radiation Physics* (New York: Prentice-Hall, Inc., 1953).
5. Behrens, C. F.: *Atomic Medicine* (Baltimore: Williams & Wilkins Company, 1954).
6. Bleuler, E., and Goldsmith, G. J.: *Experimental Nucleonics* (New York: Rinehart & Co., Inc., 1952).
7. Day, F. H.: *X-ray Calibration of Radiation Survey Meters, Pocket Chambers, and Dosimeters,* National Bureau of Standards Circular 507 (Washington, D. C.: Superintendent of Documents, Government Printing Office, 1951).
8. Sherr, R., and Gerhart, J. B.: Stabilization of photomultiplier tubes, Rev. Scient. Instruments, 23:770, 1952.
9. Birks, J. B.: *Scintillation Counters* (New York: McGraw-Hill Book Company, Inc., 1953).

PART IV

RADIATION SAFETY

CHAPTER 17

General Recommendations for Radiation Safety

THE USE OF HIGH-ENERGY RADIATION involves a health hazard unless adequate protective measures are applied according to correct operational procedures. In the medical isotope laboratory the principal sources of radiation hazard are the high-energy gamma rays which are emitted by the radioisotopes iodine-131, cobalt-60 and gold-198 and the high-energy beta rays emitted by phosphorus-32 and strontium-90. The principal types of biologic injury are: (1) direct skin injury; (2) generalized effects on the blood-forming organs, resulting in anemia and leukemias; (3) the induction of malignant tumors; (4) the induction of cataracts; (5) impaired fertility; (6) deleterious genetic effects; and (7) shortened life span. Unfortunately, it is only the skin injury that is perceptible shortly after exposure. Other injuries or their effects may not appear for years, or even generations, after exposure. Because of this delayed appearance, to newcomers in the field the strict regulations in force regarding protection and safe procedures frequently seem an unnecessary and restrictive burden. However, in view of the insidiousness of the effects, the greatest possible care is mandatory.

Radiation injuries may be received through three general types of exposure: (1) deposition of radioactive material in the body; (2) exposure of the whole body to low-level-intensity beta or gamma rays; and (3) exposures of limited areas, such as the hands, to high-level-intensity beta or gamma radiation.

Deposition in the body may occur by (1) ingestion, (2) inhalation or (3) absorption through either intact or injured body surface. Ingestion will generally be a chronic process, resulting from small amounts of contaminated material entering the mouth by way of the hands, food, drink or smoking devices, such as cigarets or pipes. The term *contamination* in this limited sense means *the presence of radioactive material where it is not wanted.* Ingestion may be an acute process, as in the event of the accidental drinking of a radioactive solution. The hazards of ingestion may be due to direct radiation of the alimentary tract or to the radiation of specific organs in which the ingested material has concentrated, such as the concentration of I^{131} in the thyroid. The longer the half-life of the ingested isotope, the more serious will be the health hazard. Therefore, the ingestion of materials such as carbon-14 and radium-226 is especially dangerous.

The inhalation of vapor, spray or dust containing radioactive material may result in deposition in the body. Inhalation may result in direct irradiation of the lung, in the absorption of active material from the lung to other parts of the body, or in the mechanical transfer of the active material to the alimentary tract.

Direct absorption would most likely result in direct radiation injury at the site of absorption, but it could also result in injury to a distant organ, where concentration might take place.

Overexposure of the whole body to low-level-intensity beta and gamma radiation could result from insufficient protective barriers for stored material; from unskilled manipulations in certain procedures, such as a too lengthy transfer of solution from one container to another; from insufficient protective barriers around large amounts of active material being instilled into a patient, such as the therapeutic instillation of Au^{198} into a body cavity; and from unawareness of the presence of contamination in frequented areas. Overexposure of limited areas, such as the hands, would in general be due to improper manipulative procedures, such as handling active material with the bare hands, especially Ra^{226} or Co^{60} needles, seeds, tubes or plaques; or their unskillful overlong insertion times could lead to chronic injury.

A. PERMISSIBLE DOSE LEVELS

The permissible dose of external radiation is specified by both the National Committee on Radiation Protection and Measurement and the Atomic Energy Commission. The permissible doses are no longer based on a time unit of 1 week but are instead based on an accumulated total dose received by a person over his entire life to the date in question and on a maximum of 3 roentgen-equivalents-man (rem) in any 13-week period. The general formula for this is:

Total dose which may be accumulated = 5 $(N - 18)$ rem

where N is the person's age in years. Thus, a person 28 years old may permissibly be exposed to, or "accumulate," a total of 5 $(28 - 18)$ = 50 rem. Further, a person under 18 years of age cannot be employed in radiation work because, below 18 years, his accumulated permissible dose is zero. The *rate* at which the total accumulated dose may be acquired is regulated by the ancillary recommendation that the total dose in any 13-week period not exceed 3 rem. The following is an example of the combined action of the two regulations: A worker, aged 22 years, enters radiation work with a history of no previous occupational exposure. He has, therefore 5 $(22 - 18)$ = 20 rem "reserve" to draw on. However, the fastest he can draw on this reserve would be at the rate of 3 rem/13-wk. period, or 12 rem/yr. At the end of the first year he would have accumulated another 5 permissible rem, or a total of 25, of which he could have used 12, leaving a balance of 13. The second year he again permissibly gains for "deposit" 5 more rem, which brings his total deposit to 18 rem. Of this, he could receive 12 during the year, leaving a balance of 6 rem. The third year he again permissibly gains 5 rem, bringing his balance to 11 rem. This third year he would not be permitted to receive 3 rem for each of four 13-week periods because, in that case, the 12 rem received that year would bring him over his permissible lifetime accumulated reserve total of 11 rem. He could receive during this third year, 3 rem for each of three 13-week periods and 2 rem the next 13-week period. At this time he now has used up his reserve; and from now on, the maximum dose he could receive would be 5 rem/yr., subject to more in any *one* year provided he had again accumulated another reserve, by receiving less than 5 rem in some intervening year or years. While the above outlined use of "banked" permissible dose is allowed, it is considered distinctly undesirable. Radiation dose should *at all times* be kept to a minimum, consistent with realistic use.

In regard to exposure to beta rays, the National Bureau of Standards, in its Handbook 47, entitled *Recommendations of the International Commission on Radiological Protection,* makes the following statement:

In the case of beta rays of high energy, the maximum exposure

TABLE 30.—PERMISSIBLE CONCENTRATIONS IN BODY, AIR AND WATER*

RADIO-ISOTOPE	PERMISSIBLE CONCENTRATION		
	In Body	In Air	In Solution
Ra^{226}	0.1 μc.	8×10^{-12} μc./ml.	4×10^{-8} μc./ml.
Sr^{90}	1.0 μc.	2×10^{-10} μc./ml.	8×10^{-7} μc./ml.
C^{14} (Fat)	250 μc.	1×10^{-6} μc./ml.	3×10^{-3} μc./ml.
(Bone)	1,500 μc.	5×10^{-7} μc./ml.	4×10^{-3} μc./ml.
Na^{24}	15 μc.	2×10^{-6} μc./ml.	8×10^{-3} μc./ml.
P^{32}	10 μc.	1×10^{-7} μc./ml.	2×10^{-4} μc./ml.
Co^{60}	3 μc.	1×10^{-6} μc./ml.	2×10^{-2} μc./ml.
I^{131}	0.3 μc.	3×10^{-9} μc./ml.	3×10^{-5} μc./ml.

* Source of data: National Bureau of Standards.

of the surface of the body in any one week shall be the energy flux of the beta radiation such that the absorption per gram of superficial tissues is equivalent to the energy absorption of 1.5 r of hard gamma rays. For purposes of calculation, the superficial tissues concerned shall be the basal layer of the epidermis, defined conventionally as lying at a depth corresponding to 7 mg./cm.^{2}

It should be noted that 7 mg./cm.^{2} corresponds to a depth of approximately 0.07 mm. in tissue.

The values of the permissible doses of internal radiation are less firmly fixed than those for external radiation. Table 30 is based on data given in National Bureau of Standards Handbook 52, entitled *Maximum Permissible Amounts of Radioisotopes in the Human Body and Maximum Permissible Concentrations in Air and Water.*

B. MEASUREMENT OF STRAY RADIATION

There are several simple methods for measuring stray radiation. They may be divided into two classes: survey instruments and personnel-monitoring devices, both of which belong under the general term of "monitoring," or "surveying." The survey meters determine: (1) the presence of contamination; (2) the radiation to which personnel are subject during processes involving the handling of radioisotopes; (3) the radiation emitted from stored radioactive material; (4) the activity level of material ready for disposal; and (5) the radiation intensity at the surface of shipping packages containing radioactive materials.

Survey meters are rate meters which can be read directly on a scale, calibrated in counts per minute or in milliroentgens per hour. The sensitive measuring volume may be either a Geiger tube crystal scintillator or an ionization chamber. When contamination is being looked for and when the amount of the contamination is of secondary importance, the Geiger crystal scintillator type of meter is usually employed. It is more sensitive qualitatively than the ionization chamber type. When accurate quantitative determinations are required, the ionization chamber type is used. Both types of meters are usually multirange, the Geiger type normally having ranges of 0–0.2, 0–2.0 and 0–20 mr./hr., whereas the ion chamber type has ranges of 0–25, 0–250 and 0–2,500 mr./hr.

The integrating ionization chamber survey meter is available in several types. It has a full scale of 20 mr. and is useful for determining the total amount of radiation reaching a given point during a known procedure or during a known elapsed time. This instrument has a built-in charging device and needs no batteries or external source of power.

All survey instruments measure gamma rays. Some instruments measure both beta and gamma rays; these meters are provided with a beta-ray discriminating shield, so that gamma rays only may be measured if so desired. A third type of meter measures alpha rays as well as beta and gamma rays. The survey meters are battery operated, with a battery life expectancy of several hundred hours.

Although survey meters serve a useful purpose in detecting radiation hazards, generally it is not possible to have the meter at the exact position of the operating personnel at all times. A second type of measurement, known as "personnel monitoring," takes over at this stage. In personnel monitoring, the individual has, attached to himself, a measuring device which integrates the total radiation he has received during the time he has worn the device.

Personnel measuring devices may be of two sorts: an ionization type meter or a film. The ionization type may be either complete electroscopes or simple ion chambers, each of which is about the size of a fountain pen. The electroscopes have a full scale of 200 mr. and are charged by a separate external charger; they may be read directly at any time. The pocket ionization chambers must be connected to an external electrometer for charging and reading and are, therefore, not as convenient as the electroscopes.

The second type of personnel monitor is known as a "film badge." It consists of a special photographic film, about an inch square, which is enclosed in a lightproof plastic case, clipped to some part of the clothing of the wearer. The badges are worn for a specified time, after which the film is processed and its density compared to the density of similar films exposed to known amounts of radiation. Various filters are inserted in the packet, above the film, to provide proper energy discrimination. The accurate dosage range includes all exposures from commonly used radioactive material, including x-rays from 30 Kev to 5 Mev, gamma rays from 30 Kev to 5 Mev and beta radiation above 400 Kev (provided the energy is known).

A modified film badge is the "ring" badge, which is a small piece of film in a plastic ring which is worn on the finger. The regular badges measure approximate total body radiation; the ring badges measure localized radiation to the hand.

C. PROTECTIVE MEASURES

In the use of radioisotopes, protective measures are required to reduce the intensity of external radiation to permissible levels and to prevent the entry of the isotope into the human body.

Protection may be secured by both direct and indirect means. Distance and absorbing barriers reduce external radiation to permissible levels, and either distance or absorbing barriers may be the dominating factor in obtaining the required reduction of intensity. The material and thickness of the absorbing medium is determined by the energy of the radiation to be attenuated.

For gamma rays the barrier material is usually lead; whereas for beta rays a plastic, such as lucite, serves adequately. For 8 hr./day protection at a distance of 1 m. against 200 mc. of I^{131}, 1.1 cm. of lead is required. For the same protection against 200 mc. of Co^{60}, 5.6 cm. of lead are necessary. A complete table, which includes the parameters of energy, amount, danger range, working time per day and absorbing material, is given in National Bureau of Standards Handbook 42, entitled *Safe Handling of Radioactive Isotopes*. (For the new gamma ray values, 1.58 half-value layers of the barrier material in question should be added to the values given for barrier thickness on page 24 of this Handbook.)

Complete protection against the beta rays from P^{32} is afforded by 6.5 mm. of lucite, 3.5 mm. of Pyrex glass or less than 1 mm. of copper. Graphs indicating the shielding from various energies of beta rays with several different materials are also given in Handbook 42.

The principal means of protecting against internal radiation and radiation from contamination is the use of procedures which will reduce these factors to a minimum. This can be accomplished by using adequate laboratory facilities and employing meticulous care in the operative techniques. The laboratory facilities were discussed in detail in Chapter 14, section B, but may be briefly listed here. Adequate facilities include: (1) a well-lighted working area; (2) remotely controlled transfer devices, such as pipettes and burettes; (3) remote handling devices, such as tongs, forceps, trays and mechanical holders; (4) adequate ventilation, including forced-draft hoods if chemical procedures are contemplated; (5) smooth, easily decontaminated laboratory bench tops; (6) smooth floors of painted concrete or linoleum, laid in one piece and without cracks; (7) adequate waste disposal facilities; and (8) monitoring instruments. The laboratory should be kept clean and neat at all times. The floors should be cleaned by dry mopping, since dry sweeping could lead to a dust hazard. Careful manipulation, neatness and cleanliness go hand and hand with these other facilities to provide a safe and contamination-free laboratory. Eating, drinking and smoking should be forbidden in any isotope laboratory, owing to the danger of carrying contamination into the mouth.

All areas of the radioisotope laboratory should be monitored regularly and frequently. A rough rule for determining undesirable amounts of contamination on a surface is that a 2 cm.^{2} flat-plate Geiger counter should show no response if passed slowly over the area. To be sure, it is important that the instrument that is used be sensitive to the type of radiation being sought. Table 31 gives a somewhat more quantitative guide to permissible contamination.

Surveys for contamination should include structural surfaces,

TABLE 31.—PERMISSIBLE CONTAMINATION*

Position	Maximum Permissible Contamination (Beta and Gamma)
Air	10^{-11} μc./ml.
Water	10^{-7} μc./ml.
Clothing	0.1 mrem./hr.
Work area surfaces	0.1 mrem./hr.
Body surfaces	0.1 mrem./hr.

* Source of data: National Bureau of Standards.

such as bench tops, hoods, floors, sinks, drainboards, drains, plumbing fixtures, furniture, radioactive waste containers and laboratory glassware, and other apparatus. In the case of patients who have received therapeutic doses of radioisotopes, post-treatment surveys should be made in the patient's room or ward. Such a survey should show less than permissible levels of external radiation to adjacent patients, and a safe contamination level of the bed, bed linens, bedpans and urinals being used by the patient under treatment.

D. PERSONNEL

Carefulness and neatness are important in keeping a radioisotope laboratory contamination-free. These attributes, therefore, should be a positive requirement of personnel. In addition, a carefully detailed physical examination should be made of prospective workers, with special attention to previous radiation history and possible present radiation effects. A complete blood count should be made at the same time of day on two successive days before employment. Periodic blood counts should be made thereafter at intervals of 3 months.

The personnel should be monitored continuously, by means of either pocket chambers, which should be read daily, or film badges, which should be processed weekly or biweekly. Ring badges should be processed weekly. A complete written record should be kept of the results of this monitoring. (See next chapter for further information regarding monitoring techniques and records.)

The hands should be washed thoroughly at all times before leaving the laboratory.

E. RADIATION ACCIDENTS

A person who has apparently been overexposed to external radiation should be immediately removed from any source of radiation and kept away from any radiation until it is evident that radiation injury has not been incurred.

In the event that a worker swallows active solutions, treatment as for ingested poisons should be instituted. The material should be removed by emetics or stomach pump, and the residue made insoluble, if possible.

When active solutions are splashed on a person, the affected parts should be thoroughly washed; and if, after washing, those parts are still contaminated, an application of titanium dioxide paste, or a saturated solution of potassium permanganate, followed by a 5 per cent sodium bisulphite solution rinse, is effective treatment.

When any part, such as the hand, is contaminated with a small spot of high specific activity, it is best not to wash the part, since this will result in spreading the contamination. The surrounding areas should be masked, and the affected spot should be cleaned with cotton-tipped applicators, dipped in suitable decontaminants.

The Atomic Energy Commission has in its official regulations a number of "reporting requirements" to be used in the case of radiation accidents. Pertinent sections of these requirements are given below:

A. Each licensee shall report by telephone *and* telegraph to the Manager of the nearest Atomic Energy Commission Operations Office (see Appended List, below), immediately after its occurrence becomes known to the licensee, any loss or theft of licensed material in such quantities and under such circumstances that it appears to the licensee that a substantial hazard may result to persons in unrestricted areas.

Appended List:

Operations Office	Mail Address	Telegraph Address
Albuquerque	P.O. Box 5400 Albuquerque, N.M.	Albuquerque, N.M.
Chicago	P.O. Box 59 Lemont, Ill.	Lemont, Ill.
Grand Junction	Grand Junction, Colo.	Grand Junction, Colo.
Hanford	P.O. Box 550 Richland, Wash.	Richland, Wash.
Idaho	P.O. Box 1221 Idaho Falls, Idaho	550 Second St. Idaho Falls, Idaho
New York	50 Columbus Ave. New York 23, N.Y.	50 Columbus Ave. New York 23, N.Y.
Oak Ridge	P.O. Box E Oak Ridge, Tenn.	Oak Ridge, Tenn.
San Francisco	518 17th St. Oakland 12, Calif.	518 17th St. Oakland 12, Calif.
Savannah River	P.O. Box A Aiken, S.C.	Augusta, Ga.
Schenectady	P.O. Box 1069 Schenectady, N.Y.	Knolls Atomic Power Laboratory Schenectady, N.Y.

B. *Immediate Notification.*—Each licensee shall immediately notify the Manager of the nearest Operations Office by telephone *and* telegraph of any incident involving licensed material possessed by him which may have caused or threatens to cause exposure of any individual to 25 rem or more of radiation, including any radioactive material taken into the body.

C. *Twenty-Four Hour Notification.*—Exposure of any individual to 3 rem or more, including any radioactive material taken into the body.

D. *Thirty-Day Reports.*—Each licensee shall make a report in writing within 30 days to the Director, Division of Civilian Application, USAEC, Washington 25, D.C., of each incident involving licensed material possessed by him, which appears to have resulted in levels of radiation or concentrations of radioactive material in excess of any applicable limits set forth in these regulations or in the licensee's license. Each report required in this paragraph shall describe the nature of the incident, the extent of exposure of persons to radiation or to radioactive material, the levels of radiation and concentrations of radioactive material involved, the cause of the incident and corrective steps taken or planned to assure against a recurrence of the incident. A copy of each report shall be transmitted to the Manager of the nearest Atomic Energy Commission Operations Office.

The entire reporting requirements may be found in the Federal Register, May 14, 1957, under Title 10, Chapter 1, Part 20. This may be obtained for a nominal sum from the Superintendent of Documents, Washington 25, D.C.

CHAPTER 18

Instructions for Laboratory Personnel

THE PERSONNEL OF THE RADIOISOTOPE LABORATORY should be aware of the precautions and practices to be observed in reducing radiation exposure to a minimum. A potential health hazard arises from the same source that enables progress to occur in this field—namely, the large amounts of energy which are expended from small amounts of radioactive material. This energy is in the form of beta and gamma rays from the clinically useful radio-isotopes. Radiation exposure to the worker may come from external sources, from contamination on the body surface or from inside the body (through inhalation, ingestion or absorption through the skin).

As a basic rule, it may be said that *any unnecessary exposure to radiation is too much* for the radioisotope worker.

A. RECOMMENDATIONS FOR REDUCTION IN EXPOSURE

1. EXTERNAL EXPOSURE

a) SHIELDING.—By using the proper thickness of dense materials between the radiation source and the working area, the total amount of radiation exposure to the worker will be reduced. Tables indicating the half-value layers for various materials for reducing the gamma radiation to a minimum level are given in

Appendix D. Lucite or glass may be used for beta shielding, whereas lead or steel is recommended for gamma shielding.

b) DISTANCE.—It follows from the laws of radiation that the dose rate from an approximately point source of radiation is inversely proportional to the square of the distance from the source, provided that the dimensions of the source are small in comparison with the distance concerned, and provided that there is no appreciable scattering or absorption of the radiation in the air through which the radiation travels. This can be explained by the following formula:

$$\frac{\text{Dose rate at } X_1}{\text{Dose rate at } X_2} = \frac{X_2{}^2}{X_1{}^2}$$

or

$$\frac{\text{mr.}_1/\text{hr.}}{\text{mr.}_2/\text{hr.}} = \frac{X_2{}^2}{X_1{}^2}$$

EXAMPLE: If we have a measurement of 50 mr./hr. at 100 cm., the dose rate at 1,000 cm. will be equal to:

$$50 \times \frac{(100)^2}{(1,000)^2} = 0.5 \ \text{mr./hr.}$$

If measurements are made at small distances or in contact with the surface of a source, the inverse square law will not hold. For accurate readings at such distances, it may be necessary to use an extrapolation chamber or any other device that will allow measurements close to the surface. These measurements can then be plotted and extrapolation made graphically back to zero distance. The considerations of scattering and absorption must also be taken into consideration at these short distances.

c) TIME.—The time spent by a worker in a *hot* area should be limited. The rate of exposure should be determined, and the worker allowed to remain no longer than the time corresponding to his maximum permissible exposure level. Each worker should be provided with personnel monitoring equipment which will indicate the exposure that he may receive. (For more details, see "Monitoring Techniques and Records," later in this chapter.)

d) CONTAMINATION.—To reduce external radiation hazards, it is necessary to remove the source of contamination. If the source is not being used, it should be removed to a segregated storage place. Contamination is easily handled if proper precautions are taken, such as the use of absorbent paper over work surfaces, or painting the surface with strippable plastic paints. An unprotected surface can be decontaminated by a washing and abrasive process. This can be done by scrubbing with a detergent, by hosing down with water—or by using acid soap agents.

Every worker in a laboratory should be provided with protective clothing in the form of a laboratory coat large enough to cover his clothing.

2. INTERNAL EXPOSURE

Internal exposure can only be controlled by preventing the entry of radioactive materials into the body and by accelerating their elimination from the body when they do enter. Inhalation protection for short periods in low concentrations of air-borne contamination may be provided by respirators which filter air to the mouth and nose. It will be found that in the usual clinical radioisotope laboratory there will be no use for such a device, since the materials employed are generally nonvolatile.

Eating and smoking in contaminated areas should not be permitted. Workers should be instructed in the use of various types of survey meters. They should request radiologic surveys when contamination exists, and should be especially careful in those situations in which the skin is broken, so that any contamination will be eliminated at an early period. Internal contamination may usually be detected by the estimation of the quantity in certain of the body fluids. Urine and blood may be assayed for such radioactivity.

3. SURFACE CONTAMINATION

Surface contamination can be reduced by the use of proper handling devices and protective clothing. Whenever radioactive materials are handled in open containers, the workers should wear rubber gloves. Absorbent paper and cloth should be readily available for the rapid absorption of surface-contaminating chemicals.

B. MONITORING TECHNIQUES AND RECORDS

1. PERSONNEL AND EQUIPMENT: RESPONSIBILITY AND SURVEYING

It is advisable that personnel be continuously monitored in the clinical radioisotope laboratory by the use of film badges. This is mainly a medicolegal protection and, in actuality, does not aid greatly in personal protection. In order to reduce the cost of this

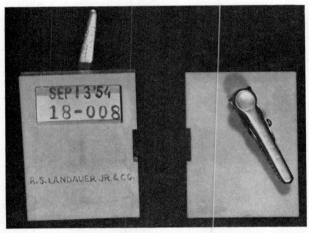

FIG. 74.—Film badge. (Courtesy: R. S. Landauer, Jr., & Co., Park Forest, Illinois.)

service, it is possible to use film badges on a biweekly service arrangement with a contracting agency. A typical film badge is shown in Figure 74. It is advisable to wear these badges at a standard location on the clothing, such as the left lapel.

The badges are generally accurate for electromagnetic radiation in the range of 30 Kev to 5 Mev. Sometimes they may be used for detection of beta radiation for energies above 400 Kev if these energies are positively known. It is recommended that each user of the film badge service calibrate his badges by exposing them to a known quantity of radiation and submitting them to the contracting agency for reading. He can then check the reading with his own calibration. It is further advisable to assign to the secretary of the radioisotope laboratory the function of collecting and dispensing film badges at periodic intervals. Some of these film badges may be worn over body areas other than that suggested, but a standard position is preferable. Other types of badges which offer certain advantages are, for example, a badge that can be worn on the wrist or a ring badge.

It is important to keep a good record as to the amounts of

TABLE 32.—FILM BADGE RECORD SHEET

Name of Participating Institution ....

Name of Person Responsible for Films ....

Number	Name of Person Wearing Badge	Date Worn	Time Worn	Position Worn	Any Unusual Use of the Film	Film Readings Shield mrep

radiation to which each individual has been exposed. Such a record sheet is illustrated in Table 32. This type of record is also valuable for medicolegal purposes.

If funds are available, it is advisable to have a number of pocket chambers handy for specialized tests which may be required in the laboratory. These chambers (see Fig. 75) offer an immediately available reading and are especially useful in procedures involving large doses of radioisotopes. Their cost is nominal, and they are convenient to read.

One of the members of the radioisotope unit should be assigned the duty of collecting and dispensing pocket chambers at regular intervals. Preferably, these chambers should be collected at the end of the week and dispensed at the beginning of the following week. The number of hours the pocket chamber has been worn and other pertinent information should be recorded (see Table 33 for a typical record sheet).

Although survey meters were described in detail in Chapter 16, it may be emphasized here that a portable Geiger counter is essential in the clinical radioisotope laboratory. In general, the calibration of a portable Geiger counter is so set that full scale

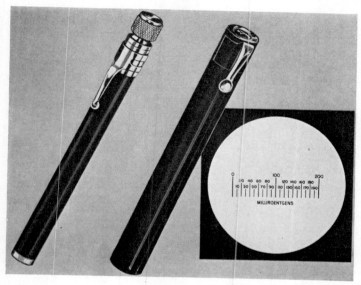

FIG. 75.—Pocket chambers: dosimeters. (Courtesy: Nuclear-Chicago.)

on the 0–20 mr./hr. scale is equivalent to 20,000 counts/min. Some meters, however, are not calibrated in this manner. When counts per minute per square centimeter are indicated as the tolerance level, this calibration will serve most purposes.

a) PERSONNEL.—Surveying of personnel should be done with the Geiger tube exposed for beta-ray measurement. If positive readings are found, it is advisable that urine samples be collected from the contaminated personnel for assay of activity. The portable Geiger counter survey meter should be employed whenever any member of the radioisotope unit believes that he may have been contaminated. No prescribed period or interval for personnel surveying is recommended. In general, personnel should wear rubber gloves whenever they handle contaminated material; thus surface body contamination will not occur frequently.

b) INSTRUMENTS.—Instruments and equipment used in the

TABLE 33.—POCKET CHAMBER RECORD

Unit							
				Period Covered			
Name	Chamber Number	Period Worn	Hours	Reading			
1.							
2.							
3.							
4.							
5.							
6.							
7.							
8.							
9.							
10.							

radioisotope laboratory should be surveyed with a portable Geiger counter whenever it is believed that these items have become contaminated. The maximum permissible contamination level is set at 1,000 cts./min. when a Geiger counter is placed over a flat square area of 2 sq. in. Obviously, this contamination level is reduced proportionately if the area is smaller. If all contamination has not been eliminated, the results of a particular test being undertaken at the laboratory may be obscured. It is important to survey thoroughly such items as syringes, needles, rubber gloves, pipettes and other items of glassware employed in the laboratory. It may be more advantageous to allow the contamination to decay rather than to try to decontaminate the items by conventional methods.

c) AREA SURVEYING.—Periodic and thorough surveys should be made of all the radioisotope laboratory facilities. These surveys should be performed at weekly intervals, using a portable

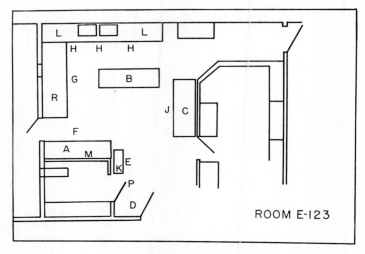

FIG. 76.—Schematic layout of area.

Geiger counter with the beta shield open. It is suggested that a schematic layout be made of the laboratory area, with particular coding assigned to various possible contaminated locales (see Fig. 76). A chart can then be kept, bearing corresponding coding, and the readings recorded (Table 34).

2. LABORATORY REGULATIONS

The regulations which follow here have been abstracted from those of the Radioisotope Unit at Hines Veterans Hospital, Hines, Illinois. They have been found to cover 99 per cent of the problems in the routine clinical laboratory.

TABLE 34.—AREA MONITORING RECORD: RADIOISOTOPE
UNIT*

Room: E123										Month _____ ,19__					
Section	Tolerance	Code	β	γ	β	γ	β	γ	β	γ	β	γ	β	γ	β	γ
Table	1 mr./hr. at surface	A														
		B														
		C														
Floor	2.5 mr./hr. at 1 in. distance	D														
		E														
		F														
		G														
		H														
		J														
Sink Drainboards	1 mr./hr. Sink L	K														
		L														
Walls	1 mr./hr. at surface	M														
Garbage pails Storage cans	2.5 mr./hr.	N														
		O														
Storage room door	2.5 mr./hr. open door	P														
Fume hood	2.5 mr./hr.	R														
Misc.																
Initials																

* β = beta ; γ = gamma .

In all rooms where radioactive materials are being used, the following regulations shall be in effect:

1. No food shall be eaten.
2. Smoking is not permitted while active material is being handled.
3. Clean outer garments shall be worn which will be left inside the laboratory whenever the worker leaves the area.
4. Film badges shall be worn at all times when working with radioactivity.
5. Pencil pocket chambers shall be worn when working with gamma emitters.
6. Rubber gloves will be worn when radioactive material in any

amount is being handled and when the wearing of gloves will not interfere with the clinical examination. In cases of biologic material containing gold-198, iodine-131 and phosphorus-32, this precaution is not necessary when the total activity is less than 0.01 μc/L., or 0.01 μc./gm. of tissue.

7. No individual shall knowingly expose himself, or cause others to be exposed, to more than 0.05 roentgens equivalent physical (rep) in any working day. In instances of unusual character and real need, an exposure not greater than 0.4 rep may be permitted provided that the individual receives no exposure during the full following week.

8. Any contaminated table tops shall be washed with carrier (or Boraxo) in water until the activity is reduced to less than 1 mr./hr., measured with the portable Geiger counter at the surface of the table.

9. Contamination of the floor with radioactivity, such that the meter readings exceed 2.5 mr./hr. at 1 ft. (when the floor cannot be decontaminated until a lower reading can be obtained), will be covered or marked off so that the area may be evacuated until the normal decay processes reduce the radiation level to the amount specified.

10. Liquid radioactive wastes may be disposed of in the usual manner when the total quantity does not exceed 5 mc. at any one instance. It is preferred that the solutions be made alkaline and the carrier be added prior to disposal.

11. Contamination of the hands shall be reduced by continuous washing with Boraxo (or carrier) and water until the activity is reduced to less than 0.1 mr./hr., measured at contact with the meter.

12. Sheets, pillow cases, rubber sheets, pajamas and other materials in contact with patients shall not be placed in the hospital laundry system if the activity exceeds 1 mr./hr. on contact. These materials shall be stored in suitable containers until the activity becomes reduced to the normal amount by decay process.

13. Gloves will be aged until the activity measured on the inside of the gloves becomes less than 0.1 mr./hr. at contact with the meter.

14. Contaminated instruments, such as three-way stopcocks, syringes, needles, forceps and scissors, shall not be used until the activity becomes less than 1 mr./hr. at contact with the unshielded probe of the Geiger survey meter.

CHAPTER 19

Instructions for Hospital Personnel Handling Patients

THIS CHAPTER IS PRESENTED in outline form in order to provide, as concisely as possible, the essentials of radioisotope techniques, including the isotope used, the effective half-life and the maximum dose usually employed, as well as rules for the care of patients receiving radioisotopes. The regulations and procedures are the results of long experience with the requirements of hospital personnel. They have been used in essentially the same form in six nursing-teaching institutions. The rationale for the rules is not presented, since this is not feasible in a technical manual, but further information can be obtained from Chapter 17. The instructions are detailed enough so that personnel untrained in the use of isotopes may be properly informed about the problem, namely, the handling of patients who have received radioisotopes.

I. TRACERS

    A. *Thyroid Tracer:* I^{131} (isotope); 6 days (effective half-life); 50 μc. (maximum dose)

        1. Purpose

            a) An oral dose of radioactive iodine is given to determine the thyroid gland avidity for iodine.

            b) Diagnosis is based on clinical history and results obtained from the thyroid uptake, 24-hour urine excretion and gland turnover of I^{131}.

        2. Preparation

            a) Examinations are to be scheduled with the radioisotope laboratory and are scheduled only in advance.

b) An examination request sheet should be sent to the radioisotope laboratory, and an instruction sheet will then be issued.

c) The patient should report to the radioisotope laboratory at the stated time in the morning. Breakfast should consist of *toast and coffee* only.

d) After having received the small dose of radioiodine, the patient should return to the nursing station. He should not eat or drink anything but water *for 3 hours* after the administration of the dose on this first day of the test. He may smoke during this period.

e) The patient should report to the radioisotope laboratory at a specified time on the *second* day after breakfast, to have a blood sample taken and a 24-hour reading made of thyroid-uptake study.

f) A 24-hour urine specimen, beginning with the time of administration of the dose, should be collected and brought to the laboratory on the second day, when indicated.

g) In some cases, special 48- or 96-hour studies are made, for which 24-hour urine specimens are saved in radioisotope bottles for the 48- and 96-hour periods. This urine must be brought daily to the radioisotope laboratory for assay.

3. Precautions

a) No special precautions are necessary in caring for the patient.

b) Proper collection of urine samples is important.

c) If the patient has been receiving iodine or thyroid medications, the tracer study should not be made until about 2 weeks after the medication has been discontinued.

d) If the patient has had gallbladder dye or the dye for an intravenous pyelograph, the radioisotope physician should be consulted before scheduling.

B. *Brain Tracer—External:* I^{131}; 1 day effective half-life; 300 μc. (maximum dose)
  1. Purpose
      a) A radioactive dye (I^{131}HSA or NaI^{131}) is given intravenously to the patient believed to have intracranial neoplasm. The dye will concentrate reasonably well in an area of suspicion.
      b) Readings are taken in 32 different positions (areas of the head), beginning 15 minutes after the radioactive injection. The examination requires about 2½ hours.
  2. Preparation
      a) The brain tracer study should be scheduled with the radioisotope laboratory two days in advance.
      b) Lugol's solution, gtts. 10, must be given to the patient for 2 days, thusly:

      1 day preceding tracer: Lugol's gtt. 10 t.i.d.
      Day of tracer: Lugol's gtt. 10 b.i.d. (i.e., after test)

      This is important to prevent the thyroid from taking up the I^{131}.
      c) The patient reports to the radioisotope laboratory on the scheduled day.
      d) The request form for brain radioisotope study must be completed by the intern and sent to the radioisotope laboratory before the examination.
  3. Precautions
      No special preparation is necessary.

C. *Brain Tumor Localization—Internal:* P^{32}; 14 days (effective half-life); 250 μc. (maximum dose)
  1. Purpose
      a) The test dose is given intravenously a day before surgery for suggested brain tumor.
      b) Phosphorus will concentrate in tumor tissue, more so than in normal tissue. With a small-sized Geiger counter, these concentrations can be determined by probing the brain tissue at the time of surgery.
  2. Preparation
      No special preparation is necessary.

3. Precautions
   a) Patient shall wear hospital pajamas or gown, which should be saved for radioisotope survey.
   b) Surgical gloves and a gown should be worn when handling the patient within 48 hours after administration of dose.
   c) Pillow should be protected in case of drainage after surgery.
   d) No other special precautions.

II. THERAPY

A. *Thyroid Therapy:* I^{131}; 6 days (effective half-life); usually 7 mc. (maximum dose)
   1. Purpose
      On the basis of clinical symptomatology and the results of the tracer dose, the patient is given a large (therapeutic) dose of radioactive iodine to reduce the thyroid gland activity. This is administered orally.
   2. Preparation
      a) The patient should not have food for 2 hours *after* having received the radioisotope dose.
      b) He will be sent to radioisotope laboratory when requested, usually in the afternoon.
   3. Precautions
      a) The patient should be in a room with other patients undergoing similar radioisotope therapy, or in a private room.
      b) There should be a rubber or plastic covering on the pillow and bed.
      c) The clothing and linen used by the patient should be saved in a linen bag in the patient's room for surveying by the radioisotope technician before they are sent to the laundry.
      d) If the patient has any dressings, these should be changed with the use of rubber gloves, and the gloves and waste material saved for surveying.
      e) During the first 48 hours after treatment, the patient should not be bathed without the use of a gown and gloves; these should be surveyed later.

If patient is ambulant, he may take a tub bath, but the tub must be thoroughly rinsed afterward.

f) If the patient uses a urinal or bedpan during the first 48 hours, these should be handled with gloves and flushed three times after each use. If the patient is ambulant, he should use the same toilet bowl at all times, and should flush it three times after each use during the first 48 hours or longer.

g) If the patient is incontinent, he should have an indwelling catheter, and the urine should be handled in the same way as above, except that the urine should be emptied frequently during the first 2 days.

h) No restrictions on visitors.

B. *Cardiac Therapy:* I^{131}; 7 days (effective half-life); 10–15 mc. (maximum dose)

1. Purpose

Some types of cardiac disease can be alleviated by reducing the thyroid function of the patient. This can be accomplished by giving a therapeutic dose of I^{131}.

2. Preparation

The patient has the same preparation and procedure as for thyroid therapy:

a) Fasting 2 hours *after* oral dose of I^{131}.

b) To radioisotope laboratory on call.

3. Precautions

These precautions are exactly the same as for thyroid therapy.

C. *Therapy of Blood Dyscrasias:* P^{32}; 14 days (effective half-life); 5 mc. (maximum dose)

1. Purpose

Radioactive phosphorus will concentrate in the bone marrow, red cells and white cells, and thereby aid in the therapy of polycythemia and certain leukemias.

2. Preparation

There is no special preparation, since the patient receives therapy by intravenous administration.

3. Precautions

a) No special room assignment is necessary.

b) The mattress and pillow should be protected by rubber or plastic covers.

c) Rubber gloves should be worn when handling the patient within the first 48 hours. Pajamas, rubber gloves and used linen should be saved for 48 hours and then surveyed by the radioisotope technician.

d) If the patient is ambulant, he may take tub baths or showers.

e) If the patient uses a urinal or bedpan during the first 48 hours, these should be handled with gloves.

f) No restrictions on visitors.

D. *Therapy for Cancer of Thyroid:* I^{131}; 2 days (effective half-life); 100 mc. (maximum dose)

1. Purpose

The patient is given a large oral dose of radioactive iodine to destroy the tumor tissue in the thyroid or elsewhere, usually after surgery for the tumor.

2. Preparation

(Same as for thyroid therapy preparation; see page 365).

3. Precautions

a) The patient should be in a private room, preferably with a private toilet.

b) All bed-care procedures should be performed before the radioisotope is administered, and they may be resumed 48 hours afterward, subject to the limitations noted hereinafter.

c) The pillow and mattress must be protected by rubber or plastic coverings.

d) Bed bathing and the changing of dressings should be performed with the personnel wearing gloves and gown up to 14 days following therapy.

e) The gloves and gown worn by personnel and the linens used by the patient should be saved in the patient's room for survey by the radioisotope technician.

POST ON OUTSIDE OF PATIENT'S ROOM

RADIOISOTOPE LABORATORY

Patient__________ Room__________ Ward__________

Radioisotope__________ Dose__________ Date Administered__________

TOLERANCE EXPOSURE HOURS PERMITTED FOLLOWING THERAPY
(Hospital Personnel and Visitors)

Site.	Day after Therapy						
	Therapy Day	1	2	3	4	5	6
Contact							
Bedside							
3 Feet							
Doorway							

RADIATION HAZARD

FIG. 77.—Radiation hazard notice and tolerance chart.

f) The urine and wastes and all specimens should be labeled "radioactive" and handled with gloves during the first 48 hours. Urinal, bedpan, thermometer and such other equipment used by the patient should be well rinsed and kept for the patient's own use.

g) If the patient is incontinent, an indwelling catheter should be used during the first 48 hours and the urine emptied frequently.

h) If the patient is ambulant, he may take tub baths if the tub is rinsed very well afterward. Also, he should use the same toilet consistently, and it should be well flushed (3 times).

i) No special handling of the food tray is required.

j) No visitors allowed in the patient's room for 48 hours; only short visits thereafter, as shown on the tolerance chart (see Fig. 77).

E. *Intracavitary Gold Application:* Au^{198}; 2.7 days (effective half-life); 100 mc. (maximum dose)

1. Purpose

Radioactive gold, administered intraperitoneally or intrapleurally, reduces the formation of fluid resulting from metastatic lesions and aids in the palliative therapy of cancer patients.

2. Preparation

The patient should be prepared by performing a paracentesis or thoracentesis at his bedside, and the radioactive gold should be immediately introduced directly into the cavity.

3. Precautions

a) All precautions are the same as for thyroid cancer therapy.

b) No special handling of food trays is required.

c) Care must also be taken to avoid a drainage from the site of the paracentesis or thoracentesis. Usually the site is sealed with collodion dressing.

d) No visitors allowed in the patient's room for 48 hours; only short visits for 14 days.

F. *Prostate Therapy:* Au^{198}; 2.7 days (effective half-life); 100 mc. (maximum dose)

1. Purpose

Radioactive gold administered into the prostate aids in destroying malignant tissue existing in this organ.

2. Preparation

No special preparation is necessary.

3. Precautions

    a) All precautions are the same as for thyroid cancer therapy, as stated above.

    b) No special handling of food trays is required.

    c) No visitors allowed in patient's room for 48 hours; only short visits for 14 days.

III. HANDLING OF RADIOISOTOPE PATIENTS AFTER DEATH

A. *Categories of Patients*

1. No special precautions are necessary in handling the bodies of patients who died shortly after receiving only *tracer* doses of radioisotopes.

2. For all patients who received *therapeutic* doses of radioisotopes within a period of 60 days previous to death, the following instructions will apply:

    a) Any personnel handling the body of the deceased in preparing it for the mortician should wear gown and gloves.

    b) All articles used by the patient, such as linen, pajamas, catheter, urinal, dressings, etc., must be surveyed by the radioisotope technician before disposal.

    c) The radioisotope laboratory must be notified of the death immediately.

    d) The pathology personnel at the morgue must be notified that the patient had had radioactive therapy, and the date on which it was administered must be reported.

    e) A report of radioactivity must be sent to the funeral director. A suggested form for the report is as follows:

RADIOISOTOPE LABORATORY

REPORT OF RADIOACTIVITY TO FUNERAL DIRECTOR

Date:_____, 19____

This certifies that the remains of _____
have been examined on this date by the Radiation Safety Officer or his deputy. Radioactivity close to the surface of the body, as determined by (Geiger counter) (ion chamber) (is) (is not) below the

rate of 30 mr./hr. that is acceptable for embalmers during their work. In all cases of positive radioactivity noted, every effort should be made to confine body fluids removed during the embalming procedures, pouring them directly into the drain, and flushing copiously with water. The maximum permissible dose rate will not be exceeded, *provided* rubber gloves are *worn,* and further precautions are observed as listed below.

Further precautions: _____

_____

_____

Signed: _____

Radiation Safety Officer

B. *Safe Handling of Cadavers Containing Radioisotopes*
   1. General Instructions
      The patients who die shortly after having received a large internal therapeutic dose of a radioisotope pose problems of exposure to the pathologist and embalmer. If, however, several days elapse between treatment and death, the hazard is considerably reduced, since Au^{198} decays 25 per cent, and I^{131} 9 per cent, each day. The patients should be hospitalized until their radioisotope content is 30 mc. or less; and if death occurs, the body should be identified as to the amount and type of isotope present and the date of administration.
   2. No Autopsy
      The hazard to the embalmer consists mainly of gamma radiation of low intensity. Several hours after administration of 150 mc. of Au^{198} and I^{131} the surface dose rate is 1.5 and 0.4 r/hr., respectively, with a reduction to 90 per cent at 50 cm. If each embalming is completed within an hour, several embalmings may be performed each week. If the body fluids are flushed into a sewer through a closed system, the contamination risk is minimal.
   3. Autopsy Performed
      The general protective measures applicable to the

body and gonads should be observed by the pathologist, but the hands require special emphasis because they are subject to relatively intense beta radiation. No autopsy should be started on a body containing more than 5 mc. of radioactive gold or iodine without consultation with the radiation safety officer, who is responsible for protection throughout his institution.

The use of double-thickness rubber autopsy gloves, which reduce the rate to a fifth of the unshielded beta radiation, is recommended. Dissections must be performed with long forceps and long-handled scissors. Organs containing high concentrations of I^{131} should be removed or avoided, and all organs should be stored several days before examination, if possible. All body fluids should be flushed directly into a sewer.

If the radiation safety officer is not available, information such as that given in Table 35 will enable the pathologist to perform an autopsy with a minimum of radiation exposure. The radioisotopes Au^{198} and I^{131} only are shown because they are gamma-ray emitters and pose the most serious hazard. Phosphorus-32 radiation can be shielded out effectively by using heavy gloves.

Generally, if large amounts of I^{131} have been used, it will have been for thyroid therapy or cancer; therefore, when performing an autopsy on a body containing I^{131} in large quantities, it is advisable to remove the thyroid and store it in a shielded can provided for that purpose.

If specimens are collected, the following information should be on the label:

Date:
Name:
Radioisotope:
Mr./hour on surface:
Safe working date (calculated at 6.25 mr./hr.):
Serial number:

TABLE 35.—A Guide for Autopsy Consideration

Key: a = probable radioactive content of body at various times after various doses; b = maximum radiation tolerance time in minutes permitted for autopsy. For values that are in italics, no precautions are necessary except wearing surgical rubber gloves; for values that are not in italics, consultation with the radiation safety officer is indicated.

Dose of Radioisotope (mc.)	1 a (mc.)	1 b (min.)	2 a (mc.)	2 b (min.)	3 a (mc.)	3 b (min.)	4 a (mc.)	4 b (min.)	6 a (mc.)	6 b (min.)	8 a (mc.)	8 b (min.)	10 a (mc.)	10 b (min.)	15 (mc.)
Au198 — Gold Remaining in Injected Cavity															
150	115	9	90	11	69	15	52	19	32	31	20	50	12	83	3
125	96	10	75	13	58	17	44	22	27	37	16	62	10	100	3
100	77	13	60	17	46	22	35	29	21	48	13	77	8	125	2
75	58	17	45	22	35	29	26	38	16	62	10	100	6	167	2
50	38	26	30	33	23	42	18	55	11	91	7	143	4	…	1
40	31	32	24	42	18	55	14	71	9	110	5	200	3	…	1
30	23	44	18	55	14	71	10	100	6	167	4		2	…	1
I131 — Iodine Remaining in Thyroid Gland Following Dose for Ablation of Normal Thyroid Tissue															
60	18		16		14		12		10		8		6		4
50	15		13		12		11		9		7		5		3
40	12		10		9		8		7		5		4		2
30	9		8		7		6		5		4		3		2
20	6		5		5		4		4		3		2		1
10	3		3		2		2		2		1		1		1
I131 — Iodine Remaining in Functioning Metastases Following Therapeutic Dose Post Thyroidectomy. (These are maximal; usually smaller.)															
100	20		18		16		14		12		9		7		4
75	15		13		12		11		9		7		5		3
50	10		9		8		7		6		5		4		2
35	7		6		5		5		4		3		2		1
20	4		4		3		3		2		2		1		1

Days Elapsed since Treatment

373

If, during autopsy or embalming, the pathologist or embalmer is injured, the work should be halted, the gloves washed and removed, the wound flushed in running water and a check made for residual contamination, and washing and checking repeated, if needed.

4. Laundry and Instruments

Laundry should be stored for a suitable decay period before it is washed. Instruments should be soaked in soap or a detergent and rinsed in running water. All disposable waste should be burned or flushed down a sewer, and special care should be taken to prevent contamination of the autopsy room floor and spread of the contamination to other parts of the institution.

5. Cremation

If cremation is performed without autopsy, there is no handling problem; otherwise autopsy precautions are in force. All Au^{198} and I^{131} is contained in the soft tissues and will pass out into the atmosphere; but to prevent any possible concentration at the base of the stack, cremation should not be performed if the radioisotope content of the body is 30 mc. or more.

6. Suggested Protective Items for Pathologist:

   a) Geiger counter.

   b) Pocket ion chambers.

   c) Plastic apron, shoe covers, eyeglasses.

REFERENCES

1. Kaplan, E., and Fields, T.: Precautions that pathologists should take in handling bodies that have received radioisotopes (editorial), Am. J. Clin. Path. 25:682, 1955.
2. Handling of radioactive cadavers (editorial), J.A.M.A. 156:773, 1954.
3. Precautions in autopsy and embalming procedures following administration of radioisotopes (editorial), Hosp. Management 74:96, 1952.
4. Precautions in Handling of Radioactive Material, U.S. Armed Forces Institute of Pathology Letter 5 (Washington, D. C.: Superintendent of Documents, Government Printing Office, April 8, 1952.)
5. Safe Handling of Radioactive Isotopes, National Bureau of Standards Handbook 42 (Washington, D. C.: Superintendent of Documents, Government Printing Office, 1949).
6. Safe Handling of Cadavers Containing Radioactive Isotopes, National Bureau of Standards Handbook 56 (Washington, D. C.: Superintendent of Documents, Government Printing Office, 1953).

APPENDIXES

A. GLOSSARY

ABSORPTION: The process by which the number of particles or quanta in a beam of radiation is reduced as it passes through some medium. The absorbed radiation may be transformed into mass, other radiation or energy by interaction with the electrons or nuclei of the atoms upon which it impinges.

ABSORPTION COEFFICIENT: Fractional decrease in the intensity of a beam of radiation per unit thickness *(linear absorption coefficient)*, per unit mass *(mass absorption coefficient)* or per atom *(atomic absorption coefficient)* of absorber.

ACTIVATED WATER: A transient chemically reactive state created in water by absorbed ionizing radiations.

ACTIVATION ANALYSIS: A method of chemical analysis, especially for small traces of material, based on the detection of characteristic radionuclides following a nuclear bombardment.

ACTIVATION ENERGY: The energy necessary to cause a particular reaction to begin. *Nuclear:* The amount of outside energy which must be added to a nucleus before a particular nuclear reaction will begin. *Chemical:* The amount of outside energy necessary to activate an atom or molecule so as to cause it to react chemically.

ACTIVITY, *see* Radioactivity.

ACUTE EXPOSURE: Term used to denote radiation exposure of short duration.

ADSORPTION: The adhesion of one substance to the surface of another.

AIR DOSE: X- or gamma-ray dose (expressed in roentgens) delivered at a point in free air. In radiologic practice, it consists only of the radiation of the primary beam and of that scattered from surrounding air.

AIR-WALL IONIZATION CHAMBER (x- or gamma rays): Ionization chamber in which the materials of the wall and electrodes are so selected as to produce ionization essentially equivalent to that in a free air ionization chamber. This is possible only over limited ranges of photon energies. Such a chamber is more appropriately termed an "air-equivalent ionization chamber."

ALPHA PARTICLE: A helium nucleus, consisting of two protons and two neutrons, with a double positive charge. Its mass is 4.002776 mass units (mu).

ALPHA RAY: Stream of fast-moving helium nuclei; a strongly ionizing and weakly penetrating radiation.

ALTERNATING CURRENT: An electric current (flow of electrons) which periodically reverses direction; Abbreviated: A.C.

ALVEOLI: The terminal air sacs of the lungs.

AMINO ACID: An organic acid; the building blocks in the formation of proteins.

AMPERE: Practical unit of electrical current; the flow of 1 coulomb per second. Abbreviated: amp.

AMPLIFICATION: As related to radiation detection instruments, the process (either gas or electronic, or both) by which ionization effects are magnified to a degree suitable for their measurement.

ANAPHASE (biologic): A stage in nuclear division, in which the paired chromosomes are separated toward opposite poles of the dividing cell.

ANEMIA: Deficiency of blood as a whole, or deficiency in the number of the red corpuscles or of the hemoglobin.

ANION: Negatively charged ion.

ANNIHILATION RADIATION: Photons produced when an electron and a positron unite and cease to exist. The annihilation of a positron-electron pair results in the production of two photons, each of at least 0.51 Mev energy.

ANODE: Positive electrode; electrode to which negative ions (anions) are attracted.

ANOXIA: Oxygen deficiency; a condition which results from a diminished supply of oxygen to the tissues.

ANTIBIOTIC: A substance, of biologic origin, which inhibits the growth of or kills micro-organisms. Common examples are penicillin, streptomycin, aureomycin, etc.

ANTIBODY: A specific substance produced in an animal (including man) as a reaction to the presence of an antigen, important in the body's defense against infectious diseases.

ANTIGEN: A foreign substance, usually protein but sometimes inorganic or polysaccharide, which on introduction into the blood or tissues causes the formation of antibodies.

ASSOCIATED CORPUSCULAR EMISSION: The full complement of secondary charged particles (usually limited to electrons) associated with an x-ray or gamma-ray beam in its passage through air. The full complement of electrons is obtained after the radiation has traversed sufficient air to bring about equilibrium between the primary photons and secondary electrons. Electronic equilibrium with the secondary photons is intentionally excluded.

ATOM: Smallest particle of an element which is capable of entering into a chemical reaction.

ATOMIC NUMBER: Number of protons in the nucleus; hence the

number of positive charges on the nucleus. Also, the number of electrons outside the nucleus of a neutral atom. Symbol: Z.

ATOMIC WEIGHT: Relative weight of the atom of an element compared with the weight of one atom of oxygen taken as 16; hence, a multiple of 1/16 the weight of an atom of oxygen.

ATROPHY: Wasting-away or diminution in the size of cell, tissue, organ or part from defect or failure of nutrition.

AUTORADIOGRAPH: Record of radiation from radioactive material in an object, made by placing its surface in close proximity to a photographic emulsion.

AVALANCHE: The multiplicative process in which a single charged particle accelerated by a strong electric field produces additional charged particles through collision with neutral gas molecules. This cumulative increase of ions is also known as "Townsend ionization" or "a Townsend avalanche."

AVERAGE LIFE (Mean Life): The average of the individual lives of all the atoms of a particular radioactive substance. It is 1.443 times the radioactive half-life.

AVOGADRO'S NUMBER: Number of molecules in a gram-molecular weight of any substance (6.03×10^{23} molecules); also, the number of atoms in a gram-atomic weight of any element.

BACKGROUND COUNTING RATE: Rate of radiation counting due to cosmic rays, to radioactive materials in the vicinity and to a slight radioactive contamination of the materials of which the instrument is made.

BACKSCATTERING: The process of scattering or reflecting into the sensitive volume of a measuring instrument radioactive radiations originally having no positive component of motion in that direction. The process is dependent on the nature of the mounting material, the nature of the sample, the type and energy of the radiations, and the particular geometrical arrangement.

BARN: Unit expressing the probability of a specific nuclear reaction taking place in terms of cross-sectional area. Numerically, it is 10^{-24} cm^2.

BASOPHIL: One of the white blood cells which takes a basic stain. It is the least abundant of the white cells.

BENIGN TUMOR: Tumor which cannot metastasize (nonmalignant).

BETA PARTICLE: Charged particle emitted from the nucleus of an atom and having a mass and charge equal in magnitude to those of the electron.

BETA RAY: A stream of high-speed electrons of nuclear origin more penetrating but less ionizing than alpha rays; a stream of high-speed electrons.

BETATRON: A device for accelerating electrons by means of magnetic induction.

BINARY SCALER: A scaler whose scaling factor is two per stage. (*See* Scaler.)

BINDING ENERGY: The energy represented by the difference in mass between the sum of the component parts and the actual mass of the nucleus.

BIOLOGIC EFFECTIVENESS OF RADIATION, *see* Relative Biologic Effectiveness of Radiation.

BIOLOGIC HALF-LIFE: The time required for the body to eliminate one half of an administered dose of any substance by regular processes of elimination. This time is approximately the same for both stable and radioactive isotopes of a particular element.

BLOOD DYSCRASIA: Any persistent change from normal of one or more of the blood components.

BONE MARROW: Soft material which fills the cavity in most bones; it manufactures most of the formed elements of the blood.

BONE SEEKER: Any compound or ion which migrates in the body preferentially into bone.

BORON COUNTER TUBE: A counter tube filled with boron trifluoride (BF_3) and/or having electrodes coated with boron or boron compounds; used for detecting slow neutrons by the (n, α) reaction of B^{10}.

BREEDER, *see* Converter.

BREMSSTRAHLUNG: Secondary photon radiation produced by deceleration of charged particles passing through matter.

CALIBRATION: Determination of variation from standard, or accuracy, of a measuring instrument, to ascertain necessary correction factors.

CALORIE (gram-calorie): Amount of heat necessary to raise the temperature of 1 gram of water 1° C. (e.g., from 14.5° to 15.5° C.). Abbreviation: cal.

CANCER: Any malignant neoplasm. (Popular usage.)

CAPACITANCE: (1) Ratio of the charge on a conductor to its potential. (2) Ratio of charge on positive plate of condenser to the potential difference across the plates. For the unit of capacitance, *see* Farad.

CAPILLARY: A small thin-walled blood vessel connecting an artery with a vein.

CAPTURE, RADIATIVE: The process by which a nucleus captures an incident particle and loses its excitation energy immediately by the emission of gamma radiation.

CAPTURE CROSS-SECTION: The probability that a nucleus will capture an incident particle. The unit of cross-section is commonly the barn (10^{-24} cm.^{2}).

CARCINOGENIC: Capable of producing cancer.

CARCINOMA: Malignant neoplasm composed of epithelial cells, regardless of their derivation.

CARRIER: (1) A quantity of an element which may be mixed with radioactive isotopes of that element giving a ponderable quantity to facilitate chemical operations. (2) A substance in ponderable amount which, when associated with a trace of another substance, will carry the trace with it through a chemical or physical process, especially a precipitation process. If the added substance is a different element from the trace, the carrier is called a "nonisotopic carrier."

CARRIER-FREE: An adjective applied to one or more radioactive isotopes of an element in minute quantity, essentially undiluted with stable isotope carrier.

CATARACT: A clouding of the crystalline lens of the eye, which obstructs the passage of light.

CATHODE: Negative electrode; electrode to which positive ions are attracted.

CATION: Positively charged ion.

CELL (biologic): The fundamental unit of structure and function in organisms.

CENTRIPETAL FORCE: Force required to keep a moving mass traveling in a circular path. The force is directed toward the axis of the circular path.

CENTROSOME (CENTRAL BODY): A minute intracellular structure from which radiate the spindle fibers during cell division.

CHAIN REACTION: Any chemical or nuclear process in which some of the products of the process or energy released by the process are instrumental in the continuation or magnification of the process.

CHARACTERISTIC (DISCRETE) RADIATION: Radiation originating from an atom following removal of an electron or excitation of the nucleus. The wavelength of the emitted radiation is specific, depending only on the element concerned and the particular energy levels involved.

CHEMICAL (ISOTOPIC) EXCHANGE: A process in which atoms (isotopes) of the same element in two different molecules exchange places.

CHROMATID: One of the sister threads of the longitudinally divided chromosome prior to nuclear division.

CHROMATIN: Nuclear protein material from which chromosomes are formed.

CHROMOSOME: A structure formed from chromatin which appears in cells during cell division; the bearer of hereditary determiners.

CHROMOSOME ABERRATION: Any rearrangement of chromosome parts as a result of breakage and reunion of broken ends.

CHROMOSOME BREAK: The transverse break of a chromosome before its longitudinal division into chromatid threads.

CHROMOSOME DELETION: Loss of a section of a chromosome.

CHROMOSOME, SEX: A chromosome which is closely bound up with the sex determination of the offspring.

CHROMOSOME, TRANSLOCATION: Change in position of a portion of a chromosome, either to different regions of the same chromosome or to another chromosome.

CHROMOSOMES, HOMOLOGOUS: Chromosomes in which the same gene loci occur in the same sequence.

CHRONIC EXPOSURE: Term used to denote radiation exposure of long duration, by fractionation or protraction. (*See* Dose, Fractionation, and Dose, Protraction.)

CILIA: Hairlike structures found on many cells, capable of a vibratory or lashing movement.

CLEAVAGE: Cell division characteristic of early stages of the embryo.

CLINICAL: Pertaining to the observed symptoms and cause of disease.

CLOUD CHAMBER: A device for observing the paths of ionizing particles, based on the principle that supersaturated vapor condenses more readily on ions than on neutral molecules.

COINCIDENCE: The occurrence of ionizing events in one or more detectors simultaneously or within an assignable time interval, as a result of the passage of a single particle or of several generically related particles.

COINCIDENCE CORRECTION: Mathematical calculation to correct observed count to the count free of coincidence losses.

COLLIMATOR: A device for confining the elements of a beam within an assigned solid angle.

COLLISION: Encounter between two subatomic particles (including photons) which changes the existing momentum and energy conditions. The products of the collision need not be the same as the initial systems.

COLLISION, ELASTIC: Collision in which kinetic energy and momentum of each colliding system are conserved.

COLLISION, INELASTIC: Collision in which at least one system gains internal excitation energy at the expense of the total kinetic energy of their center-of-gravity motion.

COMPOUND: Pure substance composed of two or more elements combined in a fixed definite proportion by weight.

COMPTON EFFECT: An absorption effect observed for x- and gamma radiation in which the incident photon interacts with an orbital electron of the absorber atom to produce a recoil electron and a photon of energy less than the incident photon.

CONDENSER R-METER: An instrument consisting of an "air-wall" ionization chamber together with auxiliary equipment for charging and measuring its voltage; it is used as an integrating instrument for measuring the quantity of x- or gamma radiation in roentgens. (See Ionization Chamber.)

CONSERVATION OF MASS-ENERGY: Energy and mass are interchangeable in accordance with the equation $E = mc^2$, where E is energy, m is mass and c is velocity of light.

CONTACT RADIATION THERAPY: X-ray therapy with specially constructed tubes in which the target-skin distance is very short (less than 2 cm.). The voltage is usually between 40 and 60 kv.

CONTAMINATION, RADIOACTIVE: Deposition of radioactive material in any place where it is not desired, and particularly in any place where its presence may be harmful. The harm may be in vitiating the validity of an experiment or a procedure, or in actually being a source of danger to personnel.

CONVERTER: A nuclear reactor that converts fertile atoms into fuel by neutron capture. Two different ways of using the words "converter" and "breeder" are in use at present: (1) A converter is a reactor that uses one kind of fuel and produces another (e.g., consumes plutonium and produces more plutonium from uranium-238). (2) A breeder is a converter that produces more fissionable atoms than it consumes.

CORIUM (DERMIS): The true skin or fibrous layer beneath the epidermis.

CORPUSCLE: A blood cell.

COSMIC RAYS: Radiation, both particulate and electromagnetic, which originates in outer space.

COULOMB: Unit of electrical charge in the practical system of units. A quantity of electricity equal to 3×10^9 electrostatic units of charge.

COUNT (radiation measurements): The external indication of a device designed to enumerate ionizing events. It may refer to a single detected event or to the total registered in a given period of time. The term often is erroneously used to designate a disintegration, ionizing event or voltage pulse.

COUNTING RATE METER: A device which gives a continuous indication of the average rate of ionizing events.

CRITICAL SIZE: For a fissionable material, the minimum amount of a material which will support a chain reaction.

CROSS-SECTION, NUCLEAR: The probability that a certain reaction between a nucleus and an incident particle or photon will occur. It is expressed as the effective "area" that the nucleus presents for the reaction. (See Barn.)

CUMULATIVE DOSE (radiation): The total dose resulting from repeated exposures to radiation of the same region or of the whole body.

CURIE: That quantity of a radioactive material having associated with it 3.7×10^{10} disintegrations per second.

CURRENT, ELECTRIC: Amount of charge flowing past a point per unit time.

CYCLOTRON: A device for accelerating charged particles to high energies by means of an alternating electric field between electrodes placed in a constant magnetic field.

CYTOPLASM: The protoplasm of a cell exclusive of that of the nucleus.

CYTOPLASMIC INHERITANCE: Inheritance which is not controlled by the genes in the nucleus but by the cytoplasm.

DEAMINATION: Removal of the amino group (NH^2) from amino acids, amines and other mono-substituted ammonia derivatives.

DECADE SCALER: A scaler whose scaling factor is a power of 10. (See Scaler.)

DECARBOXYLATION: Degrading an organic acid by removing the carboxyl group ($-COOH$) in the form of carbon dioxide.

DECAY, RADIOACTIVE: Disintegration of the nucleus of an unstable element by the spontaneous emission of charged particles and/or photons.

DECAY CONSTANT: The fraction of the number of atoms of a radioactive isotope which decay in unit time. Symbol: λ (See Disintegration Constant.)

DECAY CURVE: A curve showing the relative amount of radioactive substance remaining after any time interval.

DECONTAMINATION FACTOR: The ratio between the amount of undesired radioactive material initially present to the amount remaining after a suitable processing step has been completed. Decontamination factors may refer to the reduction of some particular type of radiation or of a gross measurable radioactivity.

DENSITOMETER: Instrument utilizing the photoelectric principle to determine the degree of darkening of developed photographic film.

DENSITY (photographic): Logarithm of opacity of exposed and processed film. Opacity is the reciprocal of transmission; transmission is the ratio of transmitted to incident intensity. Density is used to denote the degree of darkening of photographic film.

DEPOLYMERIZATION: The breaking-down of an organic compound into two or more less complex molecules.

DEPTH DOSE: The radiation dose delivered at a particular depth beneath the surface of the body. It is usually expressed as a percentage of surface dose or as a percentage of air dose.

DEUTERIUM: A heavy isotope of hydrogen having one proton and one neutron in the nucleus. Symbol: D or $_1H^2$.

DEUTERON: Nucleus of a deuterium atom, containing one proton and one neutron.

DIFFERENTIAL ABSORPTION RATIO: Ratio of concentration of an isotope in a given organ or tissue to the concentration that would be obtained if the same administered quantity of this isotope were uniformly distributed throughout the body.

DIPLOID: Having the normal paired chromosomes resulting from fertilization.

DIRECT CURRENT: Current whose flow is continual in one direction; Abbreviation: D.C.

DIRECT RADIATION (radiology): All radiation, other than the useful beam, emanating from the x-ray tube anode or the inside of the tube or tube container.

DISINTEGRATION, NUCLEAR: A spontaneous nuclear transformation (radioactivity) characterized by the emission of energy and/or mass from the nucleus. When numbers of nuclei are involved, the process is characterized by a definite half-life.

DISINTEGRATION CONSTANT: The fraction of the number of atoms of a radioactive isotope which decay in unit time; λ in the equation $N = N_0 e^{-\lambda t}$, where N_0 is the initial number of atoms present and N is the number of atoms present after some time, t.

DOMINANT CHARACTER (genetics): Of a pair of contrasted characteristics, the one which will appear in a hybrid resulting from crossbreeding of homozygous parents unlike with respect to that characteristic.

DOSE (DOSAGE): According to current usage, the radiation delivered to a specified area or volume or to the whole body. Units for dose specification are roentgens for x- or gamma rays, reps or equivalent roentgens for beta rays. In radiology the dose may be specified in air, on the skin or at some depth beneath the surface; no statement of dose is complete without specification of location. The International Congress of Radiology has specified that the rad replace the roentgen as the unit of dosage. The rad is defined as that amount of ionizing radiation which will result in the absorption in tissue of 100 ergs per gram.

DOSE, FRACTIONATION: A method of administration of radiation in which relatively small doses are given daily or at longer intervals.

DOSE, PROTRACTION: A method of administration of radiation by delivering it continuously over a relatively long period at a low dosage rate.

DOSE RATE (DOSAGE RATE): Radiation dose delivered per unit time.

DOSE-RATE METER: Any instrument which measures radiation dose rate.

DOSIMETER: Instrument used to detect and measure an accumulated dosage of radiation; in common usage, it is a pencil-sized ionization chamber with built-in self-reading electrometer; used for personnel monitoring.

DROSOPHILIA: A genus of fruit flies which has been used extensively in genetic experiments.

DYNE: The unit of force which, when acting on a mass of 1 gram, will produce an acceleration of 1 cm./sec./sec.

EDEMA: Presence of abnormally large amounts of fluid in the intercellular tissue spaces of the body or of part of the body.

EFFECTIVE ATOMIC NUMBER: A number calculated from the composition and atomic numbers of a compound or mixture. An element of this atomic number would interact with photons in the same way as the compound or mixture.

EFFECTIVE HALF-LIFE: Half-life of a radioactive isotope in a biologic organism, resulting from the combination of radioactive decay and biologic elimination.

$$\text{Effective half-life} = \frac{\text{Biologic half-life} \times \text{Radioactive half-life}}{\text{Biologic half-life} + \text{Radioactive half-life}}$$

EFFICIENCY (counters): A measure of the probability that a count will be recorded when radiation is incident on a detector. Usage varies considerably, and so it is well to make sure which factors (window transmission, sensitive volume, energy dependence, etc.) are included in a given case.

EGG CELL (OVUM): A female gamete.

ELECTRODE: Either terminal of an electric source.

ELECTROMETER: Electrostatic instrument for measuring the difference in potential between two points. Used to measure change of electric potential of charged electrodes resulting from ionization produced by radiation.

ELECTROMETER TUBE: A vacuum tube specially designed with a high input impedance and low grid current.

ELECTROMOTIVE FORCE: Potential difference across electrodes tending to produce an electric current. Abbreviation: emf.

ELECTRON: Negatively charged particle which is a constituent of every neutral atom. Unit of negative electricity equal to 4.80×10^{-10} electrostatic units. Its mass is 0.0005488 mass units (mu).

ELECTRON CAPTURE: A mode of radioactive decay involving the capture of an orbital electron by its nucleus. Capture from a particular electron shell is designated as K-electron capture, L-electron capture, etc.

ELECTRON MULTIPLIER TUBE: A tube in which small electron currents are amplified by a cascade process employing secondary emission.

ELECTRON VOLT: Amount of energy gained by a particle with a single charge in passing through a potential difference of 1 volt. Abbreviation: ev.

ELECTROSCOPE: Instrument for detecting the presence of electric charges by the deflection of charged bodies.

ELECTROSTATIC FIELD: The region surrounding an electric charge in which another electric charge experiences a force.

ELECTROSTATIC UNIT OF CHARGE (STATCOULOMB): That quantity of electric charge which, when placed in a vacuum 1 cm. distant from an equal and like charge, will repel it with a force of 1 dyne. Abbreviated: esu.

ELEMENT: Pure substance consisting of atoms of the same atomic number, which cannot be decomposed by ordinary chemical means.

EMBRYO: An early stage in the development of an organism.

EMULSION, NUCLEAR: A photographic emulsion specially designed to permit observation of the individual tracks of ionizing particles.

ENDOCRINE GLAND: A gland of internal secretion (ductless gland); a gland which produces a hormone.

ENDOERGIC REACTION: Reaction which absorbs energy.

ENDOTHELIUM: The layer of simple squamous (flat) cells lining the inner surface of the circulatory organs and certain other closed body cavities.

ENDOTHERMIC REACTION: Reaction which absorbs energy specifically in the form of heat.

ENERGY: Capacity for doing work. *Potential energy* is the energy inherent in a mass because of its position with reference to other masses. *Kinetic energy* is the energy possessed by a mass because of its motion; cgs units: gm.-cm.^{2}/sec.^{2}, or erg.

ENERGY DEPENDENCE: The characteristic response (of a radiation detector) to a given range of radiation energies (or wavelengths), as compared with the response of a standard open-air chamber.

ENRICHED MATERIAL: (1) Material in which the relative amount of one or more isotopes of a constituent has been increased. (2) Uranium in which the abundance of the U^{235} isotope is increased above normal.

ENZYME: An organic compound, frequently a protein, that accelerates (catalyzes) specific transformations of material, as in the digestion of foods.

EOSINOPHIL: A white blood cell which is readily stained by the dye eosin; a type of granulocyte.

EPIDERMIS: The outermost layer of cells of the skin.

EPILATION (DEPILATION): The temporary or permanent removal of hair.

EPIPHYSIS: In long bones, a portion of bone at each end which develops separately from the main part (the shaft) of the bone and which subsequently becomes consolidated with the main part.

EPISTAXIS: Bleeding from the nose.

EPITHELIOMA: Malignant neoplasm derived from epithelial cells lining the external and internal body surfaces. Some authorities prefer the term "carcinoma" for these growths.

EPITHELIUM: A term applied to cells that line all canals and surfaces having communication with external air and that are specialized for secretion in certain glands, such as the liver, kidneys, etc.

ERG: Unit of work done by a force of 1 dyne acting through a distance of 1 cm. Unit of energy which can exert a force of 1 dyne through a distance of 1 cm.; cgs units: dyne-cm., or gm.-cm.^{2}/sec.^{2}.

ERYTHEMA: An abnormal redness of the skin, due to distension of the capillaries with blood. It can be caused by many different agents—e.g., heat, certain drugs, ultraviolet rays, ionizing radiation.

ERYTHROCYTE: A red blood corpuscle.

ETIOLOGY: Sum of knowledge regarding causes, as of a disease.

EUGENICS: The science which deals with the influences that improve the hereditary quality of the human race.

EXCRETION: The discharge of waste materials formed in metabolism.

EXIT DOSE: Dose of radiation at the surface of body opposite to that on which the beam is incident.

EXOERGIC: That which liberates energy.

EXOTHERMIC: That which liberates energy specifically as heat.

EXTRAPOLATION IONIZATION CHAMBER: An ionization chamber with electrodes whose spacing can be adjusted and accurately determined to permit extrapolation of its reading to zero chamber volume.

FARAD: A unit of capacitance; a condenser has a capacitance of 1 farad when a potential difference of 1 volt will charge it with 1 coulomb of electricity.

FEATHER ANALYSIS: A technique established by N. Feather (1938) for the determination of the range, in aluminum, of the beta particles of a radio-element by comparison of the absorption curve with the absorption curve of a reference radio-element, usually bismuth-210 (range, 476 mg./cm.^{2}).

FERTILIZATION: The union of two gametes to form a zygote.

FILM BADGE: A pack of photographic film used for approximate measurement of radiation exposure for personnel monitoring purposes. The badge may contain two or three films of differing sensitivity, and it may contain a filter which shields part of the film from certain types of radiation.

FILM RING: A film badge in the form of a finger ring.

FILTER (radiology): *Primary:* A sheet of material, usually metal, placed in a beam of radiation to absorb, as far as possible, the less penetrating components. *Secondary:* A sheet of material of low atomic number, relative to that of the primary filter, placed in the filtered beam of radiation to remove characteristic radiation produced by the primary filter.

FISSION, *see* Nuclear Fission.

FISSION PRODUCTS: Elements resulting from fission.

FISSION YIELD: The percentage of fissions leading to a particular nuclide by direct formation and by decay of precursors.

FLUORESCENCE: The emission of radiation of particular wavelengths by a substance as a result of absorption of radiation of shorter wavelength. This emission occurs essentially only during the irradiation.

FLUORESCENT SCREEN: A sheet of material coated with a substance, such as calcium tungstate, zinc sulfide, etc., which will emit visible light when irradiated with ionizing radiation.

FLUOROGRAPHY (PHOTOFLUOROGRAPHY): Photography of an image produced on fluorescent screen by x- or gamma radiation.

FLUOROSCOPE: A fluorescent screen, suitably mounted (with respect to an x-ray tube) for ease of observation and protection, used for indirect visualization by means of x-rays of internal organs in the body or internal structures in apparatus or in masses of metal.

FOCAL SPOT (x-rays): The part of the target of the x-ray tube which is struck by the main electron stream.

FREE AIR IONIZATION CHAMBER: An ionization chamber in which a delimited beam of radiation passes between the electrodes without striking them or other internal parts of the equipment. The electric field is maintained perpendicular to the electrodes in the collecting region; as a result, the ionized volume can be accurately determined from the dimensions of the collecting electrode and the limiting diaphragm. This is the basic standard instrument for x-ray dosimetry, at least within the range from 5 to 400 kv.

FREQUENCY: Number of cycles, revolutions or vibrations completed in a unit of time, usually per second.

FUEL ROD: A long, slender fuel assembly for reactor use.

FUSION, see Nuclear Fusion.

GAMETE: A mature germ cell; sperm cell or egg.

GAMMA RAY: Short wavelength electromagnetic radiation of nuclear origin with a range of wavelengths from 10^{-9} to 10^{-12} cm., emitted from the nucleus.

GAS AMPLIFICATION: As applied to ionization radiation detecting instruments containing gas, the ratio of the charge collected to the charge produced by the initial ionizing event.

GAS-FLOW COUNTER (radiation): A counter in which an appropriate atmosphere is maintained in the counter tube by allowing a suitable gas to flow slowly through the sensitive volume.

GEIGER-MÜLLER (G-M) COUNTER TUBE: Highly sensitive, gas-filled radiation-measuring device which operates at voltages in the region of avalanche ionization.

GEIGER REGION: In an ionization radiation detector, the operating voltage interval in which the charge collected per ionizing event is essentially independent of the number of primary ions produced in the initial ionizing event.

GEIGER THRESHOLD: Minimum voltage at which a Geiger-Müller tube operates in the Geiger region.

GENE: Fundamental unit of inheritance which determines and controls hereditarily transmissible characteristics. Genes are arranged linearly at definite loci on chromosomes.

GENETIC EFFECT OF RADIATION: Inheritable changes, chiefly mutations, produced by the absorption of ionizing radiations. On the basis of present knowledge, these effects are purely additive, and there is no recovery.

GENOTYPE: The fundamental hereditary (genetic) constitution of an organism.

GEOMETRY FACTOR: The fraction of the total solid angle about the source of radiation that is subtended by the face of the sensitive volume of a detector.

GERM CELLS: The cells of an organism whose function it is to reproduce the kind. They are characteristically haploid.

GERM PLASM: The gametes and the cells from which they are formed, considered as a unit.

GESTATION: Pregnancy.

GIANT CELLS: Abnormally large multinuclear cells associated with various pathologic conditions.

GOLGI APPARATUS: A very delicate intracellular network of fibers which are thought to be associated with hormone production.

GONAD: A gamete-producing organ in animals; testis or ovary.

GRAM ATOMIC WEIGHT: A mass in grams numerically equal to the atomic weight of an element.

GRAM MOLECULAR WEIGHT (GRAM-MOLE): Mass in grams numerically equal to the molecular weight of a substance.

GRANULOCYTE: A type of white blood cell the cytoplasm of which is granular, in contrast with lymphocytes, which have clear cytoplasm (agranulocyte).

GRANULOPENIA: Decrease in number of granulocytes in the blood.

GRAVITATION: Force of attraction existing between all material bodies in the universe. The magnitude of the force between any two bodies is proportional to the product of the masses of the two bodies and inversely proportional to the square of the distance between them.

GRENZ RAYS: X-rays produced at voltages of 5–20 kv.

HALF-LIFE, RADIOACTIVE: Time required for a radioactive substance to lose 50 per cent of its activity by decay.

HALF-VALUE LAYER (HALF-THICKNESS): The thickness of any

particular material necessary to reduce the intensity of an x-ray or gamma-ray beam to one-half its original value.

HAPLOID: Having a single complete set of chromosomes, the condition of the gamete nucleus. Opposed to diploid.

HARDNESS (x-rays): A term for qualitatively specifying the relative penetrating power of x-rays. In general, the shorter the wavelength the harder the radiation.

HEALTH PHYSICS: A term in common use for that branch of radiological science dealing with the protection of personnel from harmful effects of ionizing radiation.

HEAVY WATER: Popular name for water of which the hydrogen component is deuterium.

HEMATOLOGY: The study of blood and its components.

HEMATOPOIESIS: The formation of blood or of blood cells.

HEMATOPOIETIC SYSTEM: The blood-making system; the bone marrow, spleen and lymph nodes.

HEMOGLOBIN: The oxygen-carrying pigment of the red blood corpuscles.

HEMORRHAGE: Copious bleeding.

HEPARIN: A substance which prevents the clotting of blood.

HEREDITY: Transmission of characters and traits from parents to offspring.

HETEROGENEOUS REACTOR: A nuclear reactor in which the fissionable material and moderator are arranged as discrete bodies (usually according to a regular pattern) of such dimensions that a nonhomogeneous medium is presented to the neutrons. *(See* Homogeneous Reactor.)

HETEROZYGOUS: Derived from germ cells genetically unlike.

HISTOLOGY: The study of the minute structure and composition of the tissues.

HOLD-BACK CARRIER: The inactive isotope or isotopes of a radioactive element(s), or an element of similar properties, or some reagent which may be used to diminish the amount of the radionuclide coprecipitated or adsorbed in a chemical reaction.

HOMOGENEOUS REACTOR: A nuclear reactor in which the fissionable material and the moderator (if used) are combined in a mixture such that an effectively homogeneous medium is presented to the neutrons. Such a mixture is represented either by a solution of fuel in moderator or by discrete particles having dimensions small in comparison with the neutron mean free path. *(See* Heterogeneous Reactor.)

HOMOZYGOUS: Derived from germ cells that are genetically alike.

HORMONE: A chemical regulator; a substance produced in an organ which, when transported to some other organ or tissue, produces there a specific effect.

HYPERPLASIA: The abnormal multiplication or increase in the number of normal cells in normal arrangement in a tissue.

IMMUNITY: The power which a living organism possesses to resist and overcome infection.

IMPLANT (radiology): Radioactive material in a suitable container, to be embedded in a tissue for therapeutic purposes. It may be permanent (seed) or temporary (needle).

INDUCED RADIOACTIVITY: That activity produced in a substance after bombardment with neutrons or other particles.

INHERENT FILTRATION (x-rays): The filtration introduced by the wall of the x-ray tube and any permanent tube enclosure; to be distinguished from added primary and secondary filters.

INTEGRAL DOSE (VOLUME DOSE): A measure of the total energy absorbed by a patient or any object during exposure to radiation. According to British usage, the integral dose of x- or gamma rays is expressed in gram-roentgens.

INTEGRATING CIRCUIT: Electronic circuit which records at any time an average value for the number of events occurring per unit time; or an electrical circuit which records total number of ions collected in a given time.

INTEGRATING DOSE METER: Ionization chamber and measuring system designed for determining total radiation administered during an exposure. In medical radiology the chamber is usually designed to be placed on the patient's skin. A device may be included to terminate the exposure when it has reached a desired value.

INTENSIFYING SCREEN: Sheet of cardboard or other substance coated with fluorescent material and placed in contact with the film in radiography. The x- or gamma rays excite the fluorescent substance, and the light thus emitted adds to the radiation effect on the film and produces an image of greater density for a given exposure. Sheets of thin lead may be used for the same purpose in industrial radiography with very high energy radiation. In this case, the increased effect is due largely to secondary electrons and x-rays emitted by the lead.

INTENSITY (radiology): Amount of energy per unit time passing through unit area perpendicular to the line of propagation at the point in question. Often this term is used incorrectly in the sense of dose rate.

INTERNAL CONVERSION: A mode of radioactive decay in which the gamma rays from excited nuclei cause the ejection of orbital electrons from the atom. The ratio of the number of internal conversion electrons to the number of gamma quanta emitted in the de-excitation of the nucleus is called the "conversion ratio."

INTERNAL RADIATION HAZARD: The danger to an individual from ionizing radiations originating within his body, as from radium atoms deposited in the bones.

ION: Atomic particle, atom or chemical radical (group of chemically combined atoms) bearing an electrical charge, either negative or positive.

ION EXCHANGE: A chemical process involving the reversible interchange of ions between a solution and a particular solid material, such as an ion exchange resin consisting of a matrix of insoluble material interspersed with fixed ions of opposite charge.

ION PAIR: Two particles of opposite charge, usually referring to the electron and positive atomic or molecular residue resulting after the interaction of radiation with the orbital electrons of atoms.

IONIZATION: The process or the result of any process by which a neutral atom or molecule acquires either a positive or a negative charge.

IONIZATION CHAMBER: An instrument designed to measure quantity of ionizing radiation in terms of the charge of electricity associated with ions produced within a defined volume.

IONIZATION DENSITY: Number of ion pairs per unit volume.

IONIZATION PATH (TRACK): The trail of ion pairs produced by an ionizing particle in its passage through matter.

IONIZATION POTENTIAL: The potential necessary to separate one electron from an atom, resulting in the formation of an ion pair.

IONIZING EVENT: Any occurrence of a process in which an ion or group of ions is produced.

IONIZING RADIATION: Any electromagnetic or particulate radiation capable of producing ions, directly or indirectly, in its passage through matter.

IRRADIATION: Exposure to radiation.

ISOBAR: One of two or more different nuclides having the same mass number.

ISODOSE CHART: Chart showing the distribution of radiation in a medium by means of lines or surfaces drawn through points receiving equal doses. Isodose charts have been determined for beams of x-rays traversing the body, for radium applicators used for intracavitary or interstitial therapy, and for working areas where x-rays or radioactive isotopes are employed.

ISOMER: One of several nuclides having the same number of neutrons and protons but capable of existing, for a measurable time, in different quantum states with different energies and radioactive properties. Commonly, the isomer of higher energy decays to one with lower energy by the process of isomeric transition.

ISOMERIC TRANSITION: The process by which a nuclide decays to an isomeric nuclide (i.e., one of the same mass number and atomic number) of lower quantum energy. Isomeric transitions, often abbreviated "I. T.," proceed by gamma ray and/or internal conversion electron emission.

ISOTONE: One of several different nuclides having the same number of neutrons in their nuclei.

ISOTOPE: One of several different nuclides having the same number of protons in their nuclei, and hence having the same atomic number, but differing in the number of neutrons and hence in the mass number or in energy content (isomers). Isotopes have almost identical chemical properties.

ISOTOPE DILUTION ANALYSIS: A method of chemical analysis for a component of a mixture based on the addition to the mixture of a known amount of labeled component of known specific activity, followed by isolation of a quantity of the component and measurement of the specific activity of that sample.

ISOTOPE EFFECT: The effect of the difference in the mass between isotopes on the rate and/or equilibria of chemical transformations.

ISOTOPE SEPARATION: Process in which a mixture of isotopes of an element is separated into its component isotopes or in which the abundance of isotopes in such a mixture is changed.

ISOTOPIC CARRIER, *see* Carrier.

K CAPTURE: A colloquialism for K-electron capture. Also loosely used to designate any orbital electron-capture process.

KELOID: Excessive scar formation following irradiation or other forms of skin injury.

LABELED COMPOUND: A compound consisting, in part, of labeled molecules *(see below)*. By observations of radioactivity or isotopic composition, this compound or its fragments may be followed through physical, chemical or biologic processes.

LABELED MOLECULE: A molecule containing one or more atoms distinguished by non-natural isotopic composition (with radioactive or stable isotopes).

LATENT PERIOD: The period or state of seeming inactivity between the time of exposure to an agent and the beginning of the response.

LD 50 (radiation dose), *see* Median Lethal Dose.

LEAD EQUIVALENT: The thickness of lead affording the same reduction in radiation dose rate under specified conditions as the material in question.

LESION: Any hurt, wound or local degeneration.

LETHAL MUTATION: *see* Mutation, Lethal.

LEUCOCYTE: A white blood corpuscle.

LEUCOCYTOSIS: An increase in the number of leucocytes in the blood. It occurs normally during digestion and in pregnancy, and as a response to certain pathologic conditions.

LEUKEMIA: A disease in which there is often great overproduction of white blood cells, or a relative overproduction of immature white cells, and great enlargement of the spleen. The disease is variable, at times running a more chronic course in adults than in children. It is almost always fatal. It can be produced in some animals by long-continued exposure to low intensities of ionizing radiation.

LEUKOPENIA: Abnormal diminution in the number of white cells in the blood.

LIBIDO: Sexual desire.

LINEAR ABSORPTION COEFFICIENT: A factor expressing the fraction of a beam of radiation absorbed in unit thickness of material. In the expression $I = I_0 e^{-\mu x}$, I_0 is the initial intensity, I the intensity after passage through a thickness of the material, x, and μ is the linear absorption coefficient.

LINEAR ACCELERATOR: A device for accelerating particles employing alternate electrodes and gaps arranged in a straight line, so proportioned that, when their potentials are varied in the proper amplitude and frequency, particles passing through them receive successive increments of energy.

LINEAR AMPLIFIER: A pulse amplifier in which the output pulse height is proportional to an input pulse height for a given pulse shape up to a point at which the amplifier overloads.

LINKAGE (genetics): The condition in which traits are inherited together because of the presence of their genes in the same chromosome.

LYMPH: An almost colorless fluid circulating in the lymphatic vessels of vertebrates. It closely resembles blood plasma in composition, and contains lymphocytes.

LYMPH GLAND (LYMPH NODE): Rounded masses of tissue consisting of a fibrous network in the meshes of which are numerous small circular cells. These cells, when carried off by lymph, become lymphocytes.

LYMPHOCYTE: A type of leucocyte characterized by a single sharply defined nucleus and scanty cytoplasm.

LYMPHOPENIA: Decrease in the proportion of lymphocytes in the blood.

MALIGNANT TUMOR: A tumor capable of metastasizing.

MASS ABSORPTION COEFFICIENT: The linear absorption coefficient per centimeter divided by the density of the absorber in grams per cubic centimeter. It is frequently expressed as μ/ρ, where μ is the linear absorption coefficient and ρ the absorber density.

MASS DEFECT: Difference between the mass of the nucleus as a whole and the sum of the component nucleon masses.

MASS NUMBER: The number of nucleons (protons and neutrons) in the nucleus of an atom. Symbol: A.

MATURATION (genetics): The process of gamete formation in which the number of chromosomes in the germ cells is reduced to one-half the number characteristic of the species.

MEAN FREE PATH: Average distance a particle travels between collisions.

MEDIAN LETHAL DOSE (MLD): Dose of radiation required to kill, within a specified period, 50 per cent of the individuals in a large group of animals or organisms.

MEIOSIS (biology): Nuclear division in which the members of each pair of chromosomes separate and form different nuclei, thus reducing the number of chromosomes by half. In animals, it is part of the maturation of the germ cell.

MESON: Short-lived particle carrying a positive or negative charge, or no charge, and having a variable mass in multiples of the mass of the electron. Also called "Mesotron."

METABOLISM: The sum of all the physical and chemical processes by which living organized substance is produced and maintained and by which energy is made available for the uses of the organism.

METABOLITE: Any substance produced by metabolism.

METAPHASE: A stage in nuclear division in which the divided chromosomes lie in a plane at right angles to the plane of the division spindle, and midway between its poles.

METASTABLE STATE: An excited state of a nucleus which returns to its ground state by the emission of a gamma ray over a *measurable* half-life.

METASTASIS: The transfer in the body of malignant neoplastic cells from the original or parent site to a more distant one.

MITOSIS (biology): A form of nuclear division in which the daughter nuclei come to have the same number and kinds of chromosomes as the parent nucleus, characteristic of most divisions other than those involving meiosis.

MODERATOR: Material used in a nuclear reactor to moderate (i.e., to slow down) neutrons from the high energies at which they are formed.

MOLECULE: Ultimate unit quantity of a compound which can exist by itself and retain all the properties of the original substance.

MOMENTUM: The product of the mass of a body and its velocity; cgs units: gm.-cm./sec.

MONITORING: Periodic or continuous determination of the amount of ionizing radiation or radioactive contamination present in an occupied region, as a safety measure for purposes of health protection. *Area monitoring:* Routine monitoring of the level of radiation or of radioactive contamination of any particular area, building, room or equipment. Usage in some laboratories or operations distinguishes between routine monitoring and survey activities. *Personnel monitoring:* Monitoring any part of an individual, his breath or excretions, or any part of his clothing. *(See also* Radiological Survey.)

MONOCHROMATIC RADIATION: Electromagnetic radiation of a single wave length, or in which all the photons have the same energy.

MONOCYTE: A type of large white blood cell.

MONOENERGETIC RADIATION: Particulate radiation of a given type (alpha, beta, neutron, etc.) in which all particles have the same energy.

MONSTER: A newborn who, through faulty congenital development, is incapable of properly performing vital functions or differs markedly from the normal morphology of his species.

MUCOSA: Mucous membrane lining the gastrointestinal tract and air passages; a type of epithelial tissue.

MUCOSAL GLANDS: Glands that secrete mucus.

MUTATION, GENE: A sudden and permanent change in a gene. The term "mutation" is sometimes used in a broader sense, to include chromosome aberrations as well.

MUTATION, LETHAL: Mutation leading to death of the offspring at any stage.

NATURAL SELECTION: Process leading to the survival of the best adapted (most fit) in the competition in nature.

NECROSIS: Death of a circumscribed portion of tissue.

NEOPLASM: A new growth of cells which is more or less unrestrained and not governed by the usual limitations of normal growth. *Benign*—if there is some degree of growth restraint and no spread to distant parts. *Malignant*—if the growth invades the tissues of the host, spreads to distant parts, or both.

NEUTRON: Elementary nuclear particle with a mass approximately the same as that of a hydrogen atom and electrically neutral; its mass is 1.00892 mu (mass units).

NEUTROPHIL: The most abundant type of white blood cell, a type of granulocyte.

NUCLEAR FISSION: A nuclear transformation characterized by the splitting of a nucleus into at least two other nuclei and the release of a relatively large amount of energy.

NUCLEAR FUSION: Act of coalescing two or more atomic nuclei.

NUCLEAR REACTOR: An apparatus in which nuclear fission may be sustained in a self-supporting chain reaction. The usual components of a nuclear reactor are as follows: (1) fissionable material (fuel) such as uranium or plutonium, (2) moderating material (unless it is a fast reactor), (3) usually a reflector to conserve escaping neutrons, (4) provision for heat removal and (5) measuring and control elements. The terms "pile" and "reactor" have been used interchangeably.

NUCLEIC ACID: A constituent of the cell nucleus, composed of a union between phosphoric acid, ribose or desoxyribose and the four bases: adenine, guanine, cystosine and uracil (or thymine).

NUCLEON: Common name for a constituent particle of the nucleus. At present applied to protons and neutrons, but will include any other particle found to exist in the nucleus.

NUCLEOPROTEIN: Protein conjugated with nucleic acid.

NUCLEUS (of an atom): That part of an atom in which most of the mass and the total positive electric charge are concentrated.

NUCLEUS (of a cell): A definitely delineated body within the cell, containing the chromosomes.

NUCLIDE: A general term referring to all nuclear species of the chemical elements—both stable (about 270) and unstable (about 500).

OHM: The practical unit of resistance through which a difference of potential of 1 volt will produce a current of 1 ampere.

OHM'S LAW: The current in a circuit is equal to the electromotive force in the circuit divided by the resistance. The equation is: $i = V/R$.

OÖGENESIS: The process of maturation of egg cells.

OPERATING VOLTAGE: As applied to radiation detection instruments; voltage across the electrodes in the detecting chamber required for proper detection of an ionizing event.

ORGAN: Organized group of tissues having one or more definite functions to perform.

OSMOSIS: The diffusion which proceeds through a semipermeable membrane separating two miscible solutions and tends to equalize their concentrations.

OSMOTIC: Pertaining to osmosis.

OVARY: The female reproductive organ in which eggs are produced.

OVUM: An egg; a female gamete.

PAIR PRODUCTION: An absorption process for x- and gamma radiation in which the incident photon is annihilated in the vicinity of the nucleus of the absorbing atom, with subsequent production of an electron and positron pair. This reaction does not occur for incident radiation energies of less than 1.02 Mev.

PARTICLE ACCELERATOR: Any device for accelerating charged particles.

PATHOGENIC: Disease-producing.

PERCENTAGE DEPTH DOSE: Amount of radiation delivered at a specified depth in tissue, expressed as a percentage of the amount delivered at the skin.

PERMEABLE: Affording passage or penetration.

PERMISSIBLE DOSE: The amount of radiation which may be received by an individual within a specified period with expectation of no harmful result to himself. For long-continued x- or gamma-ray exposure of the whole body, it is 0.3 r per week, measured in air.

PETECHIAE: Small dark spots seen in the skin formed by bleeding from capillaries within the skin.

PHAGOCYTE: Any cell that ingests or engulfs micro-organisms or other cells and particles.

PHANTOM (radiology): A volume of material behaving in essentially the same manner as tissue, with respect to the radiation in question, used to simulate a portion of the human body, and into which ionization chambers can be placed. Measurements made in a phantom permit the determination of the radiation dose delivered to the skin and points within the body. Materials commonly used are water, Masonite, Presdwood (unit density), beeswax.

PHOSPHORESCENCE: Emission of radiation by a substance as a result of previous absorption of radiation of shorter wavelength. In contrast with fluorescence, the emission may continue for a considerable time after cessation of the exciting irradiation.

PHOTOELECTRIC EFFECT: A process by which a photon ejects an electron from an atom. All the energy of the photon is absorbed in ejecting the electron and in imparting kinetic energy to it.

PHOTOFLUOROGRAPHY, see Fluorography.

PHOTOGRAPHIC DOSIMETRY: Determination of the accumulative dosage of radiation by use of photographic film.

PHOTON: A quantity of electromagnetic energy whose value in ergs is the product of its frequency in cycles per second and Planck's constant. The equation is: $E = h\nu$.

PHOTOSYNTHESIS: Synthesis with energy from light: specifically, the synthesis of carbohydrates by green plants in the presence of sunlight through the agency of chlorophyll.

PHYSIOLOGY: The science which treats of the function of living organisms and their parts.

PILE, see Nuclear Reactor.

PITCHBLENDE: A mineral consisting largely of uranium oxides, important as a source of uranium and radium.

PLANCK'S CONSTANT: A natural constant of proportionality (h) relating the frequency of a quantum of energy to the total energy of the quantum: $h = E/\nu = 6.6 \times 10^{-27}$ erg sec. (See Photon.)

PLATEAU: As applied to radiation detector chambers, the level portion of the counting rate-voltage curve where changes in operating voltage introduce minimum changes in the counting rate.

PLATELET (THROMBOCYTE): A small, colorless corpuscle present in large numbers in the blood of all mammals, believed to play a role in the clotting of blood.

POLYCYTHEMIA: A disease characterized by overproduction of erythrocytes.

POLYMERIZATION: Union of two or more molecules of a compound to form a more complex molecule.

POSITRON: Particle equal in mass to the electron and having an equal but opposite charge. Its mass is 0.0005488 mass units (mu).

POTENCY: The ability of the male to perform sexual intercourse.

POTENTIAL DIFFERENCE: Work required to carry a unit positive charge from one point to another.

PROMPT GAMMA: Gamma radiation emitted at the time of fission or radioactive disintegration of a nucleus.

PROPHASE: The first stages of mitosis, during which the chromosomes shorten and thicken preparatory to forming a metaphase plate.

PROPORTIONAL COUNTER: Gas-filled radiation detection tube in which the pulse produced is proportional to the number of ions formed in the gas by the primary ionizing particle.

PROPORTIONAL REGION: Voltage range in which the gas amplification is greater than 1, and in which the charge collected is proportional to the charge produced by the initial ionizing event.

PROTIUM: A name sometimes applied to the hydrogen isotope of mass 1, $(_1H^1)$ in contradistinction to deuterium $(_1H^2)$ and tritium $(_1H^3)$.

PROTON: Elementary nuclear particle with a positive electric charge equal numerically to the charge of the electron and a mass of 1.007593 mass units (mu).

PROTOPLASM: A viscid, translucent, polyphasic colloid with water as the continuous phase making up the essential living material of all plant and animal cells.

PULSE-HEIGHT SELECTOR: A circuit designed to select and pass voltage pulses in a certain range of amplitudes.

PURPURA: Large hemorrhagic spots in or under the skin or mucous tissues.

QUALITY: A term for the approximate characterization of radiation with regard to its penetrating power. It is usually expressed in terms of effective wavelengths or half-value layers.

QUANTUM: Synonymous with "Photon."

QUANTUM THEORY: The concept that energy is radiated intermittently in units of definite magnitude called "quanta," and absorbed in a like manner.

QUENCHING: The process of inhibiting continuous or multiple discharge in a counter tube which uses gas amplification.

QUENCHING VAPOR: Polyatomic gas used in Geiger-Müller counters to quench or extinguish avalanche ionization.

RABBIT: A small container propelled, usually pneumatically or hydraulically, through a tube in a nuclear reactor for exposing substances experimentally to the radiation and neutron flux of the active section; used for rapid removal of samples with very short half-lives.

RAD: The rad is that amount of ionizing radiation which will result in the absorption in tissue of 100 ergs per gram.

RADIATION SICKNESS: *In radiation therapy:* A self-limited syndrome characterized by nausea, vomiting, diarrhea and psychic depression, following exposure to appreciable doses of ionizing radiation, particularly to the abdominal region. Its mechanism is unknown, and there is no satisfactory remedy. It usually comes a few hours after a treatment and may subside within a day. It may be sufficiently severe to necessitate interrupting the treatment series or to incapacitate the patient. *In atomic bomb disaster:* A syndrome following intense acute exposure to ionizing radiations. A few hours after exposure nausea and vomiting appear, last a few hours and then subside for a variable interval. After this quiescent period, a recurrence of nausea and vomiting is accompanied by mucous or bloody diarrhea, purpura, epilation and agranulocytic infections. The illness may vary in severity and may go on to death, or partial or apparently complete recovery may ensue. The more intense the early symptoms and the shorter the period of remission, the more serious the final outcome.

RADIATION THERAPY: Treatment of disease with any type of radiation.

RADIOACTIVE EQUILIBRIUM: Among the members of a radioactive series, the state which prevails when the ratios between the amounts of successive members of the series remain constant. *Secular equilibrium:* If a parent element has a very much longer half-life than the succeeding ones, so that there is no appreciable change in its amount in the time interval required for the later products to attain equilibrium, then, after the condition is reached, equal numbers of atoms of all members of the series disintegrate in unit time. This condition is never actually attained but is essentially established in such a case as radium and its series through radium C. The half-life of radium is 1,600 years; of radon, 3.82 days; and of each of the subsequent members, a few minutes. After about a month, essentially the equilibrium amount of radon is present, and then for a long time all members of the series disintegrate the same number of atoms per unit time. *Transient equilibrium:* If the half-life of the parent is sufficiently short, so that the quantity present decreases appreciably during the period under consideration, but is still longer than that of successive members of the series, a stage of equilibrium will be reached, after which all members of the series decrease in amount exponentially with the period of the parent. An example of this is radon (half-life, 3.82 days) and the successive members of the series through radium C.

RADIOACTIVITY: Process whereby certain nuclides undergo spontaneous disintegration in which energy is liberated, generally resulting in the formation of new nuclides. The process is accompanied by the emission of one or more types of radiation, such as alpha and beta particles and gamma radiation. *(See* Curie.)

RADIOAUTOGRAPH, *see* Autoradiograph.

RADIOBIOLOGY: That branch of biology which deals with the effects of radiation on biologic systems.

RADIOGRAPHY: The making of shadow images on photographic

emulion by the action of ionizing radiation. The image is the result of the differential absorption of the radiation in its passage through the object being radiographed.

RADIOLOGIC SURVEY: Evaluation of the radiation hazards incident to the production, use or existence of radioactive materials or other sources of radiation under a specific set of conditions. Such evaluation customarily includes a physical survey of the disposition of materials and equipment, measurements or estimates of the levels of radiation that may be involved, and a sufficient knowledge of processes using or affecting these materials to predict hazards resulting from expected or possible changes in materials or equipment.

RADIOLOGY: The medical science of radioactive substances, x-rays and other ionizing radiations, and the application of the principles of this science to diagnosis and treatment of disease.

RADIORESISTANCE: Relative resistance of cells, tissues, organs or organisms to the injurious action of radiation. The term may also be applied to chemical compounds or to any substances. *(See also* Radiosensitivity.)

RADIOSENSITIVITY: Relative susceptibility of cells, tissues, organs, organisms or any substances to the injurious action of radiation. Radioresistance and radiosusceptibility are at present employed in a qualitative or comparative sense, rather than in a quantitative or absolute one.

RECESSIVE CHARACTER (genetics): Of a pair of contrasted characteristics, the one which will not appear in the hybrid from crossbreeding homozygous parents unlike with respect to this characteristic.

RECOMBINATION: The return of an ionized atom or molecule to the neutral state.

RECOVERY (radiology): the return toward normal of a particular cell, tissue or organism, after radiation injury.

RECOVERY RATE: The rate at which recovery takes place following radiation injury. It may proceed at different rates for different tissues. *Differential recovery rate:* Among tissues recovering at different rates, those having slower rates will ultimately suffer greater damage from a series of successive irradiations. This differential effect is taken advantage of in fractionated radiation therapy if the neoplastic tissues have a slower recovery rate than surrounding normal structures.

REGENERATIVE PROCESS: The process by which damaged cells are replaced by new ones of the same type.

RELATIVE BIOLOGIC EFFECTIVENESS: The ratio of x- or gamma ray dose to the dose that is required to produce the same biologic effect by the radiation in question.

RELATIVE PLATEAU SLOPE: The relative increase in the number of counts as a function of voltage expressed in percentage increase per 100 volts above the initial portion of the Geiger plateau.

RELATIVISTIC MASS: The increased mass associated with a particle when its velocity is increased. The increase in mass becomes appreciable only at velocities approaching the velocity of light $(3 \times 10^{10}$ cm./sec.).

RESOLVING TIME, COUNTER: The minimum time interval between two distinct events which will permit both to be counted. It may refer to an electronic circuit, to a mechanical indicating device or to a counter tube.

RESONANCE CAPTURE: An inelastic nuclear collision occurring when the nucleus exhibits a strong tendency to capture incident particles or photons of particular resonance energies.

RESPIRATION: The taking-in of oxygen and giving-off of carbon dioxide, and all steps involved in the process.

RESPIRATORY SYSTEM: The group of organs concerned with the exchange of oxygen and carbon dioxide in organisms. In higher animals this consists of the air passages through the mouth, nose and throat, the trachea, the bronchi, the bronchioles and the alveoli of the lungs.

RETICULAR: Pertaining to or resembling a net.

RETICULOENDOTHELIAL SYSTEM: Networks of phagocytic cells found mainly in the spleen, lymph glands, liver, lungs and bone marrow.

ROENTGEN: The quantity of x- or gamma radiation such that the associated corpuscular emission per 0.001293 grams of air produces, in air, ions carrying 1 electrostatic unit of quantity of electricity of either sign.

ROENTGEN-EQUIVALENT-MAN (rem): That quantity of radiation which, when absorbed by man, produces an effect equivalent to the absorption by man of 1 roentgen of x- or gamma radiation (400 kv). (See Rad.)

ROENTGEN-EQUIVALENT-PHYSICAL (rep): The amount of ionizing radiation which will result in the absorption in tissue of 83 ergs per gram. (Recent authors have suggested the value 93 ergs per gram.) (See Rad.)

ROENTGEN RAYS: X-rays.

ROENTGENOGRAPHY: Radiography by means of x-rays.

ROENTGENOLOGY: That part of radiology which pertains to x-rays.

ROTATION THERAPY: Radiation therapy during which either the patient is rotated before the source of radiation or the source is revolved around the patient. In this way, a larger dose is built up at the center of rotation within the patient's body than on any area of the skin.

RUTHERFORD: Quantity of a radioactive material having associated with it 10^6 disintegrations per second. Abbreviation: rd.

SARCOMA: Malignant neoplasm composed of cells imitating the appearance of the supportive and lymphatic tissues.

SCALER: An electronic device that produces an output voltage pulse whenever a prescribed number of input pulses have been received.

SCATTERED RADIATION (radiology): Radiation which, during its passage through a substance, has been deviated in direction. It may also have been modified by an increase in wavelength.

SCATTERING: Change of direction of subatomic particle or photon as a result of a collision or interaction.

SCINTILLATION COUNTER: The combination of phosphor, photomultiplier tube and associated circuits for counting light emissions produced in the phosphors by ionizing radiation.

SECONDARY RADIATION: Radiation originating as the result of absorption of other radiation in matter. It may be either electromagnetic or particulate in nature.

SELECTIVE LOCALIZATION (isotopes): In the use of radioisotopes, accumulation of a particular isotope to a significantly greater degree in certain cells or tissues. (See Differential Absorption Ratio.)

SELF-ABSORPTION: Absorption of radiation emitted by radioactive atoms by the matter in which the atoms are located; in particular, the absorption of radiation within sample being assayed.

SENSITIVE VOLUME: That portion of a counter tube or ionization chamber which responds to a specific radiation.

SEX LINKAGE: The inheritance of certain characteristics which are determined by genes located on the sex chromosomes.

SIGMOID CURVE: S-shaped curve, often characteristic of a dose-effect curve in radiobiologic studies.

SKIN DOSE (radiation therapy): Dose at center of irradiation field on skin. It is the sum of the air dose and backscatter.

SLUG: A bar-shaped piece of material prepared especially for insertion in a nuclear reactor. The term often refers to the fuel unit of a natural uranium-graphite reactor.

SOMATIC CELLS: Body cells, usually having two sets of chromosomes, as opposed to germ cells.

SPALLATION: A term used to denote a nuclear reaction induced by high-energy bombardment and involving the "chipping" of fragments off the target nucleus.

SPECIFIC ACTIVITY, GRAM ELEMENT: Total radioactivity of a given isotope per gram of element.

SPECIFIC ACTIVITY, ISOTOPE: Total radioactivity of a given isotope per gram of the radioactive isotope.

SPECIFIC IONIZATION: Number of ion pairs per unit length of path of the ionization particle in a medium; e.g., per centimeter of air or per micron of tissue.

SPERM CELL (SPERMATAZOAN): A male gamete.

SPLEEN: A large glandlike organ one of whose functions is to disintegrate the red blood corpuscles and release hemoglobin.

SPURIOUS COUNT: Count caused by any agency other than the radiation which it is desired to detect.

STABLE ISOTOPE: An isotope of an element which is not radioactive.

STEM RADIATION: X-rays given off from parts of the anode other than the target; in particular, from the target support.

STERILITY (biologic): Temporary or permanent inability to breed.

STOPPING POWER: The reciprocal of the thickness of a solid that absorbs the same amount of alpha radiation as 1 cm. of air.

STRAY RADIATION: Radiation not serving any useful purpose. It includes direct radiation and secondary radiation from irradiation objects.

SUBCRITICAL: Having an effective multiplication constant less than 1, so that a self-supporting fission-chain reaction cannot be maintained.

SULFHYDRYL: Chemical radical (SH) which is an important component of many tissue enzymes.

SYNCHROCYCLOTRON: A cyclotron in which the radio frequency of the electric field is frequency modulated to permit acceleration of particles to relativistic energies.

SYNCHROTRON: A device for accelerating particles, ordinarily electrons, in a circular orbit with frequency modulated electric fields combined with an increasing magnetic field applied in synchronism with the orbital motion.

SYNDROME: The complex of symptoms associated with any disease.

TAGGED COMPOUND, see Labeled Compound.

TARGET THEORY (HIT THEORY): Theory explaining some biologic effects of radiation on basis of ionization occurring in a very small sensitive region within the cell. One, two or more "hits" (i.e., ionizing events within the sensitive volume) may be necessary to bring about the effect.

TELETHERAPY: A method of using a radioisotope as a radiation source in which the radio-element is shielded on all sides except one, thus giving a directional beam of radiation which is directed at the area to be treated.

THIMBLE IONIZATION CHAMBER: A small cylindrical or spherical ionization chamber, usually with walls of organic material.

THRESHOLD DOSE: The minimum dose that will produce a detectable degree of any given effect.

TISSUE DOSE: Dose received by a tissue in the region of interest. In the case of x- and gamma rays, tissue doses are expressed in roentgens. At the present time, there is no generally accepted unit of tissue dose for other ionizing radiations. In radiobiologic studies it is customary to think of the tissue dose in terms of the energy absorbed per gram of tissue. Several units related to the roentgen have been suggested, such as the rep.

TISSUE-EQUIVALENT IONIZATION CHAMBER: Ionization chamber in which the material of the walls, electrode and gas are so selected as to produce ionization essentially equivalent to that characteristic of the tissue under consideration. In some cases, it is sufficient to have only tissue-equivalent walls, and the gas may be air, provided the air volume is negligibly small. The essential requisite in this case is that the contribution to the ionization in the air made by ionizing particles originating in the air is negligible, compared to that produced by ionizing particles characteristic of the wall material.

TISSUE-EQUIVALENT MATERIAL: Material made up of the same elements in the same proportions as they occur in some particular biologic tissue. Such material is important in the construction of ionization chambers for neutron measurement. In some cases the equivalence may be approximated with sufficient accuracy without exact duplication of the elemental composition of the tissue.

TOLERANCE DOSE: A term based on the assumption that an individual can receive such a dose of radiation without any harmful effect. A more acceptable term is "permissible dose."

TRACER, ISOTOPIC: The isotope or non-natural mixture of isotopes of an element which may be incorporated into a sample to make possible observation of the course of that element, alone or in combination, through a chemical, biologic or physical process. The observations may be made by measurement of radioactivity or of isotopic abundance.

TRACK: Visual manifestation of the path of an ionizing particle in a cloud chamber or nuclear emulsion.

TRITIUM ($_1H^3$ or T): The hydrogen isotope of mass number 3.

The mass is 3.0170 amu. It decays with a half-life of 12.3 years, emitting a β-ray of maximum energy 0.018 Mev. The symbol T is often used to designate tritium in compounds (or for compounds with appreciable tritium content for isotopic tracer), as HTO for molecules of that composition or for water labeled with tritium.

TUMOR: In its general sense, a swelling. The term is often synonymous with "neoplasm."

UNIT MAGNETIC POLE: A magnetic pole of such strength that it will exert a force of 1 dyne upon a pole of equal strength 1 cm. distant in a vacuum.

USEFUL BEAM (in radiology): That part of the primary radiation which passes through the aperture, cone or other collimator.

UTERUS: Womb; in female mammals an organ for containing and nourishing the young during the development previous to birth.

VACUOLE: A relatively large globule of liquid suspended in the cytoplasm of a cell.

VALENCE: Number representing the combining or displacing power of an atom; number of electrons lost, gained or shared by an atom in a compound; number of hydrogen atoms with which an atom will combine or which it will displace.

VALENCE ELECTRON: Electron which is gained, lost or shared in a chemical reaction.

VAN DE GRAAFF GENERATOR: An electrostatic generator which employs a system of conveyor belt and spray points to charge an insulated electrode to a high potential.

VOLUME DOSE, see Integral Dose.

WAVELENGTH: Distance between any two similar points of two consecutive waves; for electromagnetic radiation the wavelength is equal to the velocity of light (c) divided by the frequency of the wave (v).

WAVE MOTION: The transmission of a periodic motion or vibration through a medium or empty space. *Transverse* wave motion is that in which the vibration is perpendicular to the direction of propagation. *Longitudinal* wave motion is that in which the vibration is parallel to the direction of propagation.

WHITE BLOOD CELLS (LEUKOCYTES): A group of nucleated ameboid cells found in blood which engulf foreign particles and micro-organisms.

X-RAYS: Penetrating electromagnetic radiations having wavelengths very much shorter than those of visible light. They are usually produced by bombarding a metallic target with fast electrons in a high vacuum. In nuclear reactions it is customary to refer to photons originating in the nucleus as "gamma rays" and to those originating in the extranuclear part of the atom as "x-rays." These rays are sometimes called "roentgen rays," after their discoverer, W. C. Roentgen.

ZYGOTE: The cell resulting from the union of two gametes; the fertilized egg.

B. FORMULAS

RADIOACTIVE DECAY

The following symbols will be used in this section:

N_o = number of unstable nuclei at some original time
N = number of unstable nuclei remaining after a time interval, t
I_o = intensity of radiation at some original time
I = intensity of radiation after a time interval, t
A_o = activity of sample at some original time
A = activity remaining after a time interval, t
λ = decay constant for particular radioactive element
e = base of natural logarithms; $2.718 \ldots$
$T\frac{1}{2}$ = half-life

(1) $N = N_o e^{-\lambda t}$
(2) $A = A_o e^{-\lambda t}$
(3) $I = I_o e^{-\lambda t}$

Decay Constant:

(4) $\lambda = 0.693/T\frac{1}{2}$

Substituting equation (4) in equations (1), (2), (3):

(5) $N = N_o e^{-0.693t/T\frac{1}{2}}$
(6) $A = A_o e^{-0.693t/T\frac{1}{2}}$
(7) $I = I_o e^{-0.693t/T\frac{1}{2}}$

SPECIFIC ACTIVITY (ISOTOPIC)

Specific activity:

$\lambda N = 0.693N/T\frac{1}{2}$ = disintegrations per second per gram

where $T\frac{1}{2}$ = half-life (seconds),

N = number of atoms per gram.

RADIATION ABSORPTION

(1) *Alpha-Particle Range:*

$$R\alpha = 0.318E^{3/2}$$

where R_a = range (cm.) of air at 1 atm. and 15° C.,
   E = energy (Mev).

(2) *Beta-Particle Range:*
   Sargent's Rule $(E>0.8$ Mev):
$$R = 0.526E - 0.094$$
where R = range (gm./cm.^{2}),
   E = maximum energy (Mev).
   Feather's Rule $(E>0.6$ Mev):
$$R = 0.542E - 0.133$$
where R and E are same as in preceding equation.
Low-Energy Range—use graphic means.

(3) *Gamma-Ray Absorption* (for monoenergetic radiation):
$$I = I_0 e^{-\mu x} \text{ or } I = I_0 e^{-0.693x/x\frac{1}{2}}$$
where μ = linear absorption coefficient (cm.$^{-1}$),
   x = absorber thickness (cm.),
   $x\frac{1}{2}$ = half-value layer of absorber (cm.),
   e = base of natural logarithms (2.718 . . .),
   I_0 = original radiation exposure rate,
   I = radiation exposure rate after passing through absorber.

BETA-PARTICLE COUNTING

(1) *Self-Absorption:*
$$\frac{R}{R_0} = \frac{1}{mx}(1-e^{-mx})$$
where R = measured counting rate,
   R_0 = true counting rate,
   x = sample thickness (mg./cm.^{2}),
   m = absorption coefficient (cm.^{2}/mg.).

(See U.S. Department of Commerce, National Bureau of Standards, Handbook 51 [April, 1952], p. 26.)

(2) *Resolving-Time Determination:*
$$\tau = \frac{R_1 + R_2 - R_{12}}{2(R_1 R_2)}$$
where τ = resolving time (seconds),
   R_1 = counting rate, source 1 (cts./sec.),
   R_2 = counting rate, source 2 (cts./sec.),
   R_{12} = counting rate, combined sources 1 and 2 (cts./sec.).

(3) *Resolving-Time Correction:*
$$R = \frac{R_0}{1 - R_0\tau}$$

where R = true counting rate (cts./sec.),
R_o = observed counting rate (cts./sec.),
τ = resolving time (seconds).

STATISTICS OF COUNTING

n = number of counts, one observation,
t = counting time, one observation,
$\bar{n}$ = mean number of counts, series of observations,
$\bar{t}$ = mean counting time, series of observations,
m = number of observations,
σ = theoretical standard deviation,
S_t = observed standard deviation of the time required to record a preset number of counts,
S_n = observed mean standard deviation of the number of counts recorded in a preset time.

(1) *Theoretical Standard Deviation:*
$$\sigma_n = \sqrt{\bar{n}}$$

(2) *Observed Standard Deviation:*
a) Series of observations, preset time:
$$S_n = [\Sigma_m (n_m - \bar{n})^2 / m - 1]^{\frac{1}{2}}$$
b) Series of observations, preset count:
$$S_n = (n/\bar{t}) S_t$$
$$S_t = [\Sigma_m (t_m - \bar{t})^2 / m]^{\frac{1}{2}}$$
c) Reliability factor:
$$\text{R.F.} = \frac{S_n}{\sigma_n}$$

CALIBRATION PROCEDURES

(1) *Exposure Rate* (from point source of radium gamma radiation):
$$mr/hr = \frac{\text{Number of milligrams of radium}}{s^2}$$

where s = distance to source (yd.),
$$mr/hr = \frac{8,400 \text{ (No. of mg. of Ra)}}{s^2} \qquad (s = \text{distance [cm.]}),$$

$$r/hr = \frac{8.4 \text{ (No. of mg. of Ra)}}{s^2} \qquad (s = \text{distance [cm.]}).$$

(2) *Exposure Rate* (from any point source of radium gamma radiation):
$$r/hr = \frac{8.4 \text{ (No. of equivalent mg. of Ra)}}{s^2}$$

where s = distance to source (cm.).

(3) *Exposure Rate, Approximate* (from any gamma source):
$$r/hr \text{ at } 1 \text{ ft.} = 6(c)E$$
where c = number of curies,

E = gamma-ray energy (Mev);
$$mr/hr \text{ at } 1 \text{ ft.} = 6(mc)E$$
where mc = number of millicuries.

INTERNAL RADIATION DOSAGE

(1) *Biologic Half-Life:*

$$T_b = \frac{0.693}{\lambda_b}$$

where λ_b = biologic rate of elimination constant,
T_b = biologic half-life.

(2) *Effective Half-Life:*

$$T_{eff} = \frac{(T_{1/2})\ (T_b)}{T_{1/2} + T_b}$$

where T_{eff} = effective half-life,
$T_{1/2}$ = radioactive (physical) half-life,
T_b = biologic half-life.

(3) *Beta-Emitter Dose:*
$$D = 88ET_{eff}C(1 - e^{-\lambda t})$$
where D = dose (reps),

E = average energy of beta particle (Mev),

C = microcuries per gram of radioisotope in tissue,

λ = effective decay constant (days^{-1}),

t = time (days).

DECONTAMINATION FACTOR

$$\text{D.F.} = \frac{\text{Initial activity}}{\text{Final activity}}$$

ISOTOPIC DILUTION FACTOR

$$Q = q\left(\frac{x_1}{x_2} - 1 \right)$$

where Q = total amount of diluent material,

q = total amount of labeled material,

x_1 = specific activity of labeled material,

x_2 = specific activity of system after dilution.

C. DECAY TABLES

SODIUM-24

$T\frac{1}{2} = 14.8$ hours

λ factor (10 minutes) = 0.0078

Min. Hours	0	10	20	30 0.5	40	50	60 1	70	80	90 1.5	100	110
0	....	.9922	.9845	.9769	.9693	.9618	.9543	.9469	.9395	.9322	.9250	.9178
2	.9107	.9036	.8966	.8896	.8827	.8758	.8690	.8623	.8556	.8489	.8423	.8358
4	.8293	.8228	.8164	.8101	.8038	.7976	.7914	.7852	.7791	.7731	.7671	.7611
6	.7552	.7493	.7435	.7377	.7320	.7263	.7207	.7151	.7095	.7040	.6985	.6931
8	.6877	.6824	.6771	.6718	.6666	.6614	.6563	.6512	.6461	.6411	.6361	.6312
10	.6263	.6214	.6166	.6118	.6070	.6023	.5976	.5930	.5884	.5838	.5793	.5748
12	.5703	.5659	.5615	.5571	.5528	.5485	.5442	.5400	.5358	.5316	.5275	.5234
14	.5193	.5153	.5113	.5073	.5034	.4995	.4956	.4917	.4879	.4841	.4804	.4766
16	.4729	.4693	.4656	.4620	.4584	.4548	.4513	.4478	.4443	.4409	.4374	.4340
18	.4307	.4273	.4240	.4207	.4174	.4142	.4110	.4078	.4046	.4015	.3984	.3953
20	.3922	.3891	.3861	.3831	.3801	.3772	.3743	.3714	.3685	.3656	.3628	.3599
22	.3571	.3544	.3516	.3489	.3462	.3435	.3408	.3382	.3355	.3329	.3304	.3278
24	.3252	.3227	.3202	.3177	.3152	.3128	.3104	.3080	.3056	.3032	.3008	.2985
26	.2962	.2939	.2916	.2893	.2871	.2848	.2826	.2804	.2783	.2761	.2740	.2718
28	.2697	.2676	.2655	.2635	.2614	.2594	.2574	.2554	.2534	.2514	.2495	.2475
30	.2456	.2437	.2418	.2399	.2381	.2362	.2344	.2326	.2308	.2290	.2272	.2254
32	.2237	.2219	.2202	.2185	.2168	.2151	.2134	.2118	.2101	.2085	.2069	.2053
34	.2037		.2005		.1974		.1944		.1914		.1884	
36	.1855		.1826		.1798		.1770		.1743		.1716	
38	.1689		.1663		.1637		.1612		.1587		.1562	

SODIUM-24—(concluded)

T½ = 14.8 hours

λ factor (10 minutes) = 0.0078

Min. Hours	0	10	20	30 / 0.5	40	50	60 / 1	70	80	90 / 1.5	100	110
40	.1538		.1514		.1491		.1468		.1445		.1423	
42	.1401		.1379		.1358		.1337		.1316		.1296	
44	.1276		.1256		.1236		.1217		.1198		.1180	
46	.1162		.1144		.1126		.1108		.1091		.1074	
48	.1058		.1041		.1025		.1009		.0994		.0979	

PHOSPHORUS-32

T½ = 14.3 days

λ factor (3 hours) = 0.00606

Hours Days	0	3	6	9	12	15	18	21
0	....	.9940	.9880	.9820	.9761	.9702	.9643	.9585
1	.9527	.9469	.9412	.9355	.9299	.9243	.9187	.9131
2	.9076	.9021	.8967	.8913	.8859	.8805	.8752	.8699
3	.8646	.8594	.8542	.8491	.8439	.8388	.8338	.8287
4	.8237	.8187	.8138	.8089	.8040	.7991	.7943	.7895
5	.7847	.7800	.7753	.7706	.7659	.7613	.7567	.7521
6	.7476	.7431	.7386	.7341	.7297	.7253	.7209	.7166
7	.7122	.7079	.7036	.6994	.6952	.6910	.6868	.6826
8	.6785	.6744	.6703	.6663	.6623	.6583	.6543	.6503
9	.6464	.6425	.6386	.6348	.6309	.6271	.6233	.6196

(continued)

415

PHOSPHORUS-32—(continued)

T½ = 14.3 days

λ factor (3 hours) = 0.00606

Hours Days	0	3	6	9	12	15	18	21
10	.6158	.6121	.6084	.6047	.6011	.5974	.5938	.5902
11	.5867	.5831	.5796	.5761	.5726	.5692	.5657	.5623
12	.5589	.5555	.5522	.5488	.5455	.5422	.5390	.5357
13	.5325	.5292	.5260	.5229	.5197	.5166	.5135	.5104
14	.5073	.5042	.5012	.4981	.4951	.4921	.4892	.4862
15	.4833		.4774		.4717		.4660	
16	.4604		.4549		.4494		.4440	
17	.4386		.4333		.4281		.4230	
18	.4179		.4128		.4078		.4029	
19	.3981		.3933		.3885		.3838	
20	.3792		.3747		.3702		.3657	
21	.3613		.3569		.3526		.3484	
22	.3442		.3400		.3359		.3319	
23	.3279		.3239		.3200		.3162	
24	.3124		.3086		.3049		.3012	
25	.2976		.2940		.2905		.2870	
26	.2835		.2801		.2767		.2734	
27	.2701		.2668		.2636		.2604	
28	.2573		.2542		.2512		.2481	
29	.2451		.2422		.2393		.2364	

PHOSPHORUS-32—*(concluded)*

T½ = 14.3 days

λ factor (3 hours) = 0.00606

Hours / Days	0	3	6	9	12	15	18	21
30	.2335				.2279			
31	.2225				.2172			
32	.2120				.2069			
33	.2019				.1971			
34	.1924				.1878			
35	.1833				.1789			
36	.1746				.1704			
37	.1663				.1624			
38	.1585				.1547			
39	.1510				.1473			
40	.1438				.1404			
41	.1370				.1337			
42	.1305				.1274			
43	.1244				.1214			
44	.1185				.1156			
45	.1129				.1102			
46	.1075				.1049			
47	.1024				.1000			

417

T½ = 87 days

SULFUR-35

λ factor (½ day) = 0.003983

Days	0.0	0.5	1.0	1.5	2.0	2.5	3.0	3.5	4.0	4.5
0	.....	.9960	.9921	.9881	.9842	.9803	.9764	.9725	.9686	.9648
5	.9610	.9571	.9533	.9495	.9458	.9420	.9383	.9345	.9308	.9271
10	.9234	.9198	.9161	.9125	.9088	.9052	.9016	.8980	.8945	.8909
15	.8874	.8839	.8803	.8768	.8733	.8699	.8664	.8630	.8595	.8561
20	.8527	.8493	.8460	.8426	.8392	.8359	.8326	.8293	.8260	.8227
25	.8194	.8162	.8129	.8097	.8065	.8033	.8001	.7969	.7937	.7906
30	.7874	.7843	.7812	.7781	.7750	.7719	.7688	.7658	.7627	.7597
35	.7567	.7537	.7507	.7477	.7447	.7418	.7388	.7359	.7330	.7300
40	.7271	.7242	.7214	.7185	.7156	.7128	.7100	.7071	.7043	.7015
45	.6987	.6960	.6932	.6904	.6877	.6850	.6822	.6795	.6768	.6741
50	.6715	.6688	.6661	.6635	.6608	.6582	.6556	.6530	.6504	.6478
55	.6452	.6427	.6401	.6376	.6350	.6325	.6300	.6275	.6250	.6225
60	.6200	.6176	.6151	.6127	.6102	.6078	.6054	.6030	.6006	.5982
65	.5958	.5955	.5911	.5888	.5864	.5841	.5818	.5795	.5772	.5749
70	.5726	.5703	.5680	.5658	.5635	.5613	.5590	.5568	.5546	.5524
75	.5502	.5480	.5458	.5437	.5415	.5394	.5372	.5351	.5330	.5308
80	.5287	.5266	.5245	.5224	.5204	.5183	.5162	.5142	.5121	.5101
85	.5081	.5061	.5041	.5020	.5000	.4981	.4961	.4941	.4921	.4902
90	.4882		.4844		.4805		.4767		.4729	
95	.4692		.4654		.4617		.4581		.4545	
100	.4509		.4473		.4437		.4402		.4367	
105	.4333		.4298		.4264		.4230		.4197	
110	.4163		.4130		.4098		.4065		.4033	

SULFUR-35—(continued)

T½ = 87 days

λ factor (½ day) = 0.003983

Days	0.0	0.5	1.0	1.5	2.0	2.5	3.0	3.5	4.0	4.5
115	.4001		.3969		.3938		.3906		.3875	
120	.3845		.3814		.3784		.3754		.3724	
125	.3694		.3665		.3636		.3607		.3578	
130	.3550		.3522		.3494		.3466		.3439	
135	.3412		.3385		.3358		.3331		.3305	
140	.3278		.3252		.3227		.3201		.3176	
145	.3150		.3125		.3101		.3076		.3052	
150	.3027		.3003		.2979		.2956		.2932	
155	.2909		.2886		.2863		.2840		.2818	
160	.2796		.2773		.2751		.2730		.2708	
165	.2686		.2665		.2644		.2623		.2602	
170	.2581		.2561		.2541		.2521		.2500	
175	.2481		.2461		.2441		.2422		.2403	
180	.2384		.2365		.2346		.2327		.2309	
185	.2291		.2273		.2255		.2237		.2219	
190	.2201		.2184		.2166		.2149		.2132	
195	.2115		.2098		.2082		.2065		.2049	
200	.2033		.2017		.2001		.1985		.1969	
205	.1953		.1938		.1922		.1907		.1892	
210	.1877		.1862		.1847		.1833		.1818	
215	.1804		.1789		.1775		.1761		.1747	
220	.1733		.1720		.1706		.1692		.1679	

(continued)

SULFUR-35—(concluded)

T½ = 87 days

λ factor (% day) = 0.003983

Days	0.0	0.5	1.0	1.5	2.0	2.5	3.0	3.5	4.0	4.5
225	.1666		.1652		.1639		.1626		.1613	
230	.1601		.1588		.1575		.1563		.1550	
235	.1538		.1526		.1514		.1502		.1490	
240	.1478		.1466		.1455		.1443		.1432	
245	.1420		.1409		.1398		.1387		.1376	
250	.1365		.1354		.1343		.1333		.1322	
255	.1312		.1301		.1291		.1281		.1270	
260	.1260		.1250		.1240		.1231		.1221	
265	.1211		.1202		.1192		.1183		.1173	
270	.1164		.1155		.1145		.1136		.1127	
275	.1118		.1110		.1101		.1092		.1083	
280	.1075		.1066		.1058		.1049		.1041	
285	.1033		.1025		.1016		.1008		.1000	

420

POTASSIUM-42

T½ = 12.4 hours

λ factor (10 minutes) = 0.00932

Minutes Hours	0	10	20	30	40	50	60	70	80	90	100	110
0	.....	.9907	.9815	.9724	.9634	.9545	.9456	.9368	.9281	.9195	.9110	.9026
2	.8942	.8859	.8777	.8695	.8615	.8535	.8456	.8377	.8299	.8222	.8146	.8071
4	.7996	.7922	.7848	.7775	.7703	.7632	.7561	.7491	.7421	.7352	.7284	.7217
6	.7150	.7083	.7018	.6953	.6888	.6824	.6761	.6698	.6636	.6574	.6513	.6453
8	.6393	.6334	.6275	.6217	.6159	.6102	.6045	.5989	.5934	.5879	.5824	.5770

POTASSIUM-42—(concluded)

T½ = 12.4 hours   λ factor (10 minutes) = 0.00932

Minutes Hours	0	10	20	30	40	50	60	70	80	90	100	110
10	.5717	.5664	.5611	.5559	.5507	.5456	.5406	.5356	.5306	.5257	.5208	.5160
12	.5112	.5064	.5017	.4971	.4925	.4879	.4834	.4789	.4744	.4700	.4657	.4614
14	.4571	.4528	.4486	.4445	.4404	.4363	.4322	.4282	.4242	.4203	.4164	.4125
16	.4087	.4049	.4012	.3975	.3938	.3901	.3865	.3829	.3794	.3758	.3723	.3689
18	.3655	.3621	.3587	.3554	.3521	.3488	.3456	.3424	.3392	.3361	.3330	.3299
20	.3268	.3238	.3208	.3178	.3148	.3119	.3090	.3062	.3033	.3005	.2977	.2950
22	.2922	.2895	.2868	.2842	.2815	.2789	.2763	.2738	.2712	.2687	.2662	.2637
24	.2613	.2589	.2565	.2541	.2517	.2494	.2471	.2448	.2425	.2403	.2380	.2358
26	.2336	.2315	.2293	.2272	.2251	.2230	.2209	.2189	.2169	.2149	.2129	.2109
28	.2089	.2070	.2051	.2032	.2013	.1994	.1976	.1957	.1939	.1921	.1903	.1886
30	.1868	.1851	.1834	.1817	.1800	.1783	.1767	.1750	.1734	.1718	.1702	.1686
32	.1671	.1655	.1640	.1624	.1609	.1594	.1580	.1565	.1551	.1536	.1522	.1508
34	.1494	.1480	.1466	.1453	.1439	.1426	.1413	.1399	.1386	.1374	.1361	.1348
36	.1336	.1323	.1311	.1299	.1287	.1275	.1263	.1251	.1240	.1228	.1217	.1206
38	.1194	.1183	.1172	.1161	.1151	.1140	.1129	.1119	.1109	.1098	.1088	.1078
40	.1068	.1058	.1048	.1039	.1029	.1019	.1010	.1001	.0991			

CALCIUM-45

T½ = 152 days   λ factor (1 day) = 0.00456

Days	0	1	2	3	4	5	6	7	8	9
0	.....	.9955	.9909	.9864	.9819	.9775	.9730	.9686	.9642	.9598
10	.9554	.9511	.9467	.9424	.9382	.9339	.9296	.9254	.9212	.9170

(continued)

CALCIUM-45—(continued)

T½ = 152 days

λ factor (1 day) = 0.00456

Days	0	1	2	3	4	5	6	7	8	9
20	.9128	.9087	.9045	.9004	.8963	.8923	.8882	.8842	.8801	.8761
30	.8721	.8682	.8642	.8603	.8564	.8525	.8486	.8447	.8409	.8371
40	.8333	.8295	.8257	.8219	.8182	.8145	.8108	.8071	.8034	.7998
50	.7961	.7925	.7889	.7853	.7817	.7782	.7746	.7711	.7676	.7641
60	.7606	.7572	.7537	.7503	.7469	.7435	.7401	.7367	.7334	.7300
70	.7267	.7234	.7201	.7169	.7136	.7103	.7071	.7039	.7007	.6975
80	.6943	.6912	.6880	.6849	.6818	.6787	.6756	.6725	.6695	.6664
90	.6634	.6604	.6574	.6544	.6514	.6484	.6455	.6425	.6396	.6367
100	.6338	.6309	.6281	.6252	.6224	.6195	.6167	.6139	.6111	.6083
110	.6056	.6028	.6001	.5973	.5946	.5919	.5892	.5865	.5839	.5812
120	.5786	.5759	.5733	.5707	.5681	.5655	.5629	.5604	.5578	.5553
130	.5528	.5503	.5478	.5453	.5428	.5403	.5379	.5354	.5330	.5305
140	.5281	.5257	.5233	.5210	.5186	.5162	.5139	.5115	.5092	.5069
150	.5046	.5023	.5000	.4977	.4955	.4932	.4910	.4887	.4865	.4843
160	.4821	.4799	.4777	.4755	.4734	.4712	.4691	.4670	.4648	.4627
170	.4606	.4585	.4564	.4543	.4523	.4502	.4482	.4461	.4441	.4421
180	.4401	.4381	.4361	.4341	.4321	.4302	.4282	.4263	.4243	.4224
190	.4205	.4185	.4166	.4147	.4129	.4110	.4091	.4073	.4054	.4036
200	.4017	.3999	.3981	.3963	.3945	.3927	.3909	.3891	.3873	.3856
210	.3838	.3821	.3803	.3786	.3769	.3752	.3735	.3718	.3701	.3684
220	.3667	.3650	.3634	.3617	.3601	.3584	.3568	.3552	.3536	.3520
230	.3504	.3488	.3472	.3456	.3440	.3425	.3409	.3393	.3378	.3363
240	.3347	.3332	.3317	.3302	.3287	.3272	.3257	.3242	.3227	.3213
250	.3198	.3184	.3169	.3155	.3140	.3126	.3112	.3098	.3084	.3070

CALCIUM-45—(concluded)

λ factor (1 day) = 0.00456

Days	0	1	2	3	4	5	6	7	8	9
260	.3056	.3042	.3028	.3014	.3000	.2987	.2973	.2960	.2946	.2933
270	.2919	.2906	.2893	.2880	.2867	.2854	.2841	.2828	.2815	.2802
280	.2789	.2777	.2764	.2751	.2739	.2726	.2714	.2702	.2689	.2677
290	.2665	.2653	.2641	.2629	.2617	.2605	.2593	.2581	.2569	.2558
300	.2546	.2534	.2523	.1512	.2500	.2489	.2477	.2466	.2455	.2444
310	.2433		.2411		.2389		.2367		.2346	
320	.2324		.2303		.2282		.2261		.2241	
330	.2221		.2200		.2180		.2161		.2141	
340	.2122		.2102		.2083		.2064		.2046	
350	.2027		.2009		.1990		.1972		.1954	
360	.1937		.1919		.1902		.1884		.1867	
370	.1850		.1834		.1817		.1800		.1784	
380	.1768		.1752		.1736		.1720		.1705	
390	.1689		.1674		.1659		.1644		.1629	
400	.1614		.1599		.1585		.1570		.1556	
410	.1542		.1528		.1514		.1500		.1487	
420	.1473		.1460		.1446		.1433		.1420	
430	.1407		.1395		.1382		.1369		.1357	
440	.1345		.1332		.1320		.1308		.1297	
450	.1285		.1273		.1262		.1250		.1239	
460	.1228		.1216		.1205		.1194		.1184	
470	.1173		.1162		.1152		.1141		.1131	
480	.1121		.1110		.1100		.1090		.1080	
490	.1071		.1061		.1051		.1042		.1032	
500	.1023		.1013		.1004					

CHROMIUM-51

T½ = 26.5 days

λ factor (6 hours) = 0.00654

Hours Days	0	6	12	18	24	30	36	42	48	54	60	66
0	....	.9935	.9870	.9806	.9742	.9678	.9615	.9552	.9490	.9428	.9367	.9306
3	.9245	.9185	.9126	.9066	.9007	.8948	.8889	.8831	.8774	.8717	.8660	.8603
6	.8547	.8492	.8436	.8381	.8327	.8272	.8218	.8165	.8112	.8059	.8006	.7954
9	.7902	.7851	.7800	.7749	.7698	.7648	.7598	.7548	.7499	.7451	.7402	.7354
12	.7306	.7258	.7211	.7164	.7117	.7071	.7025	.6979	.6933	.6888	.6843	.6799
15	.6754	.6710	.6667	.6623	.6580	.6537	.6494	.6452	.6410	.6368	.6327	.6286
18	.6245	.6204	.6163	.6123	.6083	.6044	.6004	.5965	.5926	.5888	.5849	.5811
21	.5773	.5736	.5698	.5661	.5624	.5587	.5551	.5515	.5479	.5443	.5408	.5372
24	.5337	.5303	.5268	.5234	.5200	.5166	.5132	.5099	.5065	.5032	.5000	.4967
27	.4935	.4902	.4870	.4839	.4807	.4776	.4745	.4714	.4683	.4652	.4622	.4592
30	.4562	.4532	.4503	.4473	.4444	.4415	.4387	.4358	.4330	.4301	.4273	.4245
33	.4218	.4190	.4163	.4136	.4109	.4082	.4055	.4029	.4003	.3977	.3951	.3925
36	.3899	.3874	.3849	.3824	.3799	.3774	.3749	.3725	.3701	.3677	.3653	.3629
39	.3605	.3582	.3558	.3535	.3512	.3489	.3466	.3444	.3421	.3399	.3377	.3355
42	.3333	.3311	.3290	.3268	.3247	.3226	.3205	.3184	.3163	.3142	.3122	.3102
45	.3081	.3061	.3041	.3021	.3002	.2982	.2963	.2943	.2924	.2905	.2886	.2867
48	.2849	.2830	.2812	.2793	.2775	.2757	.2739	.2721	.2704	.2686	.2668	.2651
51	.2634	.2617	.2600	.2583	.2566	.2549	.2532	.2516	.2500	.2483	.2467	.2451
54	.2435	.2419	.2403	.2388	.2372	.2357	.2341	.2326	.2311	.2296	.2281	.2266
57	.2251	.2236	.2222	.2207	.2193	.2179	.2165	.2150	.2136	.2122	.2109	.2095
60	.2081	.2068	.2054	.2041	.2027	.2014	.2001	.1988	.1975	.1962	.1950	.1937

CHROMIUM-51—(concluded)

$T_{1/2}$ = 26.5 days λ factor (6 hours) = 0.00654

Hours / Days	0	6	12	18	24	30	36	42	48	54	60	66
63	.1924		.1899		.1874		.1850		.1826		.1802	
66	.1779		.1756		.1733		.1710		.1688		.1666	
69	.1645		.1623		.1602		.1581		.1561		.1541	
72	.1521		.1501		.1481		.1462		.1443		.1424	
75	.1406		.1387		.1369		.1352		.1334		.1317	
78	.1300		.1283		.1266		.1250		.1233		.1217	
81	.1202		.1186		.1171		.1155		.1140		.1125	
84	.1111		.1096		.1082		.1068		.1054		.1040	
87	.1027		.1014		.1000							

COBALT-60

$T_{1/2}$ = 5.3 years λ factor (20 days) = .007165

Days	0	20	40	60	80	100	120	140	160	180
0	....	.9928	.9857	.9787	.9717	.9648	.9579	.9511	.9443	.9375
200	.9308	.9242	.9176	.9110	.9045	.8981	.8917	.8853	.8790	.8727
400	.8665	.8603	.8541	.8480	.8420	.8360	.8300	.8241	.8182	.8124
600	.8066	.8008	.7951	.7894	.7838	.7782	.7726	.7671	.7616	.7562
800	.7508	.7454	.7401	.7348	.7296	.7244	.7192	.7140	.7089	.7039
1000	.6989	.6939	.6889	.6840	.6791	.6743	.6695	.6647	.6599	.6552
1200	.6505	.6459	.6413	.6367	.6321	.6276	.6232	.6187	.6143	.6099
1400	.6055	.6012	.5969	.5927	.5884	.5842	.5801	.5759	.5718	.5677
1600	.5637	.5596	.5556	.5517	.5477	.5438	.5399	.5361	.5322	.5285
1800	.5247	.5209	.5172	.5135	.5099	.5062	.5026	.4990	.4955	.4919

(continued)

COBALT-60—(concluded)

T½ = 5.3 years

λ factor (20 days) = .007165

Days	0	20	40	60	80	100	120	140	160	180
2000	.4884	.4849	.4815	.4780	.4746	.4712	.4679	.4645	.4612	.4579
2200	.4546	.4514	.4482	.4450	.4418	.4386	.4355	.4324	.4293	.4262
2400	.4232	.4202	.4172	.4142	.4112	.4083	.4054	.4025	.3996	.3968
2600	.3939	.3911	.3883	.3855	.3828	.3801	.3774	.3747	.3720	.3693
2800	.3667	.3641	.3615	.3589	.3563	.3538	.3513	.3487	.3463	.3438
3000	.3413	.3389	.3365	.3341	.3317	.3293	.3270	.3247	.3223	.3200
3200	.3177	.3155	.3132	.3110	.3087	.3065	.3044	.3022	.3000	.2979
3400	.2958	.2936	.2915	.2895	.2874	.2853	.2833	.2813	.2793	.2773
3600	.2753	.2733	.2714	.2694	.2675	.2656	.2637	.2618	.2599	.2581
3800	.2563	.2544	.2526	.2508	.2490	.2472	.2455	.2437	.2420	.2402
4000	.2385	.2368	.2351	.2335	.2318	.2301	.2285	.2269	.2252	.2236
4200	.2220	.2205	.2189	.2173	.2158	.2142	.2127	.2112	.2097	.2082
4400	.2067	.2052	.2037	.2023	.2008	.1994	.1980	.1966	.1952	.1938
4600	.1924	.1910	.1897	.1883	.1870	.1856	.1843	.1830	.1817	.1804
4800	.1791	.1778	.1765	.1753	.1740	.1728	.1716	.1703	.1691	.1679
5000	.1667	.1655	.1643	.1632	.1620	.1608	.1597	.1585	.1574	.1563
5200	.1552	.1541	.1530	.1519	.1508	.1497	.1486	.1476	.1465	.1455
5400	.1444	.1434	.1424	.1414	.1404	.1394	.1384	.1374	.1364	.1354
5600	.1344	.1335	.1325	.1316	.1306	.1297	.1288	.1279	.1270	.1261
5800	.1252	.1243	.1234	.1225	.1216	.1208	.1199	.1190	.1182	.1173
6000	.1165	.1157	.1148	.1140	.1132	.1124	.1116	.1108	.1100	.1092
6200	.1084	.1077	.1069	.1061	.1054	.1046	.1039	.1031	.1024	.1017
6400	.1009	.1002	.0995							

T½ = 12.8 hours

COPPER-64

λ factor (7.5 minutes) = 0.00677

Minutes Hours	0	7.5	15	22.5	30	37.5	45	52.5
0	....	.9934	.9866	.9799	.9733	.9667	.9602	.9537
1	.9473	.9409	.9345	.9282	.9220	.9158	.9096	.9034
2	.8973	.8913	.8853	.8793	.8734	.8675	.8616	.8558
3	.8500	.8443	.8386	.8329	.8273	.8217	.8162	.8107
4	.8052	.7998	.7944	.7890	.7837	.7784	.7732	.7680
5	.7628	.7576	.7525	.7474	.7424	.7374	.7324	.7275
6	.7226	.7177	.7128	.7080	.7033	.6985	.6938	.6891
7	.6845	.6798	.6753	.6707	.6662	.6617	.6572	.6528
8	.6484	.6440	.6396	.6353	.6311	.6268	.6226	.6184
9	.6142	.6101	.6059	.6018	.5978	.5937	.5897	.5858
10	.5818	.5779	.5740	.5701	.5663	.5625	.5587	.5549
11	.5511	.5474	.5437	.5401	.5364	.5328	.5292	.5256
12	.5221	.5186	.5151	.5116	.5081	.5047	.5013	.4979
13	.4946	.4912	.4879	.4846	.4813	.4781	.4749	.4717
14	.4685	.4653	.4622	.4591	.4560	.4529	.4498	.4468
15	.4438	.4408	.4378	.4349	.4319	.4290	.4261	.4233
16	.4204	.4176	.4147	.4119	.4092	.4064	.4037	.4009
17	.3982	.3955	.3929	.3902	.3876	.3850	.3824	.3798
18	.3772	.3747	.3722	.3697	.3672	.3647	.3622	.3598
19	.3573	.3549	.3525	.3501	.3478	.3455	.3431	.3408
20	.3385	.3362	.3340	.3317	.3295	.3272	.3250	.3228
21	.3207	.3185	.3164	.3142	.3121	.3100	.3079	.3058

(continued)

427

COPPER-64—(concluded)

T½ = 12.8 hours

λ factor (7.5 minutes) = 0.00677

Minutes Hours	0	7.5	15	22.5	30	37.5	45	52.5
22	.3038	.3017	.2997	.2976	.2956	.2936	.2917	.2897
23	.2877	.2858	.2839	.2820	.2801	.2782	.2763	.2744
24	.2726	.2707	.2689	.2671	.2653	.2635	.2617	.2600
25	.2582	.2565	.2547	.2530	.2513	.2496	.2479	.2463
26	.2446		.2413		.2381		.2349	
27	.2317		.2286		.2255		.2225	
28	.2195		.2165		.2136		.2107	
29	.2079		.2051		.2024		.1996	
30	.1970		.1943		.1917		.1891	
31	.1866		.1841		.1816		.1791	
32	.1767		.1744		.1720		.1697	
33	.1674		.1652		.1629		.1607	
34	.1586		.1565		.1544		.1523	
35	.1502		.1482		.1462		.1442	
36	.1423		.1404		.1385		.1366	
37	.1348		.1330		.1312		.1294	
38	.1277		.1260		.1243		.1226	
39	.1210		.1193		.1177		.1162	
40	.1146		.1130		.1115		.1100	
41	.1085		.1071		.1056		.1042	
42	.1028		.1014		.1001		.0987	

428

T½ = 250 days
ZINC-65
λ factor (2 days) = 0.005545

Days	0	2	4	6	8	10	12	14	16	18
0	....	.9945	.9890	.9835	.9781	.9727	.9673	.9619	.9566	.9513
20	.9461	.9408	.9356	.9304	.9253	.9202	.9151	.9100	.9050	.9000
40	.8950	.8901	.8852	.8803	.8754	.8706	.8658	.8610	.8562	.8514
60	.8467	.8421	.8374	.8328	.8282	.8236	.8190	.8145	.8100	.8055
80	.8011	.7966	.7922	.7879	.7835	.7792	.7749	.7706	.7663	.7621
100	.7579	.7537	.7495	.7454	.7412	.7371	.7330	.7290	.7250	.7210
120	.7170	.7130	.7091	.7051	.7012	.6973	.6935	.6897	.6859	.6821
140	.6783	.6746	.6708	.6671	.6634	.6597	.6561	.6525	.6489	.6453
160	.6417	.6382	.6346	.6311	.6276	.6242	.6208	.6173	.6139	.6105
180	.6071	.6038	.6004	.5971	.5938	.5905	.5872	.5840	.5808	.5776
200	.5744	.5712	.5680	.5649	.5618	.5587	.5556	.5525	.5494	.5464
220	.5434	.5403	.5374	.5344	.5314	.5285	.5256	.5227	.5198	.5169
240	.5141	.5112	.5084	.5056	.5028	.5000	.4972	.4945	.4918	.4890
260	.4863	.4836	.4810	.4785	.4757	.4730	.4704	.4678	.4652	.4627
280	.4601	.4576	.4550	.4525	.4500	.4475	.4450	.4426	.4401	.4377
300	.4353	.4329	.4305	.4281	.4257	.4234	.4210	.4187	.4164	.4141
320	.4118	.4095	.4073	.4050	.4028	.4005	.3983	.3961	.3939	.3918
340	.3896	.3874	.3853	.3832	.3810	.3789	.3768	.3747	.3727	.3706
360	.3686	.3665	.3645	.3625	.3605	.3585	.3565	.3545	.3526	.3506
380	.3487	.3468	.3449	.3430	.3411	.3392	.3373	.3354	.3336	.3317
400	.3299	.3281	.3263	.3245	.3227	.3209	.3191	.3173	.3156	.3138

(continued)

ZINC-65—(concluded)

T½ = 250 days

λ factor (2 days) = 0.005545

Days	0	2	4	6	8	10	12	14	16	18
420	.3121	.3104	.3087	.3070	.3053	.3036	.3019	.3002	.2986	.2969
440	.2953	.2936	.2920	.2904	.2888	.2872	.2856	.2840	.2824	.2809
460	.2793	.2778	.2763	.2747	.2732	.2717	.2702	.2687	.2672	.2657
480	.2643	.2628	.2613	.2599	.2585	.2570	.2556	.2542	.2528	.2514
500	.2500		.2473		.2445		.2418		.2392	
520	.2365		.2339		.2313		.2288		.2263	
540	.2238		.2213		.2188		.2164		.2141	
560	.2117		.2094		.2071		.2048		.2025	
580	.2003		.1981		.1959		.1937		.1916	
600	.1895		.1874		.1853		.1833		.1813	
620	.1793		.1773		.1753		.1734		.1715	
640	.1696		.1677		.1659		.1640		.1622	
660	.1604		.1587		.1569		.1552		.1535	
680	.1518		.1501		.1485		.1468		.1452	
700	.1436		.1420		.1404		.1389		.1374	
720	.1359		.1344		.1329		.1314		.1300	
740	.1285		.1271		.1257		.1243		.1229	
760	.1216		.1202		.1189		.1176		.1163	
780	.1150		.1138		.1125		.1113		.1100	
800	.1088		.1076		.1064		.1053		.1041	
820	.1030		.1018		.1007		.0996			

SELENIUM-75

T½ = 127 days   λ factor (1 day) = 0.00546

Days	0	1	2	3	4	5	6	7	8	9
0	....	.9946	.9891	.9838	.9784	.9731	.9678	.9625	.9573	.9520
10	.9469	.9417	.9366	.9315	.9264	.9214	.9164	.9114	.9064	.9015
20	.8966	.8917	.8868	.8820	.8772	.8724	.8677	.8629	.8582	.8536
30	.8489	.8443	.8397	.8351	.8306	.8260	.8215	.8171	.8126	.8082
40	.8038	.7994	.7951	.7907	.7864	.7822	.7779	.7737	.7694	.7652
50	.7611	.7569	.7528	.7487	.7446	.7406	.7366	.7326	.7286	.7246
60	.7207	.7167	.7128	.7089	.7051	.7012	.6974	.6936	.6898	.6861
70	.6824	.6786	.6749	.6713	.6676	.6640	.6604	.6568	.6532	.6496
80	.6461	.6426	.6391	.6356	.6321	.6287	.6253	.6219	.6185	.6151
90	.6118	.6084	.6051	.6018	.5986	.5953	.5921	.5888	.5856	.5824
100	.5793	.5761	.5730	.5698	.5667	.5637	.5606	.5575	.5545	.5515
110	.5485	.5455	.5425	.5396	.5366	.5337	.5308	.5279	.5250	.5222
120	.5193	.5165	.5137	.5109	.5081	.5054	.5026	.4999	.4971	.4944
130	.4917	.4891	.4864	.4837	.4811	.4785	.4759	.4733	.4707	.4681
140	.4656	.4631	.4606	.4581	.4556	.4531	.4506	.4482	.4457	.4433
150	.4409	.4385	.4361	.4337	.4313	.4290	.4267	.4243	.4220	.4197
160	.4174	.4152	.4129	.4107	.4084	.4062	.4040	.4018	.3996	.3974
170	.3953	.3931	.3910	.3888	.3867	.3846	.3825	.3804	.3784	.3763
180	.3743	.3722	.3702	.3682	.3662	.3642	.3622	.3602	.3583	.3563
190	.3544	.3524	.3505	.3486	.3467	.3448	.3430	.3411	.3392	.3374
200	.3355	.3337	.3319	.3301	.3283	.3265	.3247	.3230	.3212	.3195

(continued)

SELENIUM-75—(concluded)

T½ = 127 days   λ factor (1 day) = 0.00546

Days	0	1	2	3	4	5	6	7	8	9
210	.3177	.3160	.3143	.3126	.3109	.3092	.3075	.3058	.3041	.3025
220	.3008	.2992	.2976	.2959	.2943	.2927	.2911	.2895	.2880	.2864
230	.2848	.2833	.2818	.2802	.2787	.2772	.2757	.2742	.2727	.2712
240	.2697	.2682	.2668	.2653	.2639	.2624	.2610	.2596	.2582	.2568
250	.2554	.2540	.2526	.2512	.2499	.2485	.2472	.2458	.2445	.2431
260	.2418		.2392		.2366		.2340		.2315	
270	.2290		.2265		.2240		.2216		.2192	
280	.2168		.2144		.2121		.2098		.2075	
290	.2053		.2030		.2008		.1987		.1965	
300	.1944		.1923		.1902		.1881		.1861	
310	.1840		.1820		.1801		.1781		.1762	
320	.1743		.1724		.1705		.1686		.1668	
330	.1650		.1632		.1614		.1597		.1579	
340	.1562		.1545		.1529		.1512		.1496	
350	.1479		.1463		.1447		.1432		.1416	
360	.1401		.1386		.1370		.1356		.1341	
370	.1326		.1312		.1298		.1284		.1270	
380	.1256		.1242		.1229		.1215		.1202	
390	.1189		.1176		.1163		.1151		.1138	
400	.1126		.1114		.1102		.1090		.1078	
410	.1066		.1054		.1043		.1032		.1021	
420	.1009		.0998							

ARSENIC-76

T½ = 26.8 hours

λ factor (15 minutes) = 0.006465

Minutes Hours	0	15	30	45	60	75	90	105	120	135	150	165
0	....	.9936	.9872	.9808	.9745	.9682	.9619	.9558	.9496	.9435	.9374	.9313
3	.9253	.9194	.9135	.9076	.9017	.8959	.8901	.8844	.8787	.8730	.8674	.8618
6	.8563	.8508	.8453	.8398	.8344	.8290	.8237	.8184	.8131	.8079	.8027	.7975
9	.7924	.7873	.7822	.7771	.7721	.7671	.7622	.7573	.7524	.7476	.7428	.7380
12	.7332	.7285	.7238	.7191	.7145	.7099	.7053	.7008	.6963	.6918	.6873	.6829
15	.6785	.6741	.6698	.6655	.6612	.6569	.6527	.6485	.6443	.6401	.6360	.6319
18	.6278	.6238	.6198	.6158	.6118	.6079	.6039	.6000	.5962	.5923	.5885	.5847
21	.5810	.5772	.5735	.5698	.5661	.5625	.5589	.5553	.5517	.5481	.5446	.5411
24	.5376	.5341	.5307	.5273	.5239	.5205	.5171	.5138	.5105	.5072	.5039	.5007
27	.4975	.4943	.4911	.4879	.4848	.4816	.4785	.4755	.4724	.4693	.4663	.4633
30	.4603	.4574	.4544	.4515	.4486	.4457	.4428	.4400	.4371	.4343	.4315	.4287
33	.4260	.4232	.4205	.4178	.4151	.4124	.4098	.4071	.4045	.4019	.3993	.3967
36	.3942	.3916	.3891	.3866	.3841	.3816	.3792	.3767	.3743	.3719	.3695	.3671
39	.3647	.3624	.3601	.3577	.3554	.3531	.3509	.3486	.3464	.3441	.3419	.3397
42	.3375	.3553	.3332	.3310	.3289	.3268	.3247	.3226	.3205	.3184	.3164	.3143
45	.3123	.3103	.3083	.3063	.3044	.3024	.3004	.2985	.2966	.2947	.2928	.2909
48	.2890	.2871	.2853	.2835	.2816	.2798	.2780	.2762	.2744	.2727	.2709	.2692
51	.2674	.2657	.2640	.2623	.2606	.2589	.2573	.2556	.2540	.2523	.2507	.2491
54	.2475	.2459	.2443	.2427	.2412	.2396	.2381	.2365	.2350	.2335	.2320	.2305
57	.2290	.2275	.2261	.2246	.2232	.2217	.2203	.2189	.2175	.2161	.2147	.2133
60	.2119	.2105	.2092	.2078	.2065	.2052	.2038	.2025	.2012	.1999	.1986	.1974
63	.1961	.1948	.1936	.1923	.1911	.1898	.1886	.1874	.1862	.1850	.1838	.1826

(continued)

ARSENIC-76—(concluded)

T½ = 26.8 hours

λ factor (15 minutes) = 0.006465

Minutes Hours	0	15	30	45	60	75	90	105	120	135	150	165
66	.1814	.1803	.1791	.1780	.1768	.1757	.1745	.1734	.1723	.1712	.1701	.1690
69	.1679	.1668	.1657	.1647	.1636	.1626	.1615	.1605	.1594	.1584	.1574	.1564
72	.1554	.1544	.1534	.1524	.1514	.1504	.1495	.1485	.1475	.1466	.1456	.1447
75	.1438	.1428	.1419	.1410	.1401	.1392	.1383	.1374	.1365	.1356	.1348	.1339
78	.1331	.1322	.1313	.1305	.1296	.1288	.1280	.1272	.1263	.1255	.1247	.1239
81	.1231	.1223	.1215	.1207	.1200	.1192	.1184	.1177	.1169	.1162	.1154	.1147
84	.1139	.1132	.1125	.1117	.1110	.1103	.1096	.1089	.1082	.1075	.1068	.1061
87	.1054	.1047	.1041	.1034	.1027	.1021	.1014	.1008	.1001	.0995		

ARSENIC-77

T½ = 40 hours

λ factor (20 minutes) = 0.005776

Minutes Hours	0	20	40	60	80	100	120	140	160	180	200	220
0	....	.9942	.9885	.9828	.9772	.9715	.9659	.9604	.9548	.9493	.9439	.9384
4	.9330	.9277	.9223	.9170	.9117	.9065	.9013	.8961	.8909	.8858	.8807	.8756
8	.8706	.8656	.8609	.8556	.8507	.8458	.8409	.8361	.8313	.8265	.8217	.8170
12	.8123	.8076	.8029	.7983	.7937	.7891	.7846	.7801	.7756	.7711	.7667	.7623
16	.7579	.7535	.7492	.7449	.7406	.7363	.7321	.7279	.7237	.7195	.7153	.7112
20	.7071	.7030	.6990	.6950	.6910	.6870	.6830	.6791	.6752	.6713	.6674	.6636
24	.6598	.6560	.6522	.6484	.6447	.6410	.6373	.6336	.6300	.6263	.6227	.6192
28	.6156	.6120	.6085	.6050	.6015	.5981	.5946	.5912	.5878	.5844	.5810	.5777
32	.5744	.5710	.5678	.5645	.5612	.5580	.5548	.5516	.5484	.5453	.5421	.5390
36	.5359	.5328	.5297	.5267	.5236	.5206	.5176	.5147	.5117	.5088	.5058	.5029

ARSENIC-77—(concluded)

T½ = 40 hours λ factor (20 minutes) = 0.005776

Minutes / Hours	0	20	40	60	80	100	120	140	160	180	200	220
40	.5000	.4971	.4943	.4914	.4886	.4858	.4830	.4802	.4774	.4747	.4719	.4692
44	.4665	.4638	.4612	.4585	.4559	.4533	.4506	.4480	.4455	.4429	.4403	.4378
48	.4353	.4328	.4303	.4278	.4253	.4229	.4205	.4180	.4156	.4132	.4109	.4085
52	.4061	.4038	.4015	.3992	.3969	.3946	.3923	.3900	.3878	.3856	.3833	.3811
56	.3789	.3768	.3746	.3724	.3703	.3682	.3660	.3639	.3618	.3597	.3577	.3556
60	.3536	.3515	.3495	.3475	.3455	.3435	.3415	.3396	.3376	.3357	.3337	.3318
64	.3299	.3280	.3261	.3242	.3224	.3205	.3187	.3168	.3150	.3132	.3114	.3096
68	.3078	.3060	.3042	.3025	.3007	.2990	.2973	.2956	.2939	.2922	.2905	.2888
72	.2872	.2855	.2838	.2822	.2806	.2790	.2774	.2758	.2742	.2726	.2710	.2695
76	.2679	.2664	.2649	.2634	.2618	.2603	.2588	.2573	.2559	.2544	.2529	.2514
80	.2500	.2486	.2471	.2457	.2443	.2429	.2415	.2401	.2387	.2373	.2360	.2346
84	.2333	.2319	.2305	.2292	.2279	.2266	.2253	.2240	.2227	.2214	.2202	.2189
88	.2177	.2164	.2151	.2139	.2127	.2115	.2103	.2090	.2078	.2066	.2054	.2042
92	.2031	.2019	.2007	.1996	.1984	.1973	.1962	.1950	.1939	.1928	.1917	.1906
96	.1895	.1884	.1873	.1862	.1851	.1841	.1830	.1820	.1809	.1799	.1789	.1778
100	.1768		.1748		.1728		.1708		.1688		.1669	
104	.1650		.1631		.1612		.1593		.1575		.1557	
108	.1539		.1521		.1504		.1487		.1470		.1453	
112	.1436		.1419		.1403		.1387		.1371		.1355	
116	.1340		.1325		.1309		.1294		.1279		.1265	
120	.1250		.1236		.1222		.1208		.1194		.1180	
124	.1166		.1153		.1140		.1127		.1114		.1101	
128	.1088		.1076		.1063		.1051		.1039		.1027	
132	.1015		.1004									

IODINE-131

$T\frac{1}{2} = 8.05 \pm 0.03$ days

λ factor (2 hours) = 0.007175

Hours Days	0	2	4	6	8	10
0	.....	.9929	.9858	.9787	.9717	.9648
0.5	.9579	.9510	.9442	.9375	.9308	.9241
1.0	.9175	.9109	.9044	.8979	.8915	.8852
1.5	.8788	.8725	.8663	.8601	.8540	.8478
2.0	.8418	.8358	.8298	.8239	.8180	.8122
2.5	.8063	.8005	.7948	.7892	.7835	.7779
3.0	.7723	.7668	.7613	.7559	.7505	.7452
3.5	.7398	.7345	.7293	.7241	.7189	.7137
4.0	.7086	.7036	.6985	.6935	.6886	.6837
4.5	.6788	.6739	.6691	.6643	.6596	.6549
5.0	.6502	.6455	.6409	.6363	.6318	.6273
5.5	.6228	.6183	.6139	.6095	.6051	.6008
6.0	.5965	.5923	.5880	.5838	.5796	.5755
6.5	.5714	.5673	.5632	.5592	.5552	.5512
7.0	.5473	.5434	.5395	.5356	.5318	.5280
7.5	.5242	.5205	.5168	.5131	.5094	.5058
8.0	.5022	.4986	.4950	.4915	.4880	.4845
8.5	.4810	.4776	.4742	.4708	.4674	.4640
9.0	.4607	.4574	.4542	.4509	.4477	.4445
9.5	.4413	.4381	.4350	.4319	.4288	.4257
10	.4227	.4197	.4167	.4137	.4107	.4078
10.5	.4049	.4020	.3991	.3963	.3934	.3906

IODINE-131—(concluded)

T½ = 8.05 ± 0.03 days   λ factor (2 hours) = 0.007175

Hours Days	0	2	4	6	8	10
11.0	.3878	.3851	.3823	.3796	.3769	.3742
11.5	.3715	.3688	.3662	.3636	.3610	.3584
12.0	.3559	.3533	.3508	.3483	.3458	.3433
12.5	.3409	.3384	.3360	.3336	.3312	.3288
13.0	.3265	.3241	.3218	.3195	.3172	.3150
13.5	.3127	.3105	.3083	.3061	.3039	.3017
14.0	.2995	.2974	.2953	.2932	.2911	.2890
14.5	.2869	.2849	.2829	.2808	.2788	.2768
15.0	.2749	.2729	.2709	.2690	.2671	.2652
15.5	.2633	.2614	.2595	.2576	.2558	.2540
16.0	.2522	.2504	.2486	.2468	.2450	.2433
16.5	.2415	.2398	.2381	.2364	.2347	.2330

BARIUM-140

T½ = 8.0 days   λ factor (3 hours) = 0.00677

Hours Days	0	3	6	9	12	15	18	21
0	....	.9933	.9866	.9799	.9733	.9667	.9602	.9537
1	.9473	.9409	.9345	.9282	.9220	.9158	.9096	.9034
2	.8973	.8913	.8853	.8793	.8734	.8675	.8616	.8558
3	.8500	.8443	.8386	.8329	.8273	.8217	.8162	.8107
4	.8052	.7998	.7944	.7890	.7837	.7784	.7732	.7680

(continued)

437

BARIUM-140—(continued)

T½ = 8.0 days

λ factor (3 hours) = 0.00677

Hours / Days	0	3	6	9	12	15	18	21
5	.7628	.7576	.7525	.7474	.7424	.7374	.7324	.7275
6	.7226	.7177	.7128	.7080	.7033	.6985	.6938	.6891
7	.6845	.6798	.6753	.6707	.6662	.6617	.6572	.6528
8	.6484	.6440	.6397	.6353	.6310	.6268	.6226	.6184
9	.6142	.6101	.6059	.6018	.5978	.5938	.5898	.5858
10	.5818	.5779	.5740	.5701	.5663	.5625	.5587	.5549
11	.5511	.5474	.5437	.5401	.5364	.5328	.5292	.5256
12	.5221	.5186	.5151	.5116	.5081	.5047	.5013	.4979
13	.4946	.4912	.4879	.4846	.4813	.4781	.4749	.4717
14	.4685	.4653	.4622	.4591	.4560	.4529	.4498	.4468
15	.4438	.4408	.4378	.4349	.4319	.4290	.4261	.4233
16	.4204	.4176	.4147	.4119	.4092	.4064	.4037	.4009
17	.3982	.3955	.3929	.3902	.3876	.3850	.3824	.3798
18	.3772	.3747	.3722	.3697	.3672	.3647	.3622	.3598
19	.3573	.3549	.3525	.3501	.3478	.3455	.3431	.3408
20	.3385	.3362	.3340	.3317	.3295	.3272	.3250	.3228
21	.3207	.3185	.3164	.3142	.3121	.3100	.3079	.3058
22	.3038	.3017	.2997	.2977	.2956	.2936	.2917	.2897
23	.2877	.2858	.2839	.2820	.2801	.2782	.2763	.2744
24	.2726	.2707	.2689	.2671	.2653	.2635	.2617	.2600
25	.2582	.2565	.2547	.2530	.2513	.2496	.2479	.2463
26	.2446		.2413		.2381		.2349	
27	.2317		.2286		.2255		.2225	

BARIUM-140—(concluded)

T½ = 8.0 days

λ factor (3 hours) = 0.00677

Hours Days	0	3	6	9	12	15	18	21
28	.2195		.2165		.2136		.2107	
29	.2079		.2051		.2023		.1996	
30	.1970		.1943		.1917		.1891	
31	.1866		.1841		.1816		.1791	
32	.1767		.1744		.1720		.1697	
33	.1674		.1652		.1629		.1607	
34	.1586		.1565		.1544		.1523	
35	.1502		.1482		.1462		.1442	
36	.1423		.1404		.1385		.1366	
37	.1348		.1330		.1312		.1294	
38	.1277		.1260		.1243		.1226	
39	.1210		.1193		.1177		.1162	
40	.1146		.1130		.1115		.1100	
41	.1085		.1071		.1056		.1042	
42	.1028		.1014		.1001		.0987	

GOLD-198

T½ = 2.69 days
64.6 hours

λ factor (30 minutes) = 0.00537

Hours	0	0.5	1.0	1.5	2.0	2.5	3.0	3.5	4.0	4.5
0	....	.9946	.9893	.9840	.9787	.9735	.9683	.9631	.9579	.9528
5	.9477	.9427	.9376	.9326	.9276	.9226	.9177	.9128	.9079	.9030

(continued)

GOLD-198—(continued)

T½ = 2.69 days
64.6 hours

λ factor (30 minutes) = 0.00537

Hours	0	0.5	1.0	1.5	2.0	2.5	3.0	3.5	4.0	4.5
10	.8982	.8934	.8886	.8838	.8791	.8744	.8697	.8650	.8604	.8558
15	.8512	.8466	.8421	.8376	.8331	.8287	.8242	.8198	.8154	.8110
20	.8067	.8024	.7981	.7938	.7896	.7853	.7811	.7769	.7728	.7686
25	.7645	.7604	.7564	.7523	.7483	.7443	.7403	.7363	.7324	.7285
30	.7246	.7207	.7168	.7130	.7092	.7054	.7016	.6978	.6941	.6904
35	.6867	.6830	.6793	.6757	.6721	.6685	.6649	.6613	.6578	.6543
40	.6508	.6473	.6438	.6404	.6369	.6335	.6301	.6268	.6234	.6201
45	.6167	.6134	.6102	.6069	.6036	.6004	.5972	.5940	.5908	.5876
50	.5845	.5814	.5783	.5752	.5721	.5690	.5660	.5629	.5599	.5569
55	.5539	.5510	.5480	.5451	.5422	.5393	.5364	.5335	.5306	.5278
60	.5250	.5222	.5194	.5166	.5138	.5111	.5083	.5056	.5029	.5002
65	.4975	.4949	.4922	.4896	.4870	.4844	.4818	.4792	.4766	.4741
70	.4715	.4690	.4665	.4640	.4615	.4590	.4566	.4541	.4517	.4493
75	.4469	.4445	.4421	.4397	.4374	.4350	.4327	.4304	.4281	.4258
80	.4235	.4212	.4190	.4167	.4145	.4123	.4101	.4079	.4057	.4035
85	.4014	.3992	.3971	.3949	.3928	.3907	.3886	.3866	.3845	.3824
90	.3804	.3783	.3763	.3743	.3723	.3703	.3683	.3663	.3644	.3624
95	.3605	.3586	.3566	.3547	.3528	.3509	.3491	.3472	.3453	.3435
100	.3416	.3398	.3380	.3362	.3344	.3326	.3308	.3290	.3273	.3255
105	.3238	.3220	.3203	.3186	.3169	.3152	.3135	.3118	.3102	.3085
110	.3068	.3052	.3036	.3019	.3003	.2987	.2971	.2955	.2939	.2924

GOLD-198—(concluded)

T½ = 2.69 days
64.6 hours

λ factor (30 minutes) = 0.00537

Hours	0	0.5	1.0	1.5	2.0	2.5	3.0	3.5	4.0	4.5
115	.2908	.2892	.2877	.2862	.2846	.2831	.2816	.2801	.2786	.2771
120	.2756	.2741	.2727	.2712	.2697	.2683	.2669	.2654	.2640	.2626
125	.2612	.2598	.2584	.2570	.2556	.2543	.2529	.2516	.2502	.2489
130	.2475		.2449		.2423		.2397		.2371	
135	.2346		.2321		.2296		.2272		.2247	
140	.2223		.2200		.2176		.2153		.2130	
145	.2107		.2085		.2062		.2040		.2018	
150	.1997		.1976		.1955		.1934		.1913	
155	.1892		.1872		.1852		.1832		.1813	
160	.1794		.1774		.1755		.1737		.1718	
165	.1700		.1682		.1664		.1646		.1628	
170	.1611		.1594		.1577		.1560		.1543	
175	.1527		.1510		.1494		.1478		.1462	
180	.1447		.1431		.1416		.1401		.1386	
185	.1371		.1357		.1342		.1328		.1314	
190	.1300		.1286		.1272		.1258		.1245	
195	.1232		.1218		.1205		.1193		.1180	
200	.1167		.1155		.1142		.1130		.1118	
205	.1106		.1094		.1083		.1071		.1060	
210	.1048		.1037		.1026		.1015		.1004	
215	.0994									

441

D. HEALTH PHYSICS TABLES

THE STANDARD MAN*

TABLE 1.—Mass of Organs

Organs	Grams	Organs	Grams
Muscles	30,000	Brain	1,500
Skeleton:		Spinal cord	30
Bones	7,000	Bladder	150
Red marrow	1,500	Salivary glands	50
Yellow marrow	1,500	Eyes	30
Blood	5,000	Teeth	20
Gastrointestinal tract	2,000	Prostate	20
Lungs	1,000	Adrenals	20
Liver	1,700	Thymus	10
Kidney	300	Skin and subcutaneous	
Spleen	150	tissues	8,500
Pancreas	70	Other tissues and organs	
Thyroid	20	not separately defined	8,390
Testes	40		
Heart	300	Total body weight	70,000
Lymphoid tissue	700		

* As stated in U. S. Department of Commerce, National Bureau of Standards, Handbook 47 (1950), Appendix I.

TABLE 2.—Chemical Composition†

Element	Proportion (Per Cent)	Approximate Mass in the Body (Gm.)
Oxygen	65.0	45,500
Carbon	18.0	12,600
Hydrogen	10.0	7,000
Nitrogen	3.0	2,100
Calcium	1.5	1,050
Phosphorus	1.0	700
Potassium	0.35	245
Sulfur	0.25	175
Sodium	0.15	105
Chlorine	0.15	105
Magnesium	0.05	35
Iron	0.004	3
Manganese	0.0003	0.2
Copper	0.0002	0.1
Iodine	0.00004	0.03

† The figures for a given organ may differ considerably from these averages for the whole body. For example, the nitrogen content of the dividing cells of the basal layer of skin is probably nearer 6 per cent than 3 per cent.

TABLE 3.—APPLIED PHYSIOLOGY

Average data for normal activity in a temperate zone:

(1) *Water Balance:*

DAILY WATER INTAKE

	Liters
In food (including water of oxidation)	1.0
As fluids	1.5
Total	2.5

Calculations of maximum permissible levels for radioactive isotopes in water have been based on the total intake figure of 2.5 liters a day.

DAILY WATER OUTPUT

	Liters
Sweat	0.5
From lungs	0.4
In feces	0.1
Urine	1.5
Total	2.5

(The total water content of the body is 50 liters.)

(2) *Respiration:*

AREA OF RESPIRATORY TRACT

Respiratory interchange area	50 m.^{2}
Nonrespiratory area (upper tract and trachea to bronchioles)	20 m.^{2}
Total	70 m.^{2}

RESPIRATORY EXCHANGE

	PHYSICAL ACTIVITY	
	At Work	Not at Work
Hours per day	8	16
Tidal air in liters	1.0	0.5
Respiration per minute	20	20
Volume per 8 hours (m.^{3})	10	5
Volume per day (m.^{3})	20	20

CARBON DIOXIDE CONTENT (BY VOLUME) OF AIR

Inhaled air (dry, at sea level)	0.03%
Alveolar air	5.5 %
Exhaled air	4.0 %

TABLE 4.—MAXIMUM PERMISSIBLE TISSUE DOSE LIMITS (IN REPS PER WEEK) AGREED ON AT THE 1950 CHALK RIVER CONFERENCE

Type of Radiation	At Any Point within the Body	Relative Biologic Effectiveness	IN BASAL LAYER OF EPIDERMIS	
			Exposure of Entire Body	Exposure of Hands Only
X- and gamma rays	0.3	1	0.5	1.5
Beta rays	0.3	1	0.5	1.5
Protons	0.03	10	0.05	0.15
Alpha rays	0.015	20	0.025	0.075
Fast neutrons	0.03	10	0.05	0.15
Thermal neutrons..	0.06	5	0.1	0.3

TABLE 5.—SUGGESTED MAXIMUM PERMISSIBLE LEVELS FOR SOME RADIOISOTOPES*

Radioisotope	MPL in Total Body† (μc.)	Effective Half-Life (Days)	Permissible Daily Intake of Element by Ingestion (Gm./Day)	MPL in Air (μc./Cc.)	MPL in Liquid Media (μc./Cc.)
A^{41}	30	0.074 (physical)	....	5×10^{-7}	5×10^{-4}
Xe^{133}	300	5.27 (physical)	....	5×10^{-6}	4×10^{-3}
Xe^{135}	100	0.38 (physical)	....	2×10^{-6}	1×10^{-3}
Co^{60}	3	8.4	Trace	1×10^{-6}	2×10^{-2}
Au^{198}	10	2.6	Trace	1×10^{-7}	3×10^{-3}
Au^{199}	28	3.1	Trace	2.5×10^{-7}	7×10^{-3}
Cr^{51}	390 (kidneys)	22	Trace	8×10^{-6}	0.5
Ni^{59}	39 (liver)	8	Trace	2×10^{-5}	0.25
Mo^{99}	50	2.8	Trace	2×10^{-3}	14
Th^{234}	120	24.1	....	6×10^{-7}	3
As^{76}	10 (kidneys)	1.09	....	2×10^{-6}	0.2
Ga^{72}	8 (bone)	0.59	....	3×10^{-6}	9
Ba^{140}	5 (bone)	12	....	6×10^{-8}	2×10^{-3}
Rb^{86}	60 (muscle)	7.8	....	4×10^{-7}	3×10^{-3}
Y^{91}	15 (bone)	51	....	4×10^{-8}	0.2
Ru^{106}—Rh^{106}	4.0	19	....	3×10^{-8}	0.1
Cs^{137}—Ba^{137}	90 (muscle)	17	....	2×10^{-7}	1.5×10^{-3}
La^{140}	24 (bone)	1.59	....	1×10^{-6}	1
Ce^{144}—Pr^{144}	5.0 (bone)	177	....	7×10^{-9}	4×10^{-2}
Pm^{147}	120 (bone)	136	....	2×10^{-7}	1
Alpha emitter (where isotope is unknown)		....	....	5×10^{-12}	1×10^{-7}
Beta, gamma emitter (where isotope is unknown)		....	....	1×10^{-9}	1×10^{-7}

445

* Excerpted from National Bureau of Standards Handbook 52.
† Critical organs are listed in parentheses.

TABLE 6.—DECONTAMINATION METHODS*

Surface	Method	Advantages	Disadvantages
Paint	Water	Most practical method of gross decontamination from a distance. Contamination reduced by approximately 50 per cent.	Protection needed from contaminated spray. Runoff must be controlled. Water under high pressure should not be used on a surface covered with contaminated dust
	Steam (with detergent if available)	Most practical method for decontaminating large horizontal, vertical and overhead surfaces. Contamination reduced by approximately 90 per cent.	Same as for water
	Soapless detergents	Where effective, reduces activity to safe level in one or two applications	Mild action
	Complexing agents: oxalates, carbonates, citrates	Holds contamination in solution. Contamination on unweathered surfaces reduced by approximately 75 per cent in 4 minutes. Easily stored, nontoxic, noncorrosive	Requires application from 5 to 30 minutes for effectiveness. Has little penetrating power; hence of small value on weathered surfaces
	Organic solvents	Quick dissolving action makes solvents useful on vertical and overhead surfaces	Toxic and flammable. Requires good ventilation and fire precautions
	Caustics	Minimum contact with contaminated surface. Contamination reduced almost 100 per cent	Applicable only on horizontal surfaces. Personnel hazard. Not to be used on aluminum or magnesium
	Abrasion (wet sandblasting)	Complete removal of surface and contamination. Feasible for large-scale operations	Contaminated sand spread over large area. Method too harsh for many surfaces
Metal	Water	Contamination reduced by approximately 50 per cent	Same as for painted surfaces
	Detergents	Removal of oil or grease films	Same as for painted surfaces
	Organic solvents	Stripping of grease	Same as for painted surfaces

* Federal Civil Defense Agency Release TM-11-6, *Radiological Decontamination in Civil Defense*.

TABLE 6.—DECONTAMINATION METHODS (Cont.)

Surface	Method	Advantages	Disadvantages
Metal (Cont.)	Complexing agents: oxalates, carbonates, citrates	Holds contamination in solution	Difficult to keep in place on any but horizontal surfaces. Limited value on weathered porous surfaces
	Inorganic acids	Fast, complete decontamination	Good ventilation required; acid fumes toxic to personnel. Possibility of excessive corrosion. Acid mixture cannot safely be heated
	Acid mixtures	Action of weak acid. Reduces contamination of unweathered surfaces	Same as for inorganic acids
	Abrasion (buffers, grinders)	Useful for detailed cleaning	Follow-up procedure required to pick up powdered contamination
	Abrasion (wet sandblasting)	Same as for painted surfaces	Same as for painted surfaces
Concrete	Abrasion (vacuum blasting)	Direct removal of contaminated dust	Contamination of equipment
	Vacuum cleaning	Same as for vacuum blasting on concrete	Same as for vacuum blasting on concrete
	Flame cleaning	Only method of trapping contamination on surface	Slow and painstaking. Fire and airborne radiation hazard is great
Brick	Same as for concrete	Same as for concrete	Same as for concrete
Asphalt	Abrasion	No direct contact with surface; contamination may be reduced to safe level	Residual contamination fixed into asphalt. If road is subject to further contamination, may require recovering
Wood	Flame cleaning	Same as for flame cleaning on concrete	Same as for flame cleaning on concrete

TABLE 7.—HALF-VALUE LAYERS (IN INCHES) FOR GAMMA RADIATION

ENERGY (Mev)	MATERIAL			
	Water	Concrete	Steel	Lead
0.5	2.91	1.46	0.425	0.159
0.6	3.15 ·	1.56	0.456	0.191
0.7	3.38	1.66	0.497	0.230
0.8	3.60	1.76	0.533	0.273
0.9	3.80	1.86	0.568	0.315
1.0	4.00	1.96	0.597	0.350
1.1	4.19	2.06	0.630	0.381
1.2	4.35	2.16	0.660	0.405
1.3	4.53	2.26	0.690	0.430
1.4	4.68	2.37	0.718	0.456
1.5	4.85	2.49	0.744	0.478
1.6	4.99	2.60	0.774	0.499
1.7	5.13	2.72	0.803	0.517
1.8	5.29	2.82	0.835	0.537
1.9	5.46	2.91	0.866	0.559
2.0	5.59	2.99	0.894	0.573
2.2	5.87	3.12	0.945	0.597
2.4	6.16	3.24	0.994	0.613
2.6	6.45	3.36	1.04	0.619
2.8	6.71	3.48	1.09	0.625
3.0	7.00	3.59	1.13	0.625

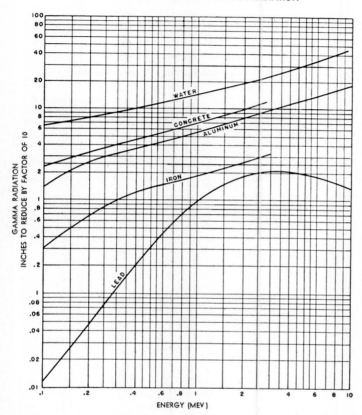

The distance to reduce gamma radiation by a factor of 10 as a function of energy in the various materials indicated. (From Stanford Research Institute Report 361, *The Industrial Uses of Radioactive Fission Products.* With permission of the Stanford Research Institute and the U. S. Atomic Energy Commission.)

449

E. EXAMPLES OF RECORD AND REPORT SHEETS

RADIOISOTOPE LABORATORY

REQUEST FOR DIAGNOSTIC THYROID TRACER

Date_____19_____

Name_____ Age_____ Admission No._____
(LAST)   (FIRST)

Room_____ SM ☐   PPI ☐   FCH ☐   Ward ☐   Previous Yes ☐
                      MRH ☐   MH ☐   PAV ☐   Private ☐   Tracer   No ☐

Attending Physician_____Resident or Intern_____

Clinical Diagnosis_____

List Present and Recent Medication_____

_____

NAME _____ Has an appointment for

A RADIOIODINE THYROID TRACER TEST

DATE _____ at _____ A.M. at Radioisotope Laboratory

Your doctor has ordered a radioiodine thyroid tracer test (uptake study) for you. This test will help him to learn more about your thyroid gland and how it is functioning. An indication of whether or not it is behaving normally is the per cent of radioiodine taken up by your thyroid and the amount found in the blood. In this test, radioiodine will be given to you on the first day, and you will be asked to return at 24 hours, and possibly at 48 hours, for testing. The report of the tests will be given to your doctor, who will discuss the results with you.

These instructions should be followed:

(1) DIET:

    (a) For *two* days prior to and during the test: Avoid all sea foods and canned fish products except fresh fish (bass, perch, carp, white fish and trout). Do not add salt except that used in cooking. Avoid all highly seasoned or salted foods such as sausage meat, salted crackers, pretzels, potato chips, snack foods. No cod liver oil.

    (b) On *each* of the mornings of the test you may only have toast, unsalted butter, jelly, coffee or tea. Cream and sugar may be added.

(2) You may smoke on the mornings of the test.

RADIOISOTOPE LABORATORY

Instructions after Radioiodine Treatment

Name _____ Date of Treatment _____

1. For two days after treatment, flush toilet 3 times after voiding.
2. No special diet is required.
3. No special handling of dishes is necessary.
4. Avoid coming closer than 3 feet to children under 5 years for one week after treatment.
5. Begin taking the prescribed medication on _____, as directed.
6. If you have any further questions, please call: CAlumet 5-5540, Ext. 404 or 405.
7. Your next appointment at the Radioisotope Laboratory is on _____

NAME (PRINT)			MRH ☐	PPI ☐	OUTPATIENT ☐
			SMH ☐	MH ☐	PRIVATE ☐
LAST		FIRST	FCH ☐	PAV ☐	WARD ☐

ATTENDING PHYSICIAN	INTERNE	Admission No.

	Normal Range	Hypothyroid Range	Hyperthyroid Range	Result
% Thyroid Uptake At 24 Hours	15-53	0-15	47-100	
PBI¹³¹ % dose/L At 24 Hours	.01-.086	.003-.054	.085-1.45	
PBI¹³¹ % dose/L At 48 Hours	.01-.098		.146-2.86	
Serum Protein-Bound Iodine (ug %)	3-8	Below 3	Above 8	
Basal Metabolic Rate	Temp.	☐ Satisfactory		(1)_____
		☐ Unsatisfactory Repeat		(2)_____

INTERPRETATION:

(OVER)

Radioisotope 1 (Thyroid Tracer PBI, BMR)	Date	Examined By

453

RADIOISOTOPE LABORATORY

THYROID EVALUATION

| NAME (Last, First) | | | AGE | M ☐
F ☐ | ADDRESS | | | DATE |

| ADMISSION No. | ROOM No. | SM ☐ | PPI ☐
FCH ☐ | OUTPATIENT ☐
PRIVATE ☐ | ATTENDING PHYSICIAN | | | REFERRING DIAGNOSIS |
| | | MRH ☐ MH ☐ | PAV ☐ | WARD ☐ | | | | |

HISTORY	YES	NO	REMARKS
NERVOUSNESS			
TREMOR			
WEAKNESS			
EASY FATIGUABILITY			
INSOMNIA			
APPETITE (INCR.) (DECR.)			
WEIGHT (GAIN) (LOSS)			
SPECIAL DIET			
SWEATING (INCR.) (DECR.)			
INTOLERANCE (HOT) (COLD)			
(DIARRHEA) (CONSTIPATION)			
PROTRUDING EYES			
SKIN CHANGES			
THYROID ENLARGEMENT			
MENSTRUAL IRREGULARITY			
PREVIOUS THYROID SURGERY			
PREVIOUS I131 TREATMENT			
RECENT IODIDES			
RECENT ANTITHYROID DRUG			
RECENT (G.B.) (I.V.P.)			

HISTORY	YES	NO	REMARKS
ANY DRUGS TAKEN NOW			
(HEART) (KIDNEY) DISEASE			
ANY OTHER ILLNESS			

ADDITIONAL HISTORY

CLINICALLY

454

PHYSICAL EXAMINATION

WEIGHT	PULSE	NECK PALPATION
B.P.	SKIN	
EYE SIGNS		

OTHER FINDINGS

THYROID SIZE

BMR	CHOLESTEROL

ECG

OTHER LAB. FINDINGS

I¹³¹ STUDIES AND PBI

DATE	% UPTAKE	PBI¹³¹	% URINE	PBI

RADIOISOTOPE LABORATORY

THERAPY RECORD

NAME (Last, First)				AGE	M ☐ F ☐	ADDRESS		DATE

ADMISSION No.	ROOM No.				OUTPATIENT ☐ PRIVATE ☐ WARD ☐	ATTENDING PHYSICIAN	REFERRING DIAGNOSIS	
		SM ☐	PPI ☐					
	MRH ☐	MH ☐	PAV ☐					

RADIOISOTOPE LABORATORY

THYROID TRACER (I¹³¹) INSTRUCTIONS

Date_____ .19____

Patient_____ Room _____ Ward _____

Follow Instructions as Checked:

Begin Thyroid Tracer Diet on_____ Until _____

I¹³¹ will be administered at_____ on _____

☐ Breakfast on first day should consist of toast, unsalted butter, jelly, and coffee with cream.

☐ First Day (after radioisotope administration):

    (1) No food or drink (except water) until _____

    (2) May smoke.

☐ Second Day:

    (1) Patient is to report to Radioisotope Laboratory at _____
    on_____ .

☐ Urine Collection:

    (1) Begin 24 hour urine collection as of time of isotope administration.
    (2) 24 hour urine specimens are to be collected on _____ (1) _____ (2)
    _____ (3) _____ (4).
    (3) Each 24 hour collection should be sent to laboratory at completion.

If in doubt call extension 420.

Per_____

457

RADIOISOTOPE LABORATORY

INSTRUCTIONS FOR I¹³¹ THERAPY (TO 30 mc.)

Date_____19____

Patient_____Room_____Ward_____

To report to Radioisotope Laboratory at_____on_____

Before Therapy: No special preparation.

After Therapy: No food until_____

(1) The patient should be in a room with other patients undergoing similar radioisotope therapy, or in a private room.

(2) There should be a rubber or plastic covering on the pillow and bed.

(3) The cothing and linen used by the patient during the 48 hours after treatment should be saved in a linen bag in the patient's room for surveying by the radioisotope technician before they are sent to the laundry.

(4) If the patient has any dressings, these should be changed using rubber gloves, and the gloves and waste material saved for surveying.

(5) During the first 48 hours after treatment, the patient should not be bathed without the use of a gown and gloves; these should be surveyed later. If patient is ambulant, he may take a tub bath, but the tub must be thoroughly rinsed afterward.

(6) If patient uses a urinal or bedpan, during the first 48 hours these should be handled with gloves and flushed three times after each use. If patient is ambulant he should use the same toilet bowl all the time, and should flush it three times after each use during the first 48 hours or longer.

(7) If patient is incontinent, he should have an indwelling catheter and the urine handled in the same way, except that the urine should be emptied frequently during the first 2 days.

(8) No restrictions on visitors.

If in doubt call extension 420.

Per_____

RADIOISOTOPE LABORATORY

INSTRUCTIONS FOR ☐ I^{131} THERAPY (100 mc.)

☐ Au^{198} THERAPY (100 mc.)

Date_____19____

Patient_____Room_____Ward_____

Isotope will be administered at_____on_____

Before Therapy: No special preparation.

After Therapy:

(1) The patient should be in a private room, preferably with private toilet.

(2) All bed care procedures should be performed before isotope administration and may be resumed 48 hours thereafter, subject to the limitations noted below.

(3) The pillow and mattress must be protected by rubber or plastic covering.

(4) Bed bathing and changing of dressings should be performed using gloves and gown up to 14 days following therapy.

(5) The gloves and gowns worn by the personnel and the linens used by the patient should be saved in patient's room for survey by the radioisotope technician.

(6) The urine and other specimens must be labelled "radioactive" and handled with gloves during the first 48 hours. Urinal, bedpan, thermometer, etc. should be well rinsed and kept for patient's own use. (I^{131} only)

(7) If patient is incontinent, an indwelling catheter must be used during the first 48 hours and the urine emptied frequently. (I^{131} only)

(8) If the patient is ambulant, he may take tub baths (if not otherwise contraindicated). The tub should be well rinsed afterward. The same toilet should be used at all times and well flushed (3 times).

(9) No special handling of food trays is necessary.

(10) No visitors in room for 48 hours; only short visits thereafter as shown on tolerance chart.

TOLERANCE EXPOSURE HOURS PERMITTED

Site	Day after Therapy						
	Therapy Day	1	2	3	4	5	6
Contact							
Bedside							
3 Feet							
Doorway							

If in doubt call extension 420.

Per_____

NAME (PRINT)			MRH ☐ PPI ☐ OUTPATIENT ☐
			SMH ☐ MH ☐ PRIVATE ☐
LAST		FIRST	FCH ☐ PAV ☐ WARD ☐

ATTENDING PHYSICIAN	INTERNE	Admission No.

	Normal Range	P.A. Range	Result
Cobalt-Vitamin B$_{12}$ Excretion (% dose)	6.2-33.4	0-3.7	
Plasma Cobalt-Vit. B$_{12}$ (% dose/L) At Hours			

INTERPRETATION:

(OVER)

Radioisotope 2	Date	Examined By

460

RADIOISOTOPE LABORATORY

INSTRUCTIONS FOR P³² THERAPY

Date_____19_____

Patient_____Room_____Ward_____

To report to Radioisotope Laboratory at_____on_____

☐ **Before Therapy:**

No special preparation.

☐ **After Therapy:**

(1) No special room assignment is necessary.

(2) The mattress and pillow should be protected by rubber or plastic covers.

(3) Rubber gloves should be worn when handling the patient within the first 48 hours. The patient's pajamas, rubber gloves and linen should be saved in patient's room for 48 hours to be surveyed by radioisotope technician.

(4) If patient is ambulant, he may take tub baths or showers.

(5) If the patient uses a urinal or bed pan during the first 48 hours, these should be handled with gloves.

(6) No restrictions on visitors.

If in doubt call extension 420.

Per_____

INSTRUCTIONS FOR BRAIN TUMOR LOCALIZATION ☐ External
☐ Internal

Date_____19____

Patient_____Room_____Ward_____

☐ **External (I[131]):**

   (1) To report to Radioisotope Laboratory at_____on_____

   (2) Day before examination: Lugol's solution 10 drops T.I.D.

   (3) May have food prior to examination.

   (4) After examination: Lugol's solution 10 drops B.I.D.

   (5) No special precautions necessary.

☐ **Internal (P[32]):**

   (1) Tracer dose will be administered at_____on_____,
   the day prior to surgery.

   (2) For 48 hours after isotope administration gloves and gown shall be worn when handling patient. Thereafter, the same procedure should be used when handling surgical dressings.

   (3) The patient's gown and dressings should be saved for survey by radioisotope technician.

   (4) Pillow should be protected in case of drainage after surgery.

If in doubt call extension 420.

Per_____

Index